"*The Essential Teachings of Sasang Medicine* is a brilliant piece of work! Not only is this book comprehensive and practical, but it is written to help the reader cultivate the proper balance of mind and body. An exciting feature of this book is specific cases showing how to apply over one hundred herbal formula for effective treatment."

—*Sande McDaniel, Publisher of* Oriental Medicine Journal

"I would like to wholeheartedly congratulate Gary Wagman on the completion of his English translation of the *Dongeui Susei Bowon*. While reviewing the manuscript, I reflected on how much effort, enthusiasm, and time this translation must have taken to complete. It is my sincere hope that Sasang medicine will spread to every corner of the earth, calming and healing the bodies and minds of more and more people."

—*Hwang Minwoo, KMD, PhD, Professor, College of Korean Medicine, Kyunghee University, Seoul, Republic of Korea, and Clinical Doctor, Sasang Medicine Clinic, Kyung Hee University Hospital at Gangdong*

*of related interest*

**Discussion of Cold Damage (Shang Han Lun)**
**Commentaries and Clinical Applications**
*Guohui Liu*
*Foreword by Dr. Henry McCann*
ISBN 978 1 84819 254 6
eISBN 978 0 85701 200 5

**Foundations of Theory for Ancient Chinese Medicine**
**Shang Han Lun and Contemporary Medical Texts**
*Guohui Liu*
*Foreword by Charles Buck*
ISBN 978 1 84819 262 1
eISBN 978 0 85701 211 1

**Essential Texts in Chinese Medicine**
**The Single Idea in the Mind of the Yellow Emperor**
*Richard Bertschinger*
ISBN 978 1 84819 162 4
eISBN 978 0 85701 135 0

# The Essential Teachings of Sasang Medicine

An Annotated Translation of
Lee Je-ma's Dongeui Susei Bowon

*Gary Wagman, PhD, LAc*

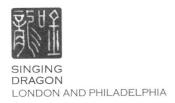

SINGING
DRAGON
LONDON AND PHILADELPHIA

First published in 2016
by Singing Dragon
an imprint of Jessica Kingsley Publishers
73 Collier Street
London N1 9BE, UK
and
400 Market Street, Suite 400
Philadelphia, PA 19106, USA

*www.singingdragon.com*

**Library of Congress Cataloging in Publication Data**
Names: Yi, Che-ma, 1837-1900, author. | Wagman, Gary, 1973- , annotator, translator. Title: The Essential Teachings of Sasang Medicine : An Annotated Translation of Lee Je-ma's Dongeui Susei Bowon / Gary Wagman. Other titles: Tongu?i suse powo?n | Dongeui susei bowon Description: London ; Philadelphia : Singing Dragon, 2016. Identifiers: LCCN 2016001947 | ISBN 9781848193178 (alk. paper) Subjects: | MESH: Yi, Che-ma, 1837-1900. Tongu?i suse powo?n. | Medicine, Korean Traditional | Longevity | Somatotypes--physiology | Yin-Yang Classification: LCC R627 | NLM WB 55.K6 | DDC 610.9519--dc23 LC record available at http://lccn.loc.gov/2016001947

**British Library Cataloguing in Publication Data**
A CIP catalogue record for this book is available from the British Library

ISBN 978 1 84819 317 8
eISBN 978 0 85701 270 8

Printed and bound in Great Britain by Bell & Bain Ltd, Glasgow

# Contents

Acknowledgments . . . . . . . . . . . . . . . . . . . . . . . . . . . . . . . . . . . . . . . 7

Introduction . . . . . . . . . . . . . . . . . . . . . . . . . . . . . . . . . . . . . . . . . . . 9

**Part I: Theory**

Chapter 1 Theories on Human Nature and Conduct (性命論) . . . . . . . . . . . . 32

Chapter 2 The Four Basic Characteristics (四端論) . . . . . . . . . . . . . . . . . 51

Chapter 3 Expanding and Fulfilling (擴充論) . . . . . . . . . . . . . . . . . . . . 67

Chapter 4 The *Zhang Fu* Organs (臟腑論) . . . . . . . . . . . . . . . . . . . . . 83

Chapter 5 The Basic Principles of Medicine (醫源論) . . . . . . . . . . . . . . . . 93

**Part II: Clinical Application**

Chapter 6 The So Eum Individual's Illness (少陰人論) . . . . . . . . . . . . . . . 104

Chapter 7 The So Yang Individual's Illness (少陽人論) . . . . . . . . . . . . . . . 203

Chapter 8 The Tae Eum Individual's Illness (太陰人論) . . . . . . . . . . . . . . 269

Chapter 9 The Tae Yang Individual's Illness (太陽人論) . . . . . . . . . . . . . . 316

**Part III: Additional Topics**

Chapter 10 The Virtuous Path—Advice for Everyday Life (廣濟說) . . . . . . . 332

Chapter 11 Four Constitutional Classification and Diagnosis
(四象人 辨證論) . . . . . . . . . . . . . . . . . . . . . . . . . . . . . . . . . . . . . . 340

Useful Resources . . . . . . . . . . . . . . . . . . . . . . . . . . . . . . . . . . . . . . . 349

Index . . . . . . . . . . . . . . . . . . . . . . . . . . . . . . . . . . . . . . . . . . . . . . . 350

# *Acknowledgments*

The following individuals played an indispensible role in the process of translating the *Dongeui Susei Bowon*. I extend my deepest gratitude…

To Dr. Lee Je-ma, who helped reignite my passion for study and practice through his profound understanding of Asian philosophy and medicine. As the originator of Sasang medicine, he contributed greatly to the start of a new era of self-empowering medicine.

To my teacher Dr. No Kyoung Mun, who never once hesitated to offer clarification, often replying to my persistent questioning via email and texting within seconds, despite thousands of miles between us. I have never met anyone with such profound patience and pure desire to share their knowledge. I extend this gratitude to his teacher, Dr. Kim Man San (Kwan Jung Sonseng Nim), who founded the Yon Kyoung Won (Institute of Classical Studies), a place where we study, discuss, eat, and drink together, blissfully embracing ancient wisdom.

To my mother, who always taught me to follow my dreams, even if it meant that I would have to travel to the other end of the world to fulfill them. She has been a constant ray of light, encouraging me every step of the way. Her unconditional love and support gave my path in life a tremendous boost.

To my wife, who epitomizes the wisdom and charm of her Korean ancestry. Without her guidance and support, this translation would have been impossible. Knowing how important this task was for me, she devoted herself to facilitating it by juggling clinic schedules and ensuring that I had enough time to contemplate and write.

To my daughter, whose joyful energy never fails to make me smile and remind me that each moment in life is precious.

To Karen Christensen, my editor and friend, whose magical touch added clarity and harmony to my translation, while respecting and preserving the essence of Lee Je-ma's writings. It was nothing short of a blessing to have worked with her.

To my patients, who I treasure as one would a family. With Sasang medicine as our vehicle, we have witnessed together time and time again the body's ability to heal from within. Not a day goes by in the clinic without being reminded of how deep our mutually enhancing relationship runs.

To Singing Dragon, who recognized the value of Lee Je-ma's teaching and graciously offered to publish this text.

Last, I would like to thank life itself, for giving me the opportunity to follow my dreams.

# Introduction

The last decade has served as a renaissance for the English translation of Chinese medical texts, adding to the integrity and depth of Eastern medical studies in the West. Most, if not all, of these translations were based on a desire to deepen the understanding of Chinese medicine outside the confines of China. While these intentions have been well received, the contributions of other Eastern medicines have yet to be given the attention they deserve. Consequently, it is of common belief in the West that the Chinese approach remains authentic and unparalleled. This text offers one example of how other countries, such as Korea, have contributed significantly to the development of Eastern medicine.

As a small country directly adjacent to and approximately 43 times smaller than China, Korea was evidently influenced by its culture and medicine. Yet China and Korea have never considered themselves one and the same, as the Yellow River divided them geographically and culturally. Korea as we know it today is shaped by a delicate balance between Chinese influences and its own intrinsic culture. Its story of creation, which offers the very first reference to herbal medicine in Korean history, involves the tale of a bear and tiger who were given the chance to become human if they survived 100 days in a chilly cave with just 20 cloves of garlic and one bundle of sage. With garlic as a herb to warm the body and sage to promote fertility, this story attests to the fact that Korea historically regarded the use of herbal medicine as a central aspect of its existence.

The first recorded Korean medical texts—*A Collection of Formulas from the Korean Elders of the Goguryeo Dynasty* (高麗老師方), written during the Goguryeo Dynasty (37 BC–668 AD), and the *Revised Collection of Baekje Formulas* (百濟新集方), written during the Baekje Dynasty (18 BC–660 AD)—both contain numerous remedies such as Mu Gua (*Fructus Chaenomelis Lagenariae*), Huang Qi (*Radix Astragali Membranacei*), and Ju Hua (*Flos Chrysanthemi Morifolii*) for lung tumors, boils, beriberi, influenza, and other ailments. Although neither of these texts survived in its entirety, what remains is a hint of the use of both Chinese and indigenous approaches to healing.

A series of epidemics during the later Silla period (668 BC–995 BC) forced Korean doctors to develop their own domestic herbal approaches, not previously given in the Chinese medical texts. To accompany this effort, the Silla government legalized the use of Ayurvedic medicine brought back by Korean scholars returning from India. The widespread use of Ayurvedic medicine in Korea paved the way for later approaches such as Sasang medicine, which emphasize the significance of one's innate emotional and physical tendencies in the healing process.

Korea's first discernible rift from an emphasis on Chinese medicine came under the rule of King Saejeong (1418–1450), who ordered a countrywide survey of native Korean plants, trees, shrubs, and flora with the belief that locally derived herbs would be more appropriate for the treating of local diseases. This survey resulted in the publication of *A Comprehensive Inventory of Local Korean Herbs* (鄉藥集成方), which includes herbal preparation methods and acupuncture techniques and consists of 30 volumes and 85 chapters. In this text, herbs such as Dang Gui (*Radix Angelicae Sinensis*) and Shi Gao (*Gypsum Fibrosum*) from China and Korea, and in some cases Japan, were given different characteristics and functions depending on their country of origin.

Following these developments came the *Mirror of Eastern Medicine* (東醫寶鑑), its authorship attributed mainly to Heo Jun (1610). This 25-volume, several-thousand-page text offers detailed herbal and acupuncture approaches to numerous health conditions and is the most comprehensive source of medical knowledge written throughout Korean history. The *Mirror of Eastern Medicine* elaborates on the medical theories and prescriptions included in *The Yellow Emperor's Classic* and teachings from the Qin and Yuan Dynasties of China. It contains, too, indigenous folk remedies, offering detailed descriptions regarding preparation, dosage, and usage.

Among the numerous contributions made by doctors of Korean medicine, the text entitled *Eastern Medical Perspectives on Longevity and Wellbeing*, or *Dongeui Susei Bowon* (東醫壽世保元), written by Lee Je-ma (1837–1900), is perhaps the most distinctive. In this text, he reignites the classical Chinese medical emphasis on Yin and Yang theory while establishing an entirely new approach referred to as Sasang Constitutional Medicine, or *Sasang Eui Hak* (四象醫學). This method stands alone as being uniquely Korean in origin and yet deeply rooted in the Eastern classics such as the *I Ching, Confucian Analects, Doctrine of the Mean, The Great Learning, Mencius*, and the *Shang Han Lun*. It breaks away from the predominant Daoist theory of *Wu Wei* (無爲), which emphasizes man's relationship with nature often at the cost of fulfilling one's societal role, and delves into the realm of Confucian theory and philosophy, which accentuate the role of social interaction. Lee Je-ma's text conveys how the Sasang approach is a medical system and philosophy in its own right.

## A Translation of the Title

A closer look at the title, *Dongeui Susei Bowon*, helps forge a deeper understanding of Lee Je-ma's desire to establish his innovative form of medicine. The characters "*Dong*" (東) and "*Eui*" (醫) translate together as Eastern medicine. The character "*Su*" (壽) translates as "longevity." Lee Je-ma was less concerned with the extension of life than with the quality of life. Yet he believed that the preservation of health will naturally lead to longer life. Hence the character for "*Bo*" (保) in the above title translates as "preservation." Health preservation according to Lee Je-ma, as will soon be shown, depends on the ability to polish one's inner self and fulfill one's purpose in life. According to Sasang medicine, polishing one's inner self can therefore be viewed as the source, or "*Won*" (元—the last character in the above title), of health and wellbeing. Finally, the third to last character, "*Sei*" (世), translates as spreading or cultivating, and refers to the action of promoting health and wellbeing in society through the above means.

## The Birth of Sasang

Lee Je-ma derived the title *Sasang* from the *I Ching*, which states: "The *Tai Qi* gives rise to Yin and Yang, which in turn become the *Sasang*" (太極生兩儀, 兩儀生四象).

The *Tai Qi*, translated as "Great Ultimate," is a vast force that permeates all things and consists of two opposing energies referred to as Yin and Yang. In their pure and isolated form, each of these energies is without significance, since all phenomena consist of varying combinations of Yin and Yang engaged in a dance of life. These combinations, in their simplest form, are referred to as Sasang or "Four Symbols." The Four Symbols are also referred to as Yin within Yin (Greater Yin), Yang within Yin (Lesser Yin), Yin within Yang (Lesser Yang), and Yang within Yang (Greater Yang). In Korean, the Four Symbols are pronounced Tae Eum (태음), So Eum (소음), So Yang (소양), and Tae Yang (태양). Lee Je-ma adapted these names for each of his four constitutions. He believed that these four combinations symbolize four fundamental differences between each person, which result from varying degrees of bodily Yin and Yang energy, where the Tae Yang (Greater Yang) type has the most abundant Yang and the Tae Eum (Greater Yin) type has the most substantial Yin energy. Furthermore, he equated the Four Symbols with the four major organ systems of the lungs, spleen, liver, and kidneys, and the heart with *Tai Chi*, since it feeds energy and blood to the entire body. Lee Je-ma's Sasang theory was heavily influenced by the *I Ching*, as this text will make further apparent.

## Comparison between Chinese and Sasang Medicine

There are as many similarities as there are differences between traditional Chinese and Sasang medicine. While the Sasang approach is a distinct medical system, it is still based on the same basic principles of Yin and Yang as traditional Chinese medicine. Without the influence of Chinese medicine, Sasang medicine would not exist. Lee Je-ma, in a sense, may therefore be considered a reformer of Chinese medicine, who examined hundreds of formulae and their herbal constituents, acknowledging their merits, criticizing their shortcomings, and adapting them to specific energetic patterns within each of the four constitutions. In situations that did not call for the use of a traditional formula, Lee Je-ma developed his own according to Sasang principles.

Sasang medicine is born from Lee Je-ma's dissatisfaction with the standard approach to medicine, emphasizing as it does the influence of external pathogens, as proposed by the most widely utilized medical text of his time, Zhang Zhongjing's *Shang Han Lun*. He believed that all illness is directly related to one's emotional wellbeing. Lee Je-ma repeatedly witnessed how the doctors of his time would often make matters worse by prescribing medicine based on symptomatic presentation rather than an imbalance of the four constitutional temperaments: sorrow, anger, joy, and calmness, which lead to imbalance of the organs. *The Yellow Emperor's Classic*, the earliest known treatise in Chinese medicine, also mentions the influence of the Seven Emotional Disorders (joy, anger, worry, contemplation, sorrow, fear, and shock), but it aimed at addressing the Six Climatic Factors (Heat, Cold, Dryness, Dampness, Summer Heat, and Wind) and balancing one's health according to the season. Hence in Chinese medicine, diseases caused by emotional imbalance were often considered difficult to treat and, although discussed, were not given precedence.

Similar to Chinese medicine, Lee Je-ma classifies illness into two major categories: Exterior and Interior. Yet he explains how the etiology of Exterior and Interior illnesses differs according to each constitution and the state of mind. In Chinese medicine, Exterior disorders are principally associated with a pathogenic attack that, if powerful enough, could penetrate the immune system of an otherwise healthy person. Exterior disorders, according to Lee Je-ma, are due to an imbalance of one's temperament, referred to as *Song* (性), while Interior disorders result from explosive and overwhelming emotion, called *Jung* (情). Sasang medicine focuses primarily on balancing the constitutionally specific *Song* nature and *Jung* emotions to enhance health and address illness—a task carried out through self-cultivation and, if necessary, herbal treatment. Lee Je-ma strongly believed that no matter how powerful a pathogenic influence may be, it would be no match against a balanced and cultivated heart and mind. The *Dongeui Susei Bowon* repeatedly gives credence to both Exterior pathogenic attack and Exterior syndromes, where the latter refers to an imbalance of the *Song* nature and the former, an external influence that takes advantage of the situation. Hence Lee Je-ma maintained that an imbalance of one's *Song* nature is what provokes illness from an External pathogenic attack.

Each of the four constitutions in Sasang medicine is born with a stronger and a weaker organ system influenced by inherent emotional inclinations. A propensity for sorrow, for example, stimulates lung development in utero, while calmness stimulates the kidneys. Excessive sorrow, however, may over-stimulate and stagnate the lung energy. Sorrow in Sasang Medicine is negatively correlated with joy, the emotion of the liver. Hence excessive sorrow decreases joy, resulting in liver deficiency, and excessive joy (ecstasy) decreases sorrow, causing lung deficiency. Although organ excess and deficiency are a central aspect of the Five Yin and Six Fu Organ (五臟六腑) Theory in Chinese medicine, emotion is not considered the source of inherent organ strength or weakness. Instead, organ strength is affected by one's *Pre-Heaven* energy within the kidneys transferred from parent to offspring. According to this principle, the health of the offspring depends primarily on the parents. Weakened *Pre-Heaven* energy causes insufficient development of the organs in utero. In Sasang medicine it is the parents' emotional not physical health that primarily influences the organ development of their offspring.

While organ theory plays a central role in both Chinese and Sasang medical diagnosis, each holds its own interpretation. In Sasang medicine, for example, each of the Four Major Organs is considered the governor of its own domain, controlling the function of other organs in its vicinity. Along with the Four Major Organs are the four sections of the body, referred to as *Cho* (焦). The Upper *Cho* is governed by the lungs and the emotion of sorrow, the Mid-Upper *Cho* is governed by the spleen and the emotion of anger, the Mid-Lower *Cho* by the liver and the emotion of joy, and the Lower *Cho* is governed by the kidneys and the emotion of calmness. Chinese medicine describes three *Jiao* (pronounced *Cho* in Korean). The Upper *Jiao* consists of the heart and lungs, Middle *Jiao* the stomach and spleen, and Lower *Jiao* the liver, small intestine, large intestine, and bladder. Although Chinese medicine associates each organ with an emotion, it doesn't emphasize the role of emotions in controlling the function of their respective organs or the *Jiao* in which they are located.

**Table I.1: The Chinese medical organ system**

| Yin organ | Location | Yang correlate | Location | Emotional correlate |
|-----------|----------|----------------|----------|---------------------|
| Lungs | Upper *Jiao* | Large intestine | Lower *Jiao* | Sorrow |
| Heart | Upper *Jiao* | Small intestine | Lower *Jiao* | Anxiety |
| Spleen | Middle *Jiao* | Stomach | Middle *Jiao* | Contemplation |
| Liver | Lower *Jiao* | Gall bladder | Lower *Jiao* | Anger |
| Kidney | Lower *Jiao* | Urinary bladder | Lower *Jiao* | Fear |

**Table I.2: The Sasang medicine organ system**

| Yin organ | Location | Yang correlate | Location | Emotional correlate |
|---|---|---|---|---|
| Lungs | Upper *Jiao* | Esophagus | Upper *Jiao* | Sorrow |
| Spleen | Mid-Upper *Jiao* | Stomach | Mid-Upper *Jiao* | Anger |
| Liver | Mid-Lower *Jiao* | Small intestine | Mid-Upper *Jiao* | Joy |
| Kidney | Lower *Jiao* | Large intestine and urinary bladder | Lower *Jiao* | Calmness/ complacency |

Lee Je-ma held that each Sasang constitution has its own specific group of herbs and formulae that promote the flow of Yin and Yang between the stronger and weaker organs. Herbs for the So Eum Individual, for example, promote upward Yang energy movement from their excessive kidneys to the deficient spleen, while the So Yang's herbs promote downward Yin energy movement from their excessive spleen to the deficient kidneys. This illustrates how, in Sasang medicine, emphasis is placed on the flow of each herb from origin to destination (i.e. kidney to spleen, lung to liver). In Chinese medicine, even though most herbs are associated with one or more organs, emphasis is given to organ destination (kidney herbs, spleen herbs, etc.). The former approach accentuates a non-static, dynamic approach to herb function, emphasizing a fundamental bond between excessive and deficient organ energies.

Most of the herbs in Sasang medicine are also used in Chinese medicine but often associated with different characteristics. In Lee Je-ma's text *Dongmu Yugo* (Lee Je-ma's Posthumous Treatise) he includes a comprehensive list of herbs utilized in Sasang medicine, categorizing them by taste, temperature, and function. In general, he incorporates the Chinese medical interpretation of the Five Flavors (Bitter, Acrid, Sweet, Salty, and Astringent) and temperature (Warm, Hot, Cool, Cold, and Neutral), but function and organ affiliation are interpreted according to Sasang standards. To illustrate, Lee Je-ma describes Da Huang (*Radix et Rhizoma Rhei*) as a herb that promotes the flow of lung energy and regulates bowel movement. Chinese medicine also associates this herb with bowel regulation, but not with lung function. In the *Dongmu Yugo*, Lee Je-ma categorizes Da Huang as a lung-affiliated herb that benefits the Tae Eum Individual, born with weaker lungs. He also describes Chuan Xiong (*Radix Ligustici Chuanxiong*) as a herb that benefits the spleen and promotes the release of pathogen from the Exterior, benefitting the So Eum Individual with External illness. Although its Exterior releasing function is the same in Chinese medicine, it does not associate Chuan Xiong with the spleen.

**Table I.3: Herb affiliation in Sasang medicine**

| Organ of primary affiliation | Prescribed for the... |
| --- | --- |
| lungs | Tae Eum Individual, since they are born with weaker lung energy |
| spleen | So Eum Individual, since they are born with weaker spleen energy |
| liver | Tae Yang Individual, since they are born with weaker liver energy |
| kidney | So Yang Individual, since they are born with weaker kidney energy |

## Sasang Constitutional Theory and the Four Humors

The concept of four humors is deeply embedded in Western medical philosophy, serving as the dominant view of medicine up to the advent of modern science. This theory, promoted by the teachings of Hippocrates (c. 460–c. 370 BC) and Galen (129–201 AD), is dismissed by mainstream Western medicine, as it adheres to a physiological vs. metaphysical view of the human body.

As far back as ancient Greece, the significance of four humors influenced which foods, exercises, and herbs were selected to improve health. Hippocrates himself claimed that it is more important to know the characteristics of the individual than the disease they present. He introduced the concept of four humors (blood, phlegm, yellow bile, and black bile) and the importance of balance between them. The four humors were later elaborated upon by Galen who associated them with psychological temperaments (blood-sanguine, black bile-melancholic, yellow bile-choleric, and phlegm-phlegmatic). This contribution was based on his belief that health depends on a balance of temperament and that disease resulted from an imbalance of humors, a concept referred to as dyscratia.

Although they came from different backgrounds and traditions, Galen and Lee Je-ma both held the four constitutional concept as the main premise of their teachings. They also shared a belief that certain foods and herbs with different characteristic temperatures could facilitate or impede balance within the body. Galen prescribed Cold-natured herbs to treat Heat-related conditions (i.e. biliary disorders) and Hot-natured herbs to address Cold-related issues (i.e. phlegmatic disorders). Lee Je-ma also applies the principle of treating Cold conditions with Hot-natured herbs and Heat-related situations with Cold-natured herbs, but adds that each constitution benefits from different temperatures. The So Yang's stronger spleen, for example, produces abundant Heat, while the So Eum's stronger kidneys produce abundant Cold. Hence the So Yang's illnesses are often Heat-related and are commonly addressed with Cold-natured herbs, while the So Eum's are Cold-related and are addressed with Hot-natured herbs.

**Table I.4: The temperature-related effects of the spleen and kidneys**

| Sasang constitution | Strongest organ | Can lead to illness caused by... | Often treated with... |
|---|---|---|---|
| So Yang | Spleen | Heat | Cold-natured herbs |
| So Eum | Kidney | Cold | Hot-natured herbs |

## Sasang and Ayurvedic Medicine

Constitutional theory and the emphasis on balancing inherently excessive and deficient energies within the body is a fundamental aspect of the approximately 3000-year tradition of Ayurvedic medicine, which introduces the concepts of *vata*, *pitta*, and *kaffa*—three aspects of human emotion and physiology, also called the Tridosha Theory. Accordingly, a single *dosha*, or combination thereof, has a profound effect on the way an individual thinks and acts throughout their lifetime. This principle is similar to the Sasang medical idea that illness and disease have constitutionally specific effects. Whereas the former includes constitutional combinations such as *vata-pitta* or *pitta-kaffa*, the latter does not consider the mutual dominance of energies within the body. Instead, it holds that an individual is born with a single stronger and weaker organ energy, and that all other organ energies fall within these parameters.

Born from a different tradition, the four constitutions mentioned in Sasang medicine do not correlate directly with the three dosha in Ayurvedic medicine and precaution should be taken when comparing them. Yet they share several general principles worth mentioning, such as the idea that the mind and body are inseparable and that each individual inherits energetic strengths and weaknesses. Each dosha in Ayurvedic medicine along with each organ system in Sasang medicine is correlated with emotional/physical characteristics and temperatures. Cooling herbs, in both medicines, for example, are prescribed to treat Heat-related issues and vice versa. The correlation of each dosha with a particular body fluid is also echoed in Sasang medicine. Vata is considered the lightest of the three dosha and therefore correlates with air, the pitta associated with the consistency of oil, and the kapha, even thicker, is as dense as bone. Sasang medicine explains how four humors, Jin (Clear Fluids), Go (Sticky Fluids), Yu (Oily Fluids), and Ek (Essence), derived from food intake, contribute to the formation of the skin, muscles, tendons, and bones, respectively.

**Table I.5: The bodily fluids in Sasang medicine**

| Bodily fluid | Produced from food inside of the... | Nourishes and engenders the... |
|---|---|---|
| Jin | Esophagus | Skin |
| Go | Stomach | Muscles |
| Yu | Small intestine | Tendons |
| Ek | Large intestine | Bones |

## Health and the Four Virtues

The *Dongeui Susei Bowon* is a text that goes beyond the confines of medicine: structured in such a way that each chapter builds a complete picture of humanity. The opening chapter, *Theories on Human Nature and Conduct*, describes the intricate and interdependent relationship between man and heaven. It also offers a philosophical anecdote of humanism according to the Confucian tradition, which emphasizes the influence of *Chon Song* (天性), the seed of heaven planted within the heart of every human being. Lee Je-ma describes how the Confucian Four Virtues of compassion (仁), humility (禮), righteousness (意), and wisdom (知), which are embedded within human nature, set humanity apart from other organisms. Health, according to Lee Je-ma, is dependent on the discovery and cultivation of these innate Virtues and thus enhancing the connection between man and heaven.

Lee Je-ma admitted that the process of manifesting virtue is a fundamental challenge that can only be accomplished through steadfast self-reflection and sincere effort. Virtue depends on the ability to balance one's temperament (sorrow, anger, joy, or calmness). These emotional tendencies either support or impede the path towards virtue and health. The manifestation of virtue, according to Confucian teachings, is primarily realized through social interaction and the ability to reflect on one's actions.

## The Che/Yong Relationship and Sasang Medicine

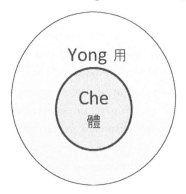

*Figure I.1: The Che/Yong relationship*

The relationship between *Che* (體) and *Yong* (用) is a common theme throughout the *Dongeui Susei Bowon*. *Che* is translated roughly as "internal aspect" or "latent nature," while *Yong* is the "external aspect" or "manifest nature." *Che* is sometimes defined as the metaphysical nature of all things, while *Yong* is the manifested or physical nature. All phenomena have both *Che* and *Yong* aspects. A seed, for example, has the potential for becoming a fruit. In this context, the seed is the *Che* aspect and the fruit is the *Yong* aspect. Conversely, a fruit has the potential for becoming a seed, in which case the fruit is the *Che* aspect and the seed is the *Yong* aspect. Depending on the context, *Che* and *Yong* can change roles just as a seed becomes a fruit and a fruit becomes a seed.

Lee Je-ma utilizes the concept of *Che* and *Yong* repeatedly throughout his treatise, initially in the title of the first chapter, *Theories on Human Nature and Conduct*. In this title, he sees human nature (*Song*, 性) as *Che* and conduct (*Myung*, 命) as *Yong*. Hence Lee Je-ma denotes how human nature manifests through conduct, and how a cultivated nature produces benevolent action. On the contrary, if one is immersed in greed or self-conceit, this will become apparent in their conduct.

Illness, according to Sasang theory, is the result of an imbalanced *Che* nature, which morphs into a *Yong* uncontrolled emotion. Anger, for example, is the *Che* nature of *Yong* sadness. Otherwise stated, if anger is not balanced, it can easily morph into uncontrolled sadness. For the same reason, imbalanced *Che* sadness can transform into *Yong* anger. In Lee Je-ma's view, uncontrolled emotions have serious health consequences.

The word for human nature, or *Song* (性), contains the radicals for "heart" and "life," and expresses how, at birth, the seed of heaven is implanted within the heart of every individual. Hence the heart, as one's connection with heaven, plays a fundamental role in health and wellbeing. Lee Je-ma classified the heart as the *Che*, internal, aspect of the Four Major Organs (lungs, spleen, liver, kidneys). Healing in Sasang medicine begins with the heart and the ability to manifest one's heavenly nature through sincerity and self-cultivation.

*Che* may also be considered the underlying aspect of disease, while *Yong* is the outer manifestation of disease. The inner aspects lurk within the body and are not easily detected, while the outer symptomatic aspects are easier to detect and may give hint to or otherwise obstruct what is lurking within the body. Without a careful examination of both *Che* and *Yong* it is easy to lose sight of disease etiology and progression. While offering a historical account of Chinese medicine, Lee Je-ma illustrates how the *Che* aspect of illness was often overlooked, resulting in mistreatment, such as the prescription of diaphoretics for internal disorders and laxatives for external disorders. He emphasizes how the recognition of an individual's *Che* nature is a fundamental aspect of addressing his/her illness.

## Metaphysics and Sasang Medicine

At the heart of Lee Je-ma's teachings is a metaphysical conception of the human body and its processes. The Greek prefix "meta" (μετά) in metaphysics is synonymous with "beyond" or "behind," where the former meaning is emphasized by philosophers such as Plato, who held that the immortal mind, capable of accessing universal truths, is "beyond" the empty and transient material body. Plato's dualistic view was perpetuated by Descartes, with his schema of the mind and body as possessing distinct roles. Rather than distinguishing between mind and body, Lee Je-ma's metaphysical approach accentuates the definition of "behind" the physical, viewing the mind as the foundation of the physical body and its movement, thus envisioning a monistic, integrated conception of the mind/body relationship. His version of monism, however, contrasts with the idealistic approach that interprets reality as nothing other than a reflection of the mind or spirit, absent of the physical. He also differs with physicalism, also known as materialistic monism, which maintains that all phenomena can be broken down into physical properties.

Lee Je-ma's definition of monism is illustrated in Chapter 2, where he compares *Ri* (理, principle) of *Hoyon Ji Ri* (浩然之理, accumulated and widespread principle) with *Gi* (氣, life-force, flow) of *Hoyon Ji Gi* (浩然之氣, accumulated and widespread flow). He shows how principle and flow are inseparable, with the former as the basis of the latter. He considers *Ri* the non-manifest aspect of all phenomena and *Gi* as the manifest, mobile aspect. This concept is expressed in his view of the mind/body relationship. Lee Je-ma's focus was on the mind's influence on the body rather than the body's effect on the mind. Similar to his view of *Ri* as the basis for *Gi*, he saw the immaterial mind as "behind" the processes of the material body, and the body as merely a reflection of the mind. Hence he maintained that the body relies on the mind for balance and healing, and the mind relies on the body for expression and movement.

Lee Je-ma developed his theory of organ function based on a metaphysical viewpoint of biology, stressing the immaterial task of each organ rather than its concrete structure and physiological function. This emphasis is illustrated in Chapter 1 where he describes the Four Major Organs as hosting the Four Human Affairs, inborn characteristics manifested through social interaction. Hence Lee Je-ma's reference to the lungs, spleen, liver, and kidneys in his *Dongeui Susei Bowon* should not be taken verbatim. An argument can be made, for example, that Lee Je-ma's use of *Bi* (脾), directly translated as spleen, should actually be interpreted as pancreas, since the latter plays a significant role in digestion, a process he closely associates with *Bi*. While such arguments can easily be justified, they fall short of considering the emphasis on metaphysical vs. physiological organ function.

## The Four Temperaments and Illness

A common theme throughout the *Dongeui Susei Bowon* is Lee Je-ma's emphasis on connection between emotion and organ health. He held that trauma and injury, in themselves, are not the only culprits behind energy blockage within the body. Actually, it is primarily the mind and body's response to trauma that inevitably determines how it affects our health.

The ability to carry out one's life mission and maintain health depends heavily on one's emotional tendencies or temperaments. The stronger lungs of the Tae

Yang Individual, for instance, correlate with sorrow, giving the Tae Yang Individual a consistent underlying feeling of sadness. When in balance, sadness is directed towards self-discovery and assisting others. The energy of the lungs can also flow smoothly to the Tae Yang Individual's weaker organs when sadness is expressed in a productive way. If the Tae Yang's sadness gets out of control, it will morph into uncontrollable anger, causing damage to the spleen, which correlates with this emotion. Herbal treatment in Sasang medicine is thus based entirely on balancing emotion and, in turn, the flow of energy from the stronger to weaker organs of each constitution.

Lee Je-ma's *Dongeui Susei Bowon* can be considered a manual of both psychology and physiology combined into a single book. It paints a detailed picture of how emotions and physiology produce mutual effects on our health, while portraying a systemized psychosomatic and bio-energetic analysis of disease pathology. Each chapter builds upon the previous one, beginning with a definition of humanity from a universal perspective, and ending with precise treatment approaches to illness according to the energetic requirements of each Sasang constitution. Despite its limited size and inclusion of case studies, each of the Sasang principles set forth by Lee Je-ma in the *Dongeui Susei Bowon* can be applied to most, if not all, clinical situations.

Sasang medicine provides a unique and practical methodology to those interested in the fields of medicine, philosophy, and/or psychology. As a medicine, the Sasang approach offers novel insight into disease epidemiology through an emphasis on intrinsic disease factors often overlooked in modern medicine. As a philosophy, the Sasang approach explores the heaven–human connection, examining the meaning of human nature and its role in health and societal harmony. From a psychological perspective, it examines the effect of emotion on one's health, discussing how each emotion has its own root and outward expression, the relationship between various emotions, and their tendency to morph into one another.

## Herb Dosage and Frequency

Herbal dosages in the *Dongeui Susei Bowon* are typically stronger that what we see in Eastern medical prescriptions of the modern day. There are several likely reasons. Even though Western medicine had already been introduced to Korea by the time Lee Je-ma became a doctor, it was rarely consulted. Hence the common people relied solely on the use of herbal medicine and acupuncture to treat illness. Herbs were prescribed much more often than they are today. It is probable that a tolerance was developed, since frequent consumption made it necessary to increase dosage to get desirable effects. Another reason may be that epidemics and other acute illnesses were rampant during Lee Je-ma's lifetime, requiring higher herbal dosages.

Traditionally, the standard single herb dosage was referred to as 1 Qian. This is equivalent to 3.75g. All other dosages were based on this amount. To illustrate, 1 Liang is 37.5g, 1 Fen is .375g, and 1 Li is .0375g. If the patient were to take two standard doses of a herb a day, they would consume 3.75 + 3.75 = 7.5g. Each herbal dosage within this text adheres to this tradition. However, for purposes of simplification, each amount was rounded to the nearest tenth (i.e. .375g = .4g, 3.75g = 4g, 37.5g = 40g).

The standard single herb amount in modern-day Eastern medicine is 9g. This would be equivalent to approximately 4g of the traditional dosage if herbs are cooked once and 2g when the herbs are re-cooked.

**Table I.6: Herb dosage equivalents**

| Traditional dosage | Equivalence in grams |
|---|---|
| 1 Liang | 37.5g |
| 1 Qian | 3.75g |
| 1 Fen | .375g |
| 1 Li | .0375g |

The bitter taste and thickness of Oriental herbal formulae may lead to compliance issues and/or digestive discomfort for sensitive patients and first timers. These patients usually respond better when given smaller and/or diluted dosages. Since most Koreans have had Oriental herbal formulae in tea form at least once, they may better tolerate higher, more concentrated dosages.

Traditionally, herbal teas were consumed three or more times a day, contrary to the current standard of twice daily. Whereas the treatment of common colds or pneumonia may require two to four doses a day, usually two doses a day is sufficient for chronic illness. Lee Je-ma occasionally prescribed smaller, more frequent doses to offer consistent support throughout the day.

When treating Western patients, it may be advantageous to convert each dose according to modern standards, where 1 Qian (3.75g) is equated with a 9g dose, 2 Qian with an 18g dose, etc. Each pack could then be cooked with enough water to last for a total of two days or a total of one day and then re-cooked the second day. When preparing herbal formulae, keep in mind that a single dose is equivalent to three-quarters of a cup of liquid tea.

## Herbal Preparation

The general rule for the decoction of each herb and formula in Sasang medicine is the same as for other forms of Eastern Medical pharmacopeia. Raw herbs are placed in a clay, glass, or stainless steel pot with a lid and one cup of water is added to the pot for each dose prescribed. For example, if four doses a day are prescribed, four cups of water are to be added. Simmer the herbs for approximately 45 minutes after bringing to the boil. The amount of water and boiling time may vary according to the formula. Lee Je-ma provides supplemental information for herbs and formulae that require special instructions.

Another method of preparing the herbs involves the use of a slow cooker or crock-pot. This method encourages further absorbency of the herbs due to longer and more consistent cooking. When using a crock-pot, add the same amount of water mentioned above. Turn the crock-pot or slow cooker setting to high and let it cook for two to three hours. For most machines, this amount of time will reduce the amount of water slightly. Add more water as the level drops below the height of the herbs.

Sasang formulae are prepared in powder, pill, or tea form. Clinically, the pill and tea forms are the most common, with tea capable of a higher concentration than pills. It is wise to keep the pill form of commonly used Sasang formulae on hand. A short-term supply of pills might be used initially to assess a patient's response before proceeding further with herbal remedies. Pills may also be given to sensitive patients or those who cannot bear the taste of herbal tea.

When administering herbs for children under the age of 12 it is necessary to adjust the dosage amount. Infants under one year old should ingest no more than 60–100ml (2 to 3.4oz) per dose. Children ages one through six should ingest no more than 150–200ml (5.1 to 6.8oz) per dose. Children ages seven through twelve should ingest no more than 200–250ml (6.8 to 8.5oz) per dose. For children, herbal tea may be mixed with juice, formula, or milk to dilute the strong taste. There are no strict guidelines as to how much juice to add since it depends on the child's preference. For younger children it may be beneficial to divide dosages into smaller portions given throughout the day. An eyedropper may prove handy with fussy toddlers/infants.

Sasang medicine is based on the principles of respecting and accommodating the unique needs of each and every patient. Each clinical situation has its own specific requirements, so the practitioner must be sensitive to the requirements of his/her patients at all times. A lack of patient compliance may be the practitioner's fault since it is easy to get discouraged and give up when a patient complains of herbal taste, odor, etc. Some situations may require that the practitioner adjust the dosage or method of preparation to suit the patient. Others may require consistent encouragement as they adjust to the herbal regime. This is simply par for the course when fulfilling the role of practitioner and making the patient's health and wellbeing one's first priority. Working through these challenges is an indispensable component of the healing process.

## An Overview of the *Dongeui Susei Bowon*

There currently exists a tendency among Sasang practitioners to overlook the rich philosophy of Sasang medicine and refer directly to the latter chapters of the *Dongeui Susei Bowon*, which focus on clinical application. Skipping through the first few chapters of this text will often lead to further confusion and lack of effective application. As illustrated in the chapter overview below, Lee Je-ma purposely structured this text in order to paint a complete picture of humanity and its energetic processes. I recommend following this process closely and reviewing content repeatedly in order to get accustomed to basic Sasang concepts before moving onwards.

### *Part I: Theory*

CHAPTER 1: THEORIES ON HUMAN NATURE AND CONDUCT (性命論)

Chapter 1 describes the four components of universal and human energy, correlating various bodily components with advantageous and disadvantageous emotional inclinations. Lastly, it offers a brief introduction to the Four *Zhang* Organs and their unique physiological and psychological Sasang-related functions.

CHAPTER 2: THE FOUR BASIC CHARACTERISTICS (四端論)

Chapter 2 discusses the difference in visceral size and strength according to each of the Four Sasang Constitutions, and examines the Four Virtues with their ability to enhance organ health and overall wellbeing. It reinforces the Confucian idea of how selfishness sets the average person apart from a Sage. Lee Je-ma states that the viscera of sage are identical to that of the average person, making it possible, through balancing one's stronger and weaker organs, to become a Sage. He also introduces the Four Temperaments and describes their biological effects.

CHAPTER 3: EXPANDING AND FULFILLING (擴充論)

Chapter 3 further discusses the different emotional/physical strengths and weaknesses of each constitution. It also elaborates on the Four Temperaments, Four Virtues, and Four Senses and how they hinder or facilitate health and wellbeing.

CHAPTER 4: THE *ZHANG FU* ORGANS (臟腑論)

Chapter 4 discusses the location and function of each Sasang bodily organ, and illustrates the pathway of *Su Kok* (digested material) and how it nourishes and engenders different areas of the body. Lee Je-ma also calls attention to how the Four Essences are stored in each of the organs, emphasizing the importance of a balancing lifestyle to preserve them.

CHAPTER 5: THE BASIC PRINCIPLES OF MEDICINE (醫源論)

This chapter includes an overview of Chinese medical history, describing how different medical scholars of the past contributed to the formation of Sasang medical theory. Lee Je-ma also credits Zhang Zhongjing with elaborating on the Six Stages of Illness, a topic he refers to throughout the *Dongeui Susei Bowon*. It was Lee Je-ma, however, who first associated the Six Stages of Illness with the Four Sasang Constitutions.

## Part II: Clinical Application

CHAPTER 6: THE SO EUM INDIVIDUAL'S ILLNESS (少陰人論)

This chapter consists of the following subtitles:

- The So Eum Individual's kidney Heat Causing Exterior Heat Syndrome

- The Seo Eum Individual's stomach Cold Causing Interior Cold Syndrome

- A Synopsis of So Eum Illness

- The So Eum Individual's 23 Formulae from Zhang Zhongjing's *Shang Han Lun*

- The So Eum Individual's 13 Formulae Presented by Doctors of the Song, Yuan, and Ming Dynasties—with Six Containing Ba Dou (*Semen Crotonis*)

- 24 Newly Discovered Formulae for the So Eum Individual (Formulated by Lee Je-ma).

CHAPTER 7: THE SO YANG INDIVIDUAL'S ILLNESS (少陽人論)

This chapter consists of the following subtitles:

- The So Yang Individual's spleen Cold Causing Exterior Cold Syndrome

- The So Yang Individual's stomach Heat Causing Interior Heat Syndrome

- A Synopsis of So Yang Illness

- The So Yang Individual's Ten Formulae from Zhang Zhongjing's *Shang Han Lun*

- The So Yang Individual's Nine Formulae Presented by Doctors of the Yuan and Ming Dynasties

- 17 Newly Discovered Formulae for the So Yang Individual (Formulated by Lee Je-ma).

CHAPTER 8: THE TAE EUM INDIVIDUAL'S ILLNESS (太陰人論)

This chapter consists of the following subtitles:

- The Tae Eum Individual's Esophageal Cold Causing Exterior Cold Syndrome

- The Tae Eum Individual's liver Heat Causing Interior Heat Syndrome

- A Synopsis of Tae Eum Illness

- The Tae Eum Individual's Four Formulae from Zhang Zhongjing's *Shang Han Lun*

- The Tae Eum Individual's Nine Formulae Presented by Doctors of the Tang, Song, and Ming Dynasties

- 24 Newly Discovered Formulae for the Tae Eum Individual (Formulated by Lee Je-ma).

CHAPTER 9: THE TAE YANG INDIVIDUAL'S ILLNESS (太陽人論)

This chapter consists of the following subtitles:

- The Tae Yang Individual's Externally Contracted Illness Affecting the Lumbar Spine

- The Tae Yang Individual's Internally Contracted Illness Affecting the small intestine

- The Tae Yang Individual's Ten Herbs from the *Ben Cao Lun*, and Two Herbs Introduced by Li Chan and Gong Xin

- Two Newly Discovered Formulae for the Tae Yang Individual (Formulated by Lee Je-ma).

*Part III: Additional Topics*

CHAPTER 10: THE VIRTUOUS PATH—ADVICE FOR EVERYDAY LIFE (廣濟說)

As the title suggests, this chapter describes the essential qualities of a virtuous person, offering advice about cultivating one's mind in order to prolong life and enhance wellbeing.

CHAPTER 11: FOUR CONSTITUTIONAL CLASSIFICATION AND DIAGNOSIS (四象人 辨證論)

The final chapter reviews core physiological and psychological characteristics of each constitution. It compares the harder to distinguish aspects between constitutions side by side in order to avoid common diagnostic pitfalls.

## Lee Je-ma (1837–1900)

Dr. Lee Je-ma, the founder of Sasang Constitutional Medicine, was a scholar of the Confucian school of thought. Shortly before his birth, Lee Je-ma's grandfather dreamed of receiving a horse from the Jeju Province. He interpreted this as an auspicious dream and named his grandson Lee Je-ma, which translates as "The Horse from Jeju." As a gifted child, Lee Je-ma quickly became well versed in history and Confucian philosophy.

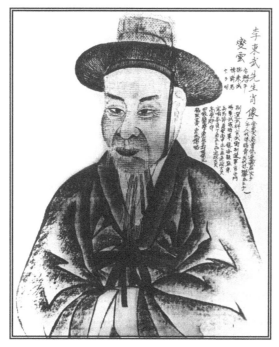

*Figure I.2: Lee Je-ma*

At age 13 he achieved the highest score on the official state examination, a test notorious for its difficulty. Afterwards he spent several years living in poverty as he traveled throughout Korea. During Lee Je-ma's lifetime, Korea was struggling internally due to political instability and externally from foreign invasion. At age 39 he joined the military and after only one year of service was promoted to general.

While serving as a military officer he was in charge of suppressing a popular uprising. In the process, he witnessed the effects of a major epidemic that spread like wildFire amongst the people, invoking his desire to find a cure. Shortly afterwards, he watched helplessly as his wife died, her condition deteriorating rapidly after she was given Cold-natured herbs to treat high fever. Even though this was the standard approach to treating fever, he concluded that other constitutional factors must also be considered. This was the catalyst for his career as a doctor, and eventually his creation of Sasang Constitutional Medicine.

In 1883, after 13 years of research and practicing medicine, Lee Je-ma authored his first book, entitled *The Attainment of Wisdom through Examining the True Nature of All Phenomena*, or *Gyeukchigo* (格致藁). This title is based on a phrase in Confucius's *The Great Learning*: "Ultimate cultivation leads to the wisdom of deciphering all phenomena" (格物致知). Lee Je-ma's *Gyeukchigo* forms the basis of Sasang medical and philosophical theory. In the first chapter, *A Summary of Confucian Teachings*, or *Yu Ryak* (儒略), he introduces the concept of "affairs, heart, body, and phenomena" (事心身物), which combines the Confucian concept of "affairs" and "phenomena" with two additional concepts, "heart" and "mind," thus uniting philosophy with physiology. The second chapter, completed in 1893, *The Practice of Sincerity through Self-Cultivation*, or *Ban Song Jam* (反誠箴), encourages awareness of one's basic nature, or *Bon Nung* (本能), and the need to balance it with one's heavenly nature, or *Chon Song* (天性), through sincerity and honesty. This chapter is divided into nine sub-sections, each devoted to the explanation of an *I Ching* hexagram. In 1883, Lee Je-ma completed the third chapter, *Advancing Along Your Life's Path*, or *Dok Heng Pyun* (獨行篇), which emphasizes the importance of embracing the Confucian Four Virtues of love, justice, respect, and wisdom, and overcoming the Four Negative Tendencies of rashness, cruelty, greed, and laziness.

One year after writing *Gyeukchigo*, Lee Je-ma completed the four-volume book entitled *Eastern Medical Perspectives on Longevity and Health Preservation*, or *Dongeui Susei Bowon* (東意壽世保元), which forms the theoretical basis and methodological structure of Sasang theory and practice. Shortly after completing the Tae Eum chapter of the *Dongeui Susei Bowon* in 1900, Lee Je-ma passed away at the age of 64.

## Translator's Note: Chinese Characters and their Meanings

In Oriental literature, a single character often has several different and sometimes contrary meanings. In order to derive the meaning of a character it is often necessary to read several interpretations beforehand while developing a clear understanding of context. This is a reflection of Oriental thought and philosophy, which places an emphasis on context rather than concrete or absolute meaning. Accordingly, all animate and inanimate objects are defined by the situation in which they exist. Instead of calling a person angry, for example, they are described as being angry about something. Without the "something" the person may not be angry and actually be quite pleasant. The same person may be happier if the "something" didn't anger them. This interpretation helps avoid the pitfalls of prejudice while enhancing a focus on relativity. Anger is an emotion that has numerous meanings depending on its context and intensity. In order to illustrate this concept further, let's take a closer look at the Four Temperaments, which are referred to periodically throughout the *Dongeui Susei Bowon*.

**Temperament**: 哀 (*Ei*)

**Translation**: Sadness, sorrow, pity

**Interpretation**: Sadness according to Oriental philosophy is not necessarily a "bad" emotion—it could encourage us to feel sorrow and compassion for others. However, if taken to the extreme it could turn into depression. The above Chinese character encompasses varying degrees of sadness and should be interpreted according to context.

**Temperament**: 怒 (*No*)

**Translation**: Anger, rage, irritability

**Interpretation**: Anger according to Oriental philosophy is not necessarily a "bad" emotion—it could encourage us to stand up for what we or others feel is right. However, if taken to the extreme it could turn into rage. The above Chinese character encompasses varying degrees of anger and should be interpreted according to context.

**Temperament**: 喜 (*Hui*)

**Translation**: Joy, happiness, giddiness, mania

**Interpretation**: Joy according to Oriental philosophy is not necessarily a "good" emotion—it could cause us to lose touch with reality and feel joy inappropriately. However, if expressed harmoniously, it could provide us and others with a sense of comfort while reducing stress. The above Chinese character encompasses varying degrees of joy and should be interpreted according to context.

**Temperament**: 樂 (*Rak*)

**Translation**: Complacency, calmness, laziness, pleasure, rapture, fun

**Interpretation**: Calmness according to Oriental philosophy is not necessarily a "good" emotion—it could cause us to become lazy and avoid responsibility. However, if expressed harmoniously, it could provide us and others with a sense of joy and freedom. The above Chinese character encompasses varying degrees of complacency and should be interpreted according to context.

Lee Je-ma took great care in capturing the essential meaning of every character in his writings. Scholars in Korea often refer to him as not just an accomplished doctor, but also a skilled philosopher and poet. The theory behind Sasang medicine is difficult to grasp and easy to misinterpret due to the various meanings that each character may present. His intricate choice of characters and their context often make it challenging even for native Korean speakers to grasp. Most of the concepts and terms to follow are also deeply embedded within Asian philosophy and Confucian tradition. Certain terms in the *Dongeui Susei Bowon* are derived by Lee Je-ma himself, based on his perspective of Confucianism and human psychophysiology. These terms are not only foreign to the Western reader, but also to scholars who are well versed in Asian philosophy. For this reason the author made a sincere effort to explain each term and portray Lee Je-ma's original intention with a consistent use of footnotes.

Moreover, certain terms, such as "Exterior," "Interior," "Heat/Hot," "Warm," "Cool," and "Cold," were purposely capitalized to emphasize their use in context with Chinese/Sasang medical principles. In Chinese medicine, Interior and Exterior refer to the source of disease pathology, where the former indicates disease of Internal origin and the latter of External origin. In Sasang medicine, all illness stems from an imbalance of the Four Temperaments and, hence, is considered to be of Internal origin. Exterior disease is therefore considered a result of Song nature imbalance rather than an attack from an External pathogenic influence.

In Chinese/Sasang medicine, the capitalization of "Warm," "Hot," Cool," and "Cold" refers to energetic, or metaphysical, attributes rather than actual temperature, for which the lower case version is provided. When discussing the Organ Systems (lungs, spleen, liver, and kidneys), for example, these terms are capitalized, but presented in lower case when describing the palpable temperature of the abdomen, hands, feet, etc.

Part I ————————————————

# THEORY

Chapter 1 ——————————————————

# 性命論

# Theories on Human Nature and Conduct[1]

天機 有四하니 一曰地方이오 二曰人倫이오 三曰世會이오 四曰天時이니라.

*Chon Ki* (Heavenly Affairs)[2] consists of four aspects.[3] The first aspect is *Ji Bang* (the

---

1 The title of this chapter is pronounced *Song Myung*. The character for *Song* (性) consists of two radicals, translating as "heart/mind" and "birth/life." According to the principles of Sasang medicine, human life begins when the energy of heaven descends, enters the heart, and embeds the Four Virtues (love, humility, righteousness, and wisdom). When combined, these two radicals can be defined as "human nature." The recognition of one's *Song* is equivalent to discovering his or her connection with the heavens. The second character, *Myung* (命), contains the radical for "distinguish/discern" and signifies the ability to discern one's divine mission and purpose in life. The preservation of health and manifestation of virtue are dependent upon discovering one's *Song* and carrying out one's *Myung*.

2 The *Chon Ki* (Heavenly Affairs) are universal aspects that connect heaven and all mankind. They serve as a foundation of *In Sa* (Human Affairs) and the basis of human existence. *Chon Ki* is considered *Che* (internal aspect), while *In Sa* is considered *Yong* (external/manifest aspect—please see introduction for *Che/Yong* explanation). Hence the ability to engage *In Sa* depends on the discovery and implementation of *Chon Ki*.

3 Throughout the *Dongeui Susei Bowon*, Lee Je-ma introduced most of his concepts in groups of four, the common denominator of all natural phenomena, mentioned in Confucius's commentary on the *I Ching* entitled the *Ten Wings*. In this text, Confucius shows how all existence is derived from a single source, the *Tai Chi*, which separates into latent, or *Che* (non-manifest), aspects of Yin and Yang, and then into manifest, or *Yong*, aspects, which are Yin within Yin and Yang within Yin, Yang within Yang, and Yin within Yang. The latter four concepts are also referred to as "*Sasang*" (as in Sasang medicine), which translates as "Four Symbols." Whereas latent Yin and Yang do not manifest into matter, the Four Symbols do, and are correlated with the four seasons, four directions, the four phases (birth, growth, fruition, death), and the four Sasang body types (Tae Yang, Tae Eum, So Yang, So Eum).

existence of all things),[4] the second is *In Ryun* (social skills and talents),[5] the third is *Sei Wei* (society at large),[6] and the fourth is *Chon Shi* (the ebb and flow of nature).[7]

人事 有四하니 一日居處이오 二日黨與이오 三日交遇이오 四日事務이니라.

*In Sa* (Human Affairs)[8] consists of four aspects. The first aspect is *Ko Cho* (knowing the proper place to reside),[9] the second aspect is *Dang Yo* (establishing group responsibilities),[10] the third aspect is *Kyo Uh* (associating with others one on one),[11] and the fourth is *Sa Mu* (fulfilling one's mission and work).[12]

---

4    *Ji Bang*: *Ji* (地): Earth + *Bang* (方): Direction, the Way or "Dao," path—*Ji Bang* consists of two characters, land and direction. Direction in this sense may be further defined as "action" or "manifestation"; land refers to one's current position. When interpreted together, these characters refer to the ability to know the proper place to take action. *Ji Bang* is concerned with determining the right "place," *In Ryun* is concerned with determining the right "thing to do," *Sei Wei* is concerned with determining the right "time," and *Chon Shi* is concerned with determining the right "meaning." *Ji Bang* correlates with and is expressed through the Virtue of love.

5    *In Ryun*: *In* (人): Human, humanity, person + *Ryun* (倫): Morality, humaneness—*In Ryun* refers to the talent or skill of governing or controlling one's surroundings and to talent or skill in general. In order to carry out *In Ryun* it is necessary to decipher between what is right and wrong. Therefore, *In Ryun* correlates with the Virtue of righteousness. *Sei Wei* correlates with the ability to unite, while *In Ryun* is the ability to separate or decipher. These are opposing aspects of *Chon Ki* (Heavenly Affairs).

6    *Sei Wei*: *Sei* (世): Era, generation + *Wei* (會): Meeting, interaction—*Sei Wei* describes the ability to bring people together according to the right time. Lee Je-ma equates this ability with a heightened understanding of time and the cyclical nature of all phenomena. *Sei Wei* corresponds with the Virtue of humility, which entails the ability to unite or bring people together.

7    *Chon Shi*: *Chon* (天): Heaven, divine + *Shi* (時): Time, voice, meaning—*Chon Shi* has several interpretations. It signifies the "voice" or the "divine meaning" of heaven, which manifests as time here on earth. It may also translate as the ebb and flow of nature and be referred to as the four seasons. *Chon Shi* corresponds to the Virtue of wisdom.

8    *In Sa* (人事, Human Affairs) manifests through social interaction. How successful and harmonious these actions are depends on one's awareness of their *Myung* (divine mission) and *Chon Ki* (their connection with heaven). Human Affairs also depend on the Four Virtues (love, humility, justice, and wisdom), which are embedded within the heart. According to Confucius, one has to cleanse the heart, strive for achievement, prioritize, and control/cultivate one's mind to carry out virtue. Lee Je-ma viewed heaven and human as intricately connected. One is seen as a reflection of the other. *Chon Ki* is embedded equally within the heart of each person, while *In Sa* manifests differently according to the action of the individual.

9    *Ko Cho*: *Ko* (居): Dwelling, live, seat oneself, settle + *Cho* (處): Arrange, consider—*Ko Cho* is the first of four *In Sa*, which correlates with the first of four *Chon Ki*, referred to as *Ji Bang*. *Ko Cho* is the effort one makes to establish a firm foundation in life by incorporating *Ji Bang* (the appropriate place for action). *Ji Bang* and *Ko Cho* are carried out through the Virtue of *In* 仁 (love).

10   *Dang Yo*: *Dang* (黨): A group, company, village, neighborhood, become familiar with + *Yo* (與): To give, aid, assist, share, participate—*Dang Yo* is the second *In Sa*, which correlates with the second *Chon Ki*, referred to as *In Ryun*. It represents the effort to find similar qualities in others and overcome one's own prejudice through the incorporation of *In Ryun* (one-on-one interaction). *In Ryun* and *Dang Yo* are carried out through the Virtue of *Eui* (義, righteousness), which according to Confucius is the ability to prioritize and decipher between right and wrong. When socializing, *Eui* is the ability to distinguish the strengths and weaknesses of others.

11   *Kyo Uh*: *Kyo* (交): Exchange, make friends, mix, pair up with, together + *Uh* (遇): To meet, assemble, treat with respect, opportunity, chance—*Kyo Uh* is the third *In Sa*, which correlates with the third *Chon Ki*, referred to as *Sei Wei*. It is the effort one makes to show humility and respect through the incorporation and adaptation of *Sei Wei* (society and social duty). *Sei Wei* and *Kyo Uh* are carried out through the Virtue of *Ye* (禮, humility).

12   *Sa Mu*: *Sa* (事): Affairs, work, devotion, serve, rule (over), administer + *Mu* (務): Do one's best, strive, help, aid, assist, one's duty—*Sa Mu* is the fourth *In Sa*, which correlates with the fourth *Chon Ki*, referred to as *Chon Shi*. *Sa Mu* is the adaptation and incorporation of *Chon Shi* (divine meaning) in societal affairs and the ability to know the appropriate, or meaningful, time to take action. *Chon Shi* and *Sa Mu* are carried out through the Virtue of *Ji* (知, wisdom).

**Table 1.1: The correlation between Heavenly and Human Affairs**

| Heavenly Affair | Human Affair |
|---|---|
| *Chon Shi* | *Sa Mu* |
| *Sei Wei* | *Kyo Wu* |
| *In Ryun* | *Dang Yo* |
| *Ji Bang* | *Ko Cho* |

耳聽天時하며 目視世會하며 鼻嗅人倫하며 口味地方이니라

The ears can hear the sound of *Chon Shi*, the eyes can see *Sei Wei*, the nose can smell *In Ryun*, and the mouth can taste *Ji Bang*.[13]

天時는 極蕩也오 世會는 極大也오 人倫은 極廣也오 地方은 極邈也니라

The current[14] of *Chon Shi* is extremely swift and forceful, *Sei Wei* is extremely large and vast, *In Ryun* is extremely broad, and *Ji Bang* is boundless.[15]

肺達事務하며 脾合交遇하며 肝立黨與하며 腎定居處니라.

The lungs circulate *Sa Mu*.[16] The spleen harmonizes and unites *Kyo Wu*.[17] The liver deciphers and divides *Dang Yo*.[18] The kidneys calm and root *Ko Cho*.[19,20]

---

13    According to Lee Je-ma, the ears, eyes, nose, and mouth are mankind's closest connection to the heavens. From his perspective, they are more than just sense organs, but metaphysical aspects of the spirit that provide insight and the ability to interpret our surroundings.

14    Lee Je-ma took great care in selecting every character in the *Dongeui Susei Bowon*, often applying several meanings to each. The character for "current" (蕩) contains the radical for water and the radical for Yang. Water, in ancient Chinese philosophy, correlates with danger as well as life. Since water flows downwards, so does the energy of the heavens. Yang correlates with heaven, while Yin correlates with earth. Hence within the character for "current" is both heaven and water, representing water or rain falling from the sky. Hence, *Chon Shi* can be compared to a flood that brings about strife as well as renewed life.

15    The above phrase refers to the incomprehensible and infinite nature of *Chon Ki* (Heavenly Affairs).

16    As mentioned earlier, all phenomena form a *Che* (internal/latent) and *Yong* (external/manifest) relationship. The four *In Sa* and the four *Chon Ki* also form a *Che/Yong* relationship, whereas *In Sa* is considered *Yong* while the four *Chon Ki* are considered *Che*. Hence, *Sa Mu* is the *Yong* aspect of *Chon Shi* (divine meaning). The function of the lungs is to circulate *Chon Shi* (divine meaning) through *Sa Mu* (one's individual mission and work).

17    The function of the spleen is to harmonize and bring together *Sei Wei* (society) through establishing *Kyo Uh* (personal relationships).

18    The function of the liver is to divide and decipher *Dang Yo* (group responsibility) through *In Ryun* (social skills and talents).

19    The function of the kidneys is to arrange *Ji Bang* (the appropriate place for action) through *Ko Cho* (establishing a firm foundation in life).

20    The energy of *Chon Ki* (Heavenly Affairs) is transmitted through the senses (ears, eyes, nose, and mouth) and then to the organ systems (lung, spleen, liver, and kidney). It then takes the form of *In Sa* (Human Affairs).

事務는 克修也오 交遇는 克成也오 黨與는 克整也오 居處는 克治也니라.
居處克治也

*Sa Mu* must be polished and cultivated, *Kyo Uh* must be obtained through sincerity, *Dang Yo* must be refined, and *Ko Cho* must be planned and schemed out correctly.[21]

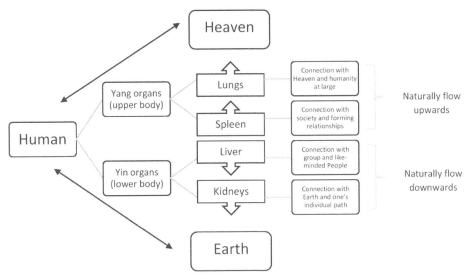

*Figure 1.1: The relationship between heaven, man, and earth*

The Three Poles Theory, or San Ji Zhi Dao (三極之道), denotes man's role as the connection between heaven and earth, and his existence as the outward manifestation of heaven above and earth below. The Three Poles Theory also relates to the flow of energy within the body, whereas the energy of the upper body organs (lung and spleen) flow upward towards heaven, and the lower body organs (liver and kidney) flow downward towards the earth. Hence, each of the Four Major Organs (lungs, spleen, liver, kidneys) in Sasang medicine are also influenced by the energy of heaven and earth, whereas the lungs, associated with *Sa Mu*, have the closest affiliation, among the four organs, to heaven, and the kidneys, associated with *Ko Cho*, have the closest affiliation with the earth.

---

21 Even though the four aspects of *In Sa* (*Sa Mu, Kyo Uh, Dang Yo,* and *Ko Cho*) exist within the heart of all human beings, they manifest only through self-cultivation, sincerity, refinement, and planning.

頷有籌策하고 臆有經綸하고 臍有行檢하고 腹有度量이니라.

*Ju Chek* (the ability to calculate profit from loss)[22] resides in the chin, *Kyung Ryun* (the government and administration of affairs)[23] in the chest, *Heng Gom* (the ability to reflect on one's actions)[24] in the umbilical area, and *Do Ryang* (the ability to embrace and tolerate others)[25] in the lower abdomen.[26]

籌策은 不可驕也오 經綸은 不可矜也오 行檢은 不可伐也오 度量은 不可夸也니라

*Ju Chek* prevents excessive pride and haughtiness,[27] *Kyung Ryun* guards against self-conceit,[28] *Heng Gom* prevents self-praise,[29] and *Do Ryang* thwarts overreaction.[30]

---

22  *Ju Chek*: *Ju* (籌): Calculate, evaluate + *Chek* (策): Plan—*Ju Chek* is the intuitive ability to evaluate one's circumstances and make sound judgment. It is also the ability to comprehend the mystical or metaphysical nature of existence, a trait derived from *Chon Shi*. Since this intuition is powerful and instinctive, it is necessary to manifest the Virtue of wisdom to carry it out.

23  *Kyung Ryun*: *Kyung* (經): To teach, reason, principle + *Ryun* (綸): Rule, reign, govern—*Kyung Ryun* is the ability to govern and administer affairs. In order to perform this ability, it is necessary to manifest the Virtue of humility and respect for others. To show humility and respect for others, it is necessary to understand the transient and ever-transforming nature of man and nature, a trait derived from *Sei Wei*.

24  *Heng Gom*: *Heng* (行): Actions, deeds, movement + *Gom* (檢): Sparing, generous—*Heng Gom* is the ability to reflect on one's actions. In order to reflect on one's actions it is necessary to manifest the Virtue of righteousness (deciphering between right and wrong). In order to decipher between right and wrong, it is necessary to have a strong sense of justice and fairness, a trait derived from *In Ryun*.

25  *Do Ryang*: *Do* (度): Laws, regulations, manners, system, organization, consider + *Ryang* (量): Consider, ponder—*Do Ryang* is the ability to embrace and tolerate others. In order to embrace and tolerate others, it is necessary to manifest the Virtue of love and compassion. Love and compassion come from the ability to comprehend the basis and root of human existence, a trait derived from *Ji Bang*.

26  *Ju Chek*, *Kyung Ryun*, *Heng Gom*, and *Do Ryang* are associated with *Song* (性, heavenly endowed nature). *Shik Kyun*, *Wi Eui*, *Jae Gan*, and *Bang Ryak* are associated with *Myung* (命, divine mission). *Song* is the *Che* (internal/latent) aspect of *Myung*, while *Myung* is the *Yong* (external/manifest) aspect of *Song*. The cultivation of one's heavenly endowed nature provides the ability to carry out his/her divine mission.

27  Only when an effort is made to carry out *In Sa* can selfishness be overcome. According to Lee Je-ma, each aspect of the anterior and posterior body houses both benevolent and malevolent tendencies. *Ju Chek* isn't the only characteristic that resides in the chin. Excessive pride and haughtiness reside there too. Therefore, the cultivation of *Ju Chek* is what overrides pride and haughtiness.

28  *Kyung Ryun* isn't the only characteristic that resides in the chest. Self-conceit resides there too. Therefore, the cultivation of *Kyung Ryun* is what overrides self-conceit.

29  *Heng Gom* isn't the only characteristic that resides in the umbilical area. Self-praise resides there too. Therefore, the cultivation of *Heng Gom* is what overrides self-praise.

30  *Do Ryang* isn't the only characteristic that resides in the lower abdomen. Overreaction resides there too. Therefore, the cultivation of *Do Ryang* is what overrides overreaction.

頭有識見하고 肩有威儀하고 腰有材幹하고 臀有方略이니라.

*Shik Kyun* (knowing the right time to take action)[31] resides in the head, *Wi Eui* (the ability to show respect and discipline towards others)[32] resides in the shoulders, *Jae Gan* (manners and skills)[33] resides in the lower back, and *Bang Ryak* (strategic planning and tactics)[34] resides in the buttocks.

識見은 必無奪也오 威儀는 必無侈也오 材幹은 必無懶也오 方略은 必無竊也니라

In order to manifest *Shik Kyun* one must never take from others;[35] in order to manifest *Wi Eui* one must never be excessively extravagant;[36] in order to manifest *Jae Gan* one must never be too lazy;[37] in order to manifest *Bang Ryak* one must never be too sneaky.[38]

---

31  *Shik Kyun*: *Shik* (識): To recognize, know, wisdom, intelligence + *Kyun* (見): Sight, vision—*Shik Kyun* is the wisdom of understanding when to act. It resides in the back of the head (occipital area), is derived from *Ju Chek* (the ability to calculate profit from loss) and correlates with *Myung* (命, divine mission or path), while *Ju Chek* correlates with *Song* (性, heavenly endowed nature). As mentioned above, *Myung* is the *Yong* aspect of *Song*. All people are endowed with *Ju Chek*, but *Shik Kyun* manifests through the realization of one's *Myung*. This realization is what provides the ability to carry out *Sa Mu* (taking action at the appropriate time).

32  *Wi Eui*: *Wi* (威): Dignity, influence, force, power + *Eui* (儀): Conduct, behavior, model, consider—*Wi Eui* is the ability to show dignity and respect towards others. It resides in the shoulders and is derived from *Kyung Ryun* (the ability to govern and administrate affairs). *Wi Eui* is *Myung* (命), while *Kyung Ryun* is *Song* (性). All people are endowed with *Kyung Ryun*, but *Wi Eui* manifests through the realization of one's *Myung*. This realization is what provides the ability to carry out *Kyo Uh* (associating with others one on one) with dignity and influence.

33  *Jae Gan*: *Jae* (材): Ability, talent, genius, propriety, duty, consider + *Gan* (幹): Ability, capability, gift—*Jae Gan* is equated with manners and skills. It resides in the lower back and is derived from *Heng Gom* (the ability to reflect on one's actions). *Jae Gan* is *Myung* (命), while *Heng Gom* is Song (性). All people are endowed with *Heng Gom*, but *Jae Gan* is manifested through the realization of one's *Myung*. This realization is what provides the ability to carry out *Dang Yo* (establishing group responsibilities) with talent and skill.

34  *Bang Ryak*: *Bang* (方): Direction, angle, share, distribute, the "way" + *Ryak* (略): Govern, control, regulate, survey—*Bang Ryak* is equated with strategic planning and tactics; it resides in the buttocks and is derived from *Do Ryang* (the ability to embrace and tolerate others). *Bang Ryak* is *Myung* (命), while *Do Ryang* is *Song* (性). All people are endowed with *Do Ryang*, but *Bang Ryak* is manifested through the realization of one's *Myung*. This realization is what provides the ability to carry out *Ko Cho* (knowing the proper place to reside and take action).

35  The Virtue of wisdom is needed to carry out *Shik Kyun*. Without wisdom, one has the tendency to use *Shik Kyun* for selfish reasons. One who knows the right time to act, but does so without wisdom, will eventually lead others astray. A cult leader is an example of one who uses *Shik Kyun* to their personal advantage or takes away the opportunity for others to utilize their own *Shik Kyun*.

36  The Virtue of humility is needed to carry out *Wi Eui*. Without humility one has the tendency to use *Wi Eui* selfishly. One who portrays dignity and respect on the surface but does so for selfish reasons eventually comes across as being shallow and/or extravagant. The use of social skills to display authority is another example of selfishly utilizing *Wi Eui*.

37  The Virtue of righteousness is needed to carry out *Jae Gan*. Without righteousness one has the tendency to use *Jae Gan* selfishly. One who disregards their talents and skills, or utilizes them for selfish reasons, eventually becomes lazy and unproductive. Righteousness is the ability to decipher between Yin and Yang, right and wrong, value and demerit.

38  The Virtue of love is needed to carry out *Bang Ryak*. Without love one has the tendency to take advantage of *Bang Ryak* for his or her own pleasure. One who makes plans and devises tactics for their own pleasure will eventually come across as being sneaky and devious.

**Table 1.2: The relationship between *Chon Ki*, *In Sa* and the anterior/pos=terior body**

| Che | | | Yong | | |
|---|---|---|---|---|---|
| Che ◄─────► Yong | | Che ◄─────► Yong | | | |
| Song | | Myung | | | |
| **Chon Ki** | Chin, chest, umbilical area, lower abdomen | Head, shoulders, lower back, buttocks | *In Sa* | | |
| Chon Shi | Ju Chek | Shik Kyun | Sa Mu | | |
| Sei Wei | Kyung Ryun | Wi Eui | Kyo Uh | | |
| In Ryun | Heng Gom | Jae Gan | Dang Yo | | |
| Ji Bang | Do Ryang | Bang Ryak | Ko Cho | | |
| Self-reflection ◄─────► Action | | | | | |

耳目鼻口는 觀於天也오 肺脾肝腎은 立於人也오
頷臆臍腹은 行其知也오 頭肩腰臀은 行其行也니라.

The ears, eyes, nose, and mouth perceive and connect with the energy of the heavens.[39] The lungs, spleen, liver, and kidneys carry out Human Affairs[40] through this connection. The chin, chest, umbilical area, and lower abdomen[41] bring forth inner wisdom. The head, shoulders, lower back, and buttocks[42] provide the ability to take action.[43]

天時는 大同也오 事務는 各立也오 世會는 大同也오 交遇는 各立也오
人倫은 大同也오 黨與는 各立也오 地方은 大同也오 居處는 各立也니라.

All mankind is subject to the influence of *Chon Shi* (divine intention). Each person, however, has his/her own *Sa Mu* (unique mission). All mankind is subject to the influence of *Sei Wei* (societal duty) and everyone has their own level of *Kyo Wu* (showing respect). All mankind is influenced by human interaction (*In Ryun*). However, *Dang Yo* (how one chooses to interact) varies amongst each individual. All

---

39 The energy of the heavens (or *Chon Ki*, Heavenly Affairs) consists of *Ji Bang*, *In Ryun*, *Sei Wei*, and *Chon Shi*.

40 Human Affairs (or *In Sa*) consist of *Ko Cho*, *Dang Yo*, *Kyo Uh*, and *Sa Mu*.

41 The chin, chest, umbilical area, and lower abdomen house *Ju Chek*, *Kyung Ryun*, *Heng Gom*, and *Do Ryang* respectively.

42 The head, shoulders, lower back, and buttocks house *Shik Kyun*, *Wi Eui*, *Jae Gan*, and *Bang Ryak* respectively.

43 Both heaven and man exhibit a *Che* (internal)/*Yong* (external) relationship, whereas heaven is the *Che* (internal aspect of man), and man is the *Yong* (external aspect) of heaven. Otherwise stated, the seed of heaven embedded within the human heart manifests through Human Affairs, or actions. Wisdom (知) and action (行) also have an internal/external relationship. Wisdom is the root of virtuous action, and virtuous action is the manifestation of wisdom. Action based in wisdom is how we manifest *In Sa* (Human Affairs), which is derived from *Chon Ki* (Heavenly Affairs).

mankind has *Ji Bang* (a place to reside). Yet, *Ko Cho* (how one functions within his/her dwelling place) differs according to the individual.[44]

籌策은 博通也오 識見은 獨行也오 經綸은 博通也오 威儀는 獨行也오
行檢은 博通也오 材幹은 獨行也오 度量은 博通也오 方略은 獨行也니라.

*Ju Chek* (the potential to calculate profit from loss) is bestowed equally within each individual, but *Shik Kyun* (the ability to distinguish and decipher) is derived through effort. *Kyung Ryun* (the government and administration of affairs) is bestowed equally within each individual, but *Wi Eui* (the ability to show respect and humility) comes through effort. *Heng Gom* (the potential to reflect on one's actions) is bestowed equally within each individual, but *Jae Gan* (manners and skills) is derived solely through effort. *Do Ryang* (the potential to embrace and tolerate) is bestowed equally within each individual, but *Bang Ryak* (strategic planning and tactics) is derived solely through effort.[45]

大同者 天也오 各立者 人也오 博通者 性也오 獨行者 命也니라.

Heaven distributes all things[46] without discrimination. Yet each individual has his/her own unique path.[47] *Song* (性) indicates the bestowal of heaven's influence far and wide. *Myung* (命) indicates the actions we take individually.

耳好善聲하고 目好善色하고 鼻好善臭하고 口好善味ㅣ니라.

The ears like to hear pleasant sounds. The eyes like to see pleasant colors. The nose likes to smell pleasant scents. The mouth likes to taste pleasant flavors.[48]

---

44  Heavenly Affairs (*Chon Shi*, *Sei Wei*, *In Ryun*, and *Ji Bang*) are endowed within the heart of each person through the ears, eyes, nose, and mouth. The manifestation of Human Affairs (*Sa Mu*, *Kyo Wu*, *Dang Yo*, and *Ko Cho*), on the other hand, depends on human interaction.

45  *Ju Chek*, *Kyung Ryun*, *Heng Gom*, and *Do Ryang* correlate with *Song* (性), the aspect of our spirit/mind that is equally endowed within each person. It represents the pure, untethered connection between man and heaven. *Shik Kyun*, *Wi Eui*, *Jae Gan*, and *Bang Ryak* correlate with *Myung* (命), or divine mission, which is cultivated through effort and discovering/utilizing our relationship with heaven, or *Song*.

46  "All things" in this context refers to the bestowal of *Chon Ki* (天機), the four Heavenly Affairs (*Ji Bang*, *In Ryun*, *Sei Wei*, and *Chon Shi*).

47  "Different path" in this context refers to the carrying out of *In Sa* (人事), the four Human Affairs (*Ko Cho*, *Dang Yo*, *Kyo Uh*, and *Sa Mu*).

48  As mentioned earlier, the senses receive *Chon Ki* (Heavenly Affairs). Pleasant sounds, sights, smells, and tastes are a reflection of the benevolent nature of heaven and thus appeal to the senses. Each of the four sensory organs has a natural desire to connect with heaven through hearing, seeing, smelling, and tasting. When in balance, the sensory organs desire sensory stimuli that encourage the smooth flow of energy within the body. Yet when they are not balanced, the organs will crave stimuli that instigate more imbalance.

善聲은 順耳也오 善色은 順目也오 善臭는 順鼻也오 善味는 順口也니라.

Pleasant sounds promote the smooth flow[49] of energy to and from the ears. Pleasant colors promote the smooth flow of energy to and from the eyes. Pleasant scents promote the smooth flow of energy to and from the nose. Pleasant tastes promote the smooth flow of energy to and from the mouth.

肺惡惡聲하고 脾惡惡色하고 肝惡惡臭하고 腎惡惡味니라.

The lungs have an aversion to unpleasant sounds. The spleen has an aversion to unpleasant colors. The liver has an aversion to unpleasant odors. The kidney has an aversion to unpleasant tastes.[50]

惡聲은 逆肺也오 惡色은 逆脾也오 惡臭는 逆肝也오 惡味는 逆腎也니라.

Unpleasant sounds cause the reversal of lung Qi. Unpleasant colors cause the reversal of spleen Qi. Unpleasant odors reverse the liver Qi. Unpleasant taste causes the reversal of kidney Qi.[51]

頷有驕心하고 臆有矜心하고 臍有伐心하고 腹有夸心이니라.

*Kyo Shim*[52] (haughtiness) resides in the chin. *Gung Shim* (self-conceit) resides in the chest. *Bol Shim* (self-praise) resides in the umbilical area. *Gwa Shim* (boastfulness) resides in the lower abdomen.[53]

---

49    The words "smooth flow" in the above sentence is a rough translation of the character *Sun* (順), which depicts the downward flow of heaven's energy. It can also be interpreted as "providence" or "divinity." The opposite character *Yok* (逆), or "reverse flow," describes upward movement, the direction of earth's energy as it naturally rises towards the heavens. The flow of *Sun* and *Yok* is what forms the basic upward and downward flow within the body, since according to *San Ji Zhi Dao* Theory (三極, Three Poles Theory—see Figure 1.1), humanity is a blend of heaven above and earth below. Pleasant sounds, sights, smells, and tastes assist the downward flow, or *Sun*, within the body. Self-reflection and virtuous action are what promote the harmonious flow of *Yok* upwards.

50    As mentioned earlier, the senses directly receive *Chon Ki* (Heavenly Affairs), and are, by nature, pure and untarnished. The organs receive *Chon Ki* through the senses. Hence, the organs rely on the senses to bring them pleasant sounds, colors, smells, and tastes. Pleasant sounds, colors, smells, and tastes bring harmony, whereas unpleasant ones result in impurity and imbalance of the organs.

51    Each organ system has its naturally balanced direction of flow. Unpleasant sounds, sights, smells, and tastes reverse the natural flow of organ energy, leading to sickness and disease.

52    Haughtiness, self-conceit, self-praise, and boastfulness each contain the character *Shim* (心). This character, which literally means "heart," signifies the place where moment-to-moment emotions are processed. Haughtiness, self-conceit, self-praise, and boastfulness are a result of quick, unreflective emotion and action.

53    As mentioned earlier, the chin, chest, umbilical area, and lower abdomen house our heavenly endowed virtuous nature (*Ju Chek*, *Kyung Ryun*, *Heng Kom*, and *Do Ryang*). In this section, Lee Je-ma illustrates how *Kyo Shim*, *Gung Shim*, *Bol Shim*, and *Gwa Shim*, which represent selfishness, also reside in these areas of the body. The dual nature of the chin, chest, umbilical area, and lower abdomen illustrates how the human heart is just as capable of being influenced by selfish desire as it is towards carrying out its innately virtuous behavior.

驕心은 驕意也요 矜心은 矜慮也요 伐心은 伐操也요 夸心은 夸志也니라.

*Kyo Shim* refers to having too much pride in knowing (the way of heaven). *Gung Shim* indicates the act of showing off one's ability to consider and yield to others. *Bol Shim* refers to the act of showing off one's moral character and integrity. *Gwa Shim* expresses the act of showing off one's integrity and willpower.[54]

**Table 1.3: Metaphysical aspects of the anterior body**

| Location (anterior) | If one discovers their *Song* then… | | If one neglects their *Song* then… | |
|---|---|---|---|---|
| Chin | *Ju Chek* | Manifests via the expression of one's *divine nature* | *Kyo Shim* | Manifests due to the ignorance of one's innate virtuous potential and connection to heaven |
| Chest | *Kyung Ryun* | | *Gong Shim* | |
| Umbilical area | *Heng Gom* | | *Bol Shim* | |
| Lower abdomen | *Do Ryang* | | *Gwa Shim* | |

頭有擅心하고 肩有侈心하고 腰有懶心하고 臀有欲心이니라.

*Chon*[55] *Shim*[56] resides in the head. *Chi*[57] *Shim* resides in the shoulders, *Na*[58] *Shim* in the lower back, while *Yok*[59] *Shim* resides in the buttocks.[60]

---

54 Knowing (the way of heaven) is a heavenly bestowed ability, while haughtiness is the abuse of this ability. The ability to consider and yield to others is a heavenly bestowed gift, whereas self-conceit is the abuse of this gift. Moral character and integrity is a heavenly bestowed characteristic, whereas self-praise is the abuse of this characteristic. Integrity and willpower are heavenly bestowed facilities, while boastfulness is the abuse of these facilities.

55 *Chon* (擅): To do as one pleases without considering others.

56 *Chon Shim*, *Chi Shim*, *Na Shim*, and *Yok Shim* each contain the character *Shim* (心). As mentioned above, this character literally means "heart" but also refers to selfish desire. Selfishness in this sense is a result of quick, unreflective emotion and action.

57 *Chi* (侈): Extravagance, excess, immoderation, disorderly conduct.

58 *Na* (懶): Laziness, languor, lack of volition, refusal to carry out or ignorance of one's divine mission.

59 *Yok* (欲): To want, desire, commence. When *Shim* (心, heart) is added to this character, the definition is changed to "selfishness." In this text, Lee Je-ma often uses *Yok* and *Jul* (竊) interchangeably.

60 As mentioned above, the head, shoulders, lower back, and buttocks house the potential for virtuous action via *Shik Kyun*, *Wi Eui*, *Jae Gan*, and *Bang Ryak*. Yet, they are also home to *Chon Shim*, *Chi Shim*, *Na Shim*, and *Yok Shim*, which represent selfish and ignorant behavior. The head, shoulders, lower back, and buttocks, similar to the chin, chest, umbilical area, and lower abdomen, host both benevolent and malevolent potential.

擅心은 奪利也오 侈心은 自尊也오 懶心은 自卑也오 欲心은 竊物也니라.

*Chon Shim* deprives others of virtuous conduct or wisdom. *Chi Shim* is the expression of an elevated self-image. *Na Shim* is the possession of a low self-image and a lack of dignity. *Yok Shim* is the desire to steal objects from others.[61]

**Table 1.4: Metaphysical aspects of the posterior body**

| Location (posterior) | If one carries out their *Myung* then… | | If one neglects their *Myung* then… | |
|---|---|---|---|---|
| Head | *Shik Kyun* | Manifests via the action based on carrying out one's *divine nature* | *Tal/Chon Shim* | Manifests as a result of refusing to carry out of ignoring one's *divine mission* |
| Shoulders | *Wi Eui* | | *Chi Shim* | |
| Lower back | *Jae Gan* | | *Na Shim* | |
| Buttocks | *Bang Ryak* | | *Jul Shim* | |

人之耳目鼻口는 好善이 無雙也오 人之肺脾肝腎은 惡惡이 無雙也오
人之頷臆臍腹은 邪心이 無雙也오 人之頭肩腰臀은 怠心이 無雙也니라.

The ears, eyes, nose, and mouth each have an unsurpassed[62] desire for benevolence, and the lungs, spleen, liver, and kidneys have an unsurpassed desire to avoid malevolence. The chin, chest, umbilicus, and lower abdomen have an unsurpassed tendency towards malicious intent, and the head, shoulders, lower back, and buttocks have an unsurpassed tendency towards laziness and negligence.[63]

---

61  *Chon Shim* and *Yok Shim* oppose one another, with the former involving immaterial affairs and the latter involving material objects. *Chi Shim* and *Na Shim* also oppose one another, as the former involves an inflated self-image and the latter involves a lower self-image. These relationships are another example of *Che* (internal, latent aspect) and *Yong* (external, manifest aspect) correlation. Based on this principle, it may also be said that a low self-image is the root (*Che*) of an elevated one (*Yong*), and vice versa. Moreover, the desire to deprive others of virtue (*Chon Shim*) may be the result of a need to take (steal) something substantial (*Yok Shim*) from them, and vice versa.

62  The word "unsurpassed" may also be translated as "most influenced by." The ears, eyes, nose, and mouth, for example, are most influenced by benevolence since they are our closest connection with the heavens. The chin, chest, umbilical area, lower abdomen, head, shoulders, lower back, and buttocks are most influenced by malevolence because they are "farther" from the heavens and are therefore prone to negative inclination.

63  As our closest connection to the heavens, the senses and organs are the purest aspects of the human body and psyche. They desire benevolence and have an aversion to malevolence. Despite this desire, we cannot totally free ourselves from the influence of evil intent or negligence, which resides in the chin, chest, umbilical area, lower abdomen, head, shoulders, lower back, and buttocks.

堯舜之行仁이 在於五千年前而至于今天下之稱善者 皆曰堯舜則人之好
善이 果無雙也오

Emperor Yao and Emperor Shun[64] were compassionate leaders who lived approximately 5000 years ago. Even today when a person carries out benevolent acts, they are compared to Emperors Yao and Shun. Thus, the desire for benevolence transcends the test of time.

桀紂之行暴 在於四千年前而至于今天下之稱惡者 皆曰桀紂則人之惡惡이
果無雙也오

Emperor Jie of the Xia Dynasty and Emperor Zhou[65] of the Shang Dynasty were barbaric leaders who lived approximately 4000 years ago. Even today when a person acts brutally, they are compared to Emperors Jie and Zhou. Therefore, the aversion to injustice and malevolence transcends the test of time.

以孔子之聖으로 三千之徒 受敎而惟顏子三月不違仁하고 其餘는 日月至
焉而心悅誠服者 只有七十二人則人之邪心이 果無雙也.

Even though the ancient sage Confucius had 3000 followers, An Zi was the only one who took just three months to fully grasp his teachings and embrace the Virtue of *In* (benevolence). An Zi steadfastly followed the teachings of his mentor and not for a day, let alone a month, did he even slightly falter. Out of 3000 disciples, only 72 others were capable of obtaining a true sense of joy through sincerely practicing his teachings. Yet even these disciples could not free themselves from negativity. Here we see that the tendency towards negativity transcends the test of time.[66]

---

64 Emperor Yao and Emperor Shun are known as two of the Five Legendary Emperors of China. They are believed to have ruled China with utmost virtue and benevolence. Confucian scholars, historians, and the common people alike often refer to these emperors as being the perfect example of self-reflection and virtuous behavior. The aged Emperor Yao enthroned Emperor Shun based on his moral conduct rather than family lineage. Emperor Shun was raised in humble circumstances and showed unfaltering devotion to his parents despite being treated unfairly by them.

65 Both of the above emperors were the last in a series of rulers of their dynasty, and were eventually overthrown. Vulgar action and authoritarian behavior made them historical examples of non-virtue and malevolence. As mentioned above, the lungs, spleen, liver, and kidneys have an aversion to malevolence. Even if one isn't benevolent themselves, they will have an aversion to malevolence in others because of this natural trait. This aversion comes from the organs, while malevolence comes from a lack of cultivating virtue.

66 Confucius said that An Zi was the only disciple to have truly grasped his teachings. Upon hearing of An Zi's death, Confucius felt such a deep sense of grief that he pounded the ground, screaming: "The heavens have finally destroyed me." Afterwards, when one of his disciples praised Confucius by claiming that he was the embodiment of *In* (benevolence), he declined and said that An Zi was the only one who was capable of fulfilling such a role.

以文王之德으로 百年而後崩하사대 未洽於天下러시니 武王周公이 繼
之然後에 大行而管叔蔡叔이 猶以至親으로 作亂則人之怠行이 果無雙
也니라.

Even though Wen's[67] virtuous life lasted 100 years, he himself never made it to
the status of King. His legacy was carried on by his sons King Wu and Zhu Gong
(the Duke of Zhou) who ruled over the entire kingdom of China. However, it was
the negligent actions of Zhu Gong's own siblings Guan Shu and Cai Shu[68] that
eventually led the empire astray. This attests to the fact that even in times of great
benevolence, the seeds of negligence and carelessness[69] still lurk.

耳目鼻口는 人皆可以爲堯舜이오 頷臆臍腹은 人皆自不爲堯舜이오
肺脾肝腎은 人皆可以爲堯舜이오 頭肩腰臀은 人皆自不爲堯舜이니라.

The ears, eyes, nose, and mouth are capable of obtaining the same stature as Emperor
Yao and Emperor Shun. However, the chin, chest, umbilicus, and lower abdomen
are not capable of obtaining this stature on their own. The lungs, spleen, liver, and
kidneys are capable of obtaining the same stature as Emperor Yao and Emperor
Shun. Yet the head, shoulders, lower back, and buttocks are not capable of attaining
this stature on their own.[70]

人之耳目鼻口好善之心은 以衆人耳目鼻口論之而堯舜이 未爲加一鞭也오

The ears, eyes, nose, and mouth desire benevolence. There is no difference
between the ears, eyes, nose, and mouth of Emperors Yao and Shun and the senses
of an average person.

---

67 Wen, the founder of the Zhou Dynasty (1046–256 BC), was said to be a man of great virtue. He lived during
the reign of the malevolent King Zhou of the Shang Dynasty. As governor of Zhou, Wen gained immense
popularity, catching the eye of King Zhou, who eventually incarcerated him. Yet upon his release, the aged
Wen and his son Wu overthrew King Zhou and started the Zhou Dynasty. King Wen is also credited with
the establishment of the 64 hexagrams from the Eight Trigram Theory and their explanations, written in the
I Ching.

68 King Wu died only two years after he and his father, King Wen, founded the Zhou Dynasty. His oldest
brother, Guan Shu, who as the eldest son regretted not being appointed king by his father, saw Wu's passing
as an opportunity. Accompanying his younger brother, Cai Shu, he tried unsuccessfully to attain the throne.
The Duke of Zhou, who was appointed king by the late King Wu, therefore maintained his status as the new
king of Zhou.

69 As mentioned above, the tendency towards negligence and carelessness exists in the chin, chest, umbilical area,
lower abdomen, head, shoulders, lower back, and buttocks, which are influenced by impulsive emotions.

70 The chin, chest, umbilicus, lower abdomen, head, shoulders, lower back, and buttocks represent the
vulnerability of the human mind because they possess both benevolent and ambivalent qualities. They cannot
achieve the stature of Emperors Yao and Shun automatically or without self-cultivation. The ears, eyes, nose,
and mouth directly connect with the energy of heaven. The lungs, spleen, liver, and kidneys receive the energy
of heaven directly from the senses. Both the senses and the organs are therefore, by nature, the same stature as
Emperors Yao and Shun.

人之肺脾肝腎惡惡之心은 以堯舜肺脾肝腎論之而衆人이 未爲一少鞭也니 人皆可以爲堯舜者 以此오

The lungs, spleen, liver, and kidneys of the average person hate malevolence, as did the lungs, spleen, liver, and kidneys of Emperors Yao and Shun. This is why the average person could attain the same stature as Emperors Yao and Shun.

人之頷臆臍腹之中에 誣世之心이 每每隱伏也니 存其心養其性然後에 人 皆可以爲堯舜之知也오

Deep within the chin, chest, umbilical area, and lower abdomen lurks the tendency towards confusion and deception.[71] Only after the heartfelt cultivation of one's heavenly nature[72] can the average person gain the wisdom of Emperors Yao and Shun.

人之頭肩腰臀之下에 罔民之心이 種種暗藏也니 修其身立其命然後에 人 皆可以爲堯舜之行也니 人皆自不爲堯舜者 以此니라.

Lurking within the head, shoulders, lower back, and buttocks is the tendency towards exploiting and enslaving[73] others. Only through polishing one's heart and carrying out his or her divine mission[74] can the average person achieve the same merit as Emperors Yao and Shun. This is the reason why not all people can obtain the stature of Emperors Yao and Shun.

---

71  The chin, chest, umbilicus, and lower abdomen correlate with the imperfect aspects of the mind, hence they harbor the tendency towards emotional and spiritual confusion and deceiving others.

72  The "heartfelt cultivation of one's heavenly nature" is a rough translation of *Jon Gi Shim Yang Gi Song* (存其心養其性). *Jong Gi Shim* literally translates as "to reside in" or "to focus on" the heart, while *Yang Gi Song* means to "nourish" one's *Song* (heavenly nature). As mentioned above, the head, shoulders, lower back, and buttocks correlate with *Song*, while the chin, chest, umbilical area, and lower abdomen correlate with *Myung* (divine mission).

73  The head, shoulders, lower back, and buttocks correlate with the material aspect of the body, hence the tendency towards "physically" exploiting or enslaving oneself and/or others. The chin, chest, umbilical area, and lower abdomen correlate with the immaterial aspect of the body, hence the tendency towards emotionally exploiting oneself and/or others.

74  To "polish one's heart and carry out his or her divine mission" is a rough translation of *Su Gi Shin Ip Gi Myung* (修其身立其命). *Su Gi Shin* (修其身) translates literally as "to polish" or "to cleanse" the mind, while *Ip Gi Myung* (立其命) means "to carry out" or "to stand up for" one's *Myung* (divine mission). This phrase includes the Chinese character for "body" (*Shin*, 身), translated here as "mind." Actually, Lee Je-ma interprets this character as both "body" and "mind." The mention of *Song* (heavenly nature) in "heartfelt cultivation of one's heavenly spirit" (*Jon Gi Shim Yang Gi Song*) emphasizes one's discovery and awareness of his or her heart-rooted heavenly nature, and the inclusion of *Myung* in "polish one's heart and carry out his or her divine mission" (*Su Gi Shin Ip Gi Myung*) refers to action, or carrying out one's mission, based on this awareness. Hence the awareness of one's heavenly endowed nature is considered *Che* (internal aspect) and the action based on this discovery is considered *Yong* (external manifestation).

耳目鼻口之情은 行路之人이 大同於協義故로 好善也니 好善之實이 極公
也니 極公則亦極無私也오

All people are born with the capacity to work together for the sake of justice and
righteousness because it is the nature of the ears, eyes, nose, and mouth to desire
benevolence. If the desire is taken to the limit, then one will become exceptionally
fair, with no room left for selfishness.

肺脾肝腎之情은 同室之人이 各立於擅利故로 惡惡也니 惡惡之實이 極無
私也니 極無私則亦極公也니라

It is the nature of the lungs, spleen, liver, and kidneys to hate malevolence.
Especially when it involves members of the same family that selfishly protect their
own profit and arbitrarily lose their morality. If the hatred of malevolence is taken to
the extreme, there is no room for selfishness and exceptional fairness will naturally
manifest to its fullest.[75]

頷臆臍腹之中에 自有不息之知 如切如磋하나 而驕矜伐夸之私心이 卒然
敗之하면 則自棄其知而不能博通也오

Deep within the chin, chest, umbilicus, and lower abdomen lies an inherently
unceasing wisdom, which must be sincerely and systematically manifested through
self-cultivation. *Kyo Shim, Gung Shim, Bol Shim,* and *Gwa Shim*[76] can quickly and
easily block the expression of wisdom.

頭肩腰臀之下에 自有不息之行이 赫兮┌兮하나 而奪侈懶竊之慾心이 卒然
陷之하면 則自棄其行而不能正行也니라.

Within the head, shoulders, lower back, and buttocks exists an unceasingly bright
and praiseworthy potential for manifesting one's virtue. Yet *Chon Shim, Chi Shim,
Na Shim,* and *Jul Shim*[77] can quickly suppress the potential to carry out one's virtue.
The inability to manifest one's inner potential leads to unjust behavior.

---

75  In the previous sentence, Lee Je-ma explains how the desire for benevolence leads to fairness and a lack of
selfishness. In the current sentence, he continues by stating that the hatred of selfishness leads to fairness and
benevolence. The desire for benevolence comes from the ears, eyes, nose, and mouth, while the hatred of
malevolence comes from the lungs, spleen, liver, and kidneys. The senses are associated with heaven and the
organs are associated with humanity. Hence, the heaven-related senses and the humanity-related organs form
a *Che* (latent internal)/*Yong* (manifest external) relationship, where the *Che* desire for benevolence manifests
as the *Yong* hatred of malevolence.

76  As *Kyo Shim, Gong Shim, Bol Shim,* and *Gwa Shim* also lurk within the chin, chest, umbilical area, and lower
abdomen respectively, they equally influence the heart and mind.

77  *Chon Shim, Chi Shi, Na Shim,* and *Jul Shim* also lurk within the head, shoulders, lower back, and buttocks
respectively and therefore equally influence the heart and mind.

耳目鼻口는 人皆知也오 頷臆臍腹은 人皆愚也오
肺脾肝腎은 人皆賢也오 頭肩腰臀은 人皆不肖也니라.

The ears, eyes, nose, and mouth are easily capable of attaining wisdom. The chin, chest, umbilicus, and lower abdomen easily succumb to foolishness. The lungs, spleen, liver, and kidneys have the capacity for benevolence and gentleness. The head, shoulder, lower back, and buttocks easily succumb to rudeness and unworthiness.[78,79]

人之耳目鼻口는 天也니 天이 知也오 人之肺脾肝腎은 人也니 人이 賢
也오
我之頷臆臍腹은 我自爲心而未免愚也니 我之免愚는 在我也오
我之頭肩腰臀은 我自爲身而未免不肖也니 我之免不肖는 在我也니라.

The ears, eyes, nose, and mouth correlate directly with heaven and thus are endowed with wisdom. The lungs, spleen, liver, and kidneys correlate with humanity, making them capable of benevolence and gentleness. The chin, chest, umbilicus, and lower abdomen correlate with the imperfect aspects of the mind, and are susceptible to foolishness and stupidity. Overcoming foolishness and stupidity depends on the effort of the individual. The head, shoulders, lower back, and buttocks correlate with the material aspect of the body, easily succumbing to rudeness and unworthiness. Overcoming rudeness and unworthiness depends on the individual's effort.[80]

天生萬民에 性以慧覺하니 萬民之生也 有慧覺則生하고 無慧覺則死ㅣ니
慧覺者는 德之所由生也니라.

All people receive life from heaven along with wisdom and knowledge, which are embedded within *Song* (heavenly endowed nature). Survival is dependent on the recognition of one's heavenly endowed wisdom and knowledge. If they are not discovered, life will be cut short. Virtue is the result of recognizing and acting upon one's heavenly endowed wisdom and knowledge.[81]

---

78  *Bul Cho* (不肖) translates literally as "rudeness and unworthiness." From the standpoint of Confucius's teachings, it also translates as lacking in filial obligation to one's parents.

79  The senses are considered a reflection of heaven within the human body. They serve as a vehicle or pathway to connect humanity with heaven. The organs receive their energy directly from the senses and are therefore capable of benevolence. The chin, chest, umbilicus, and lower abdomen, and the head, shoulders, lower back, and buttocks, are associated with human inclination more than heavenly energy, and are thus prone to foolishness and rudeness.

80  This paragraph summarizes the relationship between heaven (天), man (人), heart (心), and body (身), with heaven and man considered *Che* (latent aspect) and the heart and body considered *Yong* (manifest aspect). In other words, the intentions of heaven with humanity are carried out through the heart and body. This relationship can be broken down further in respect to heaven—human—and heart—body. In comparison to man, heaven is considered *Che* while man is *Yong*, since man is capable of carrying out the will of heaven. Furthermore, the heart is also considered *Che*, and the body *Yong*, since thought and emotion are manifested by the actions of the body.

81  *Song* is considered the *Che* (internal) aspect and wisdom is the *Yong* (external) aspect of human nature, whereas *Song* is the foundation of wisdom. Without tapping into our connection with heaven, life itself cannot be sustained.

天生萬民에 命以資業하니 萬民之生也 有資業則生하고
無資業則死니 資業者는 道之所由生也니라.

All people receive life from heaven along with their individual task, or *Myung*. Life is dependent on the discovery of one's task, or divine mission. If it is not discovered, life will be cut short. The Way is born from the discovery of one's mission in life.[82]

仁義禮智忠孝友悌諸般百善은 皆出於慧覺이오
士農工商田宅邦國諸般百用은 皆出於資業이니라.

The Virtues of love, humility, justice, wisdom, loyalty, filial piety, friendship, and respect come from wisdom and knowledge.[83] All mankind is capable of attaining wisdom and knowledge. The work and practice of scholars, agriculturists, artisans, merchants, fieldworkers, homemakers, and politicians all involve carrying out one's *Myung* (divine deed). All mankind is capable of carrying out their deed through the activation of their wisdom and knowledge.

慧覺은 欲其兼人而有敎오 資業은 欲其廉己而有功也니 慧覺私小者 雖有
其傑이나 巧如曹操而不可爲敎也오 資業橫濫者 雖有其雄이나 猛如秦王
而不可爲功也니라.

Wisdom and knowledge are derived from the human desire to teach and bring others to one's level of understanding. Deed is derived from the desire for self-cultivation and helping others succeed. If the desire to teach is based on selfishness, then even with certain superior qualities, there is nothing worth teaching. This can be compared to the cunning teachings of General Cao Cao[84] during the Three Kingdoms Period of China. If one's effort to carry out his/her deed is taken to the extreme, then even with certain superior qualities, failure follows. Such extreme ways were apparent in the harsh and ferocious ways of Emperor Qin[85] of the Qin Dynasty, who inevitably lost his life at 49 years of age.

---

82  *Myung* (divine mission) is considered the *Che* (internal) aspect, and carrying out one's divine mission is the *Yong* (external aspect): the discovery of our mission in life (*Che*) is the basis for carrying it out (*Yong*).

83  As stated above, wisdom and knowledge are rooted in *Song* (heavenly endowed nature).

84  Cao Cao (曹操, 155–220 AD) was a military strategist and general who lived during the end of the Han Dynasty, which is also referred to as the Three Kingdoms Period. His military tactics eventually earned him the posthumous title of Emperor Wu. The majority of his life was spent in battle against other opposing factions. He harbored the selfish desire of conquering other factions to ultimately rule over all of China. Power rather than morality was the driving force behind his actions.

85  Emperor Qin (秦始皇, 260–210 BC) was fixated on the idea of immortality and attempted to find every possible way to prolong his life through ingesting numerous remedies. One of these remedies contained mercury and eventually killed him. He was a harsh and ferocious Emperor who put to death many scholars and ordered the burning of all educational and philosophical texts. He did succeed in unifying all of China under a legalist system but not in prolonging his life.

人之善而我亦知善者 至性之德也오 惡人之惡而我必不行者 正命之道
也라 知行이 積則道德也오 道德이 成則仁聖也니 道德이 非他라 知行
也오 性命이 非他라 知行이니라.

To appreciate the benevolent nature of others and to manifest one's own benevolent nature is referred to as *Ji Song* (至性, Mastering One's Heavenly Endowed Nature). To dislike the malevolent nature of others and to avoid negativity is referred to as *Jung Myung* (正命, Refining One's Heavenly Endowed Mission). Virtue is accumulated through wisdom and conduct, which leads to the expression of divine love. Virtue is nothing other than wisdom and conduct; *Ji Song* and *Jung Myung* are nothing but wisdom and conduct.[86]

或曰擧知而論性은 可也而擧行而論命은 何義耶아 曰命者는 命數也니 善
行則命數 自美也오 惡行則命數 自惡也니 不待卜筮而可知也라 詩云永言
配命이 自求多福이라하니 卽此義也니라.

Someone once asked me: "What does it actually mean when you say that wisdom is associated with *Song* and conduct is associated with *Myung*?" I responded that *Myung* correlates with *Myung Su* (命數, destiny/fortune). If one becomes aware of and carries out their *Myung* through benevolent deed, then their *Myung Su* will naturally become favorable. If one chooses to carry out malevolent action, then one's *Myung Su* will naturally become unpleasant. There is no need to have one's fortune told to figure this out. Rather, through carrying out one's *Myung*, one attains the wisdom needed to predict the effect of their actions. The *Shijing* (*Classic of Poetry*)[87] illustrates this point by stating that if one conducts benevolence through the realization of their *Myung*, then they will accumulate good fortune on their own accord.

或曰吾子之言에 曰耳聽天時하며 目視世會하며 鼻嗅人倫하며 口味地
方이라하니 耳之聽天時와 目之視世會則可也이 鼻 何以嗅人倫하며 口
何以味地方乎아 曰處於人倫하야 察人外表하야 「探各人才行之賢不肖者
此非嗅耶아 處於地方하여 均嘗各處人民生活之地利者 此非味耶아

Someone once asked me: "How can the ears hear the sound of *Chon Shi*, the eyes see *Sei Wei*, the nose smell *In Ryun*, and the mouth taste *Ji Bang*?" I responded by saying: "How could it not be the sense of smell, associated with *In Ryun* (social

---

86  As mentioned earlier, wisdom is derived from *Song* (heavenly endowed nature) and conduct is based in *Myung* (divine mission). Even though all people are uniformly bestowed with a *Song* nature and *Myung* mission, some do not recognize these aspects at all. Still others may only sporadically and inconsistently recognize them. *Ji Song* and *Jung Myung* are the result of consistent self-reflection and the firm, unshakable realization of one's connection with heaven and his or her divine mission in life.

87  The *Shijing* (詩經, *Classic of Poetry*) consists of 305 poems written from the 11th to the 7th centuries BC. As one of the Five Classics (*Classic of Poetry*, *Book of Documents*, *Book of Rites*, *I Ching*, and the *Spring and Autumn Annals*), it is considered the oldest collection of poems in Chinese history.

skills and talents), that silently investigates the conduct of others and determines the capability of carrying out benevolent or unworthy action? How could it not be the sense of taste, which is directly affiliated with *Ji Bang* (establishing the appropriate time and place for action), that impartially determines the place where profit and advantage exist?"[88]

存其心者는 責其心也라 心體之明暗이 雖若自然而責之者 淸하고 不責者 濁이니 馬之心覺이 點於牛者는 馬之責心이 點於牛也오 鷹之氣勢 猛於 鴟者는 鷹之責氣 猛於鴟也니 心體之淸濁과 氣宇之强弱이 在於牛馬鴟鷹 者 以理推之而猶然커든 況於人乎아 或相倍ㄷ하며 或相千萬者 豈其生而 輒得하야 茫然不思하며 居然自至而然哉아.

In order to preserve the ability to smell and taste, it is important to always reflect upon and modify one's way of thinking. The brightness and darkness of one's heart[89] also depends on the reflection upon and modification of one's way of thinking. Those who are able to reflect have a bright outlook, while those who do not have a dark outlook. A horse is able to come to such realization more quickly than a cow. This is because a horse's ability to reflect is greater than the cow's. Since the stern nature of a hawk is fiercer than the nature of a kite, the ability of a hawk to reflect on its action too is obviously greater than a kite's [which is simply controlled by the direction of the wind]. The bright and dark, clear and turbid,[90] strong and weak nature of the heart can be compared to that of a horse, cow, hawk, and kite. It goes without saying that these qualities also manifest in human beings, which may be displayed two times, five times, 1000 times, or even 10,000 times more depending on the person. How could anyone imagine that self-reflection can spontaneously manifest without thought or effort?[91]

---

88  According to Lee Je-ma the senses (hearing, seeing, smelling, and tasting) have integrative physical and metaphysical functions. Separating the physical from the metaphysical would be like separating Yin and Yang or earth and heaven, which simply could not be done. He explains how the nose not only inhales fragrance but also "smells" the conduct or merit of others (*In Ryun*), and the tongue not only registers the flavor of food or drink but also "tastes" the proper time and place for action (*Ji Bang*).

89  In Sasang medicine, the *Shim* (心, heart) is considered the center of both psychological and physiological function, and is where *Chon Song* (天性, the seed of heaven) is implanted. Emotional and physical health depend entirely on the purity of one's heart, which depends upon self-reflection and sincerity in one's affairs.

90  When the energy of the heart flows smoothly it is said to be "clear"; when it is stagnant or blocked, it is referred to as "turbid." A lack of self-reflection and the inability to carry out one's path in life will lead to turbid heart energy, which has both emotional and physical repercussions.

91  Self-reflection is a central component of Confucian teachings and Sasang medicine alike. Lee Je-ma asserts that humans have the highest capacity to reflect and cultivate their virtue, even though other animals such as a cow, horse, or hawk also have varying degrees of virtuous potential. Yet an individual who doesn't reflect on or cultivate themselves is no different than a kite—an inanimate object completely controlled by its environment. Through self-reflection and virtue, humans can preserve and enhance the ability to distinguish smell and taste.

## Chapter 2

# The Four Basic Characteristics

四<br>端<br>論

人稟臟理에 有四不同하니 肺大而肝小者를 名曰太陽人이오 肝大而肺小者를 名曰太陰人이오 脾大而腎小者를 名曰少陽人이오 腎大而脾小者를 名曰少陰人이니라.

Each Sasang constitution is born with relatively different organ sizes.[1] The Tae Yang Individual is born with larger lungs and a smaller liver and the Tae Eum Individual is born with smaller lungs and a larger liver. The So Yang Individual is born with a larger spleen and smaller kidneys, while the So Eum Individual is born with larger kidneys and a smaller spleen.

**Table 2.1: The smaller and larger organs of each Sasang constitution**

| Sasang constitution | "Smallest" organ | "Largest" organ |
| --- | --- | --- |
| Tae Yang | Lungs | Liver |
| So Yang | Spleen | Kidneys |
| Tae Eum | Liver | Lungs |
| So Eum | Kidneys | Spleen |

---

1   The reference to organ size isn't meant to be taken literally. As mentioned previously, Sasang theory emphasizes the metaphysical function of each organ. Hence Lee Je-ma's reference to "larger" and "smaller" more closely relates to levels of innate strength. The largest organ of each Sasang constitution is generally the strongest and most active. But strength, in this sense, isn't to be confused with health. It is often the case that the stronger organs, associated with *Jung* emotion, become hyperactive, hoard the body's energy, and turn out to be the culprit behind illness. The smallest organ of each Sasang constitution is considered to be the weakest. But weakness is not to be confused with a lack of health since the smallest organs are not always the culprit behind the onset of illness. Actually, the discovery and cultivation of one's smaller organ provides the opportunity to protect and nourish it, optimizing overall emotional and physical health.

人趨心慾에 有四不同하니 棄禮而放縱者를 名曰鄙人이오
棄義而偸逸者를 名曰懦人이오 棄智而飾私者를 名曰薄人이오
棄仁而極慾者를 名曰貪人이니라.

Humans cannot escape the inclination towards selfishness, which manifests in four different ways according to one's constitution. The first form of selfishness [associated with the Tae Yang Individual] involves reckless behavior and disregard for the Virtue of humility, which is seen as dirty and vulgar. The second form of selfishness [associated with the So Eum Individual] involves stealing or hiding things, disregarding the Virtue of righteousness, which is considered feeble and timid. The third form of selfishness [associated with the So Yang Individual] involves adorning and decorating oneself and disregarding the Virtue of wisdom, which is considered frivolous and superficial. The fourth form of selfishness [associated with the Tae Eum Individual] involves disregarding the Virtue of love, which is considered greedy and self-centered.[2]

五臟之心은 中央之太極也오 五臟之肺脾肝腎은 四維之四象也니 中央之
太極은 聖人之太極이 高出於衆人之太極也오 四維之四象은 聖人之四
象이 旁通於衆人之四象也니라.

The heart is the central force, or *Tai Chi*,[3] of the four *Zhang*[4] organs. The four *Zhang* organs are the Sasang[5] of the four cardinal directions. The *Tai Chi* of the commoner is the same as the *Tai Chi* of the Sage. The *Tai Chi* of the Sage, however, has achieved a higher level of self-discovery than the *Tai Chi* of the common person. The Sasang of the Sage flows endlessly within the Sasang of a commoner.

---

2   Each of the four Sasang constitutions has a propensity towards one of the above aspects of selfishness. However, selfishness arises only in those who do not make an effort to grow spiritually and challenge their own negative tendencies. Lee Je-ma, in accordance with Confucian teachings, refers to this type of person as *So In* (小人), or "uncultivated person." The *So In* of the Tae Yang constitution succumbs to the first type of selfishness, which lacks humility and carries out reckless action. The Tae Eum constitution succumbs to the second type of selfishness, lacking righteousness and hiding their feelings from others. The So Yang constitution succumbs to the third type of selfishness, which lacks wisdom and engages in self-adornment. The So Eum constitution succumbs to the fourth type of selfishness, lacking love and being self-centered.

3   As mentioned in the previous chapter, *Tai Chi* splits into Yin and Yang, and is the mother of all existence. Within the context of the human body, it is the heart, and hence the reference to *Tai Chi* in this sentence simultaneously means the human heart.

4   The Four Major *Zhang* Organs in Sasang medicine are the lungs, spleen, liver, and kidneys. The Four Major *Zhang* Organs correlate with Yin, while the Four Major *Fu* Organs (esophagus, stomach, small intestine, large intestine) correlate with Yang.

5   Sasang (四象), literally translated as "Four Symbols," represents the four basic categories of all phenomena. In this sentence it refers to the four organs that surround the heart, located in the center. Sasang also refers to the four constitutions: Tae Yang, Tae Eum, So Yang, and So Eum.

太少陰陽之臟局短長은 四不同中에 有一大同하니 天理之變化也라 聖人
與衆人이 一同也오 鄙薄貪懦之心之淸濁은 四不同中에 有萬不同하니 人
欲之闊狹也라 聖人與衆人이 萬殊也니라.

The relative size of each organ differs with each Sasang constitution. Yet the connection with heaven and its natural law (of change) is shared among all of the constitution types and Sages alike. Each of the four constitutions also displays different malevolent tendencies such as ruthlessness, self-adornment, greediness, and laziness. Whether we manifest our connection with heaven or succumb to malevolence depends on how clear or turbid our heart is. There are a thousand differences when comparing the extent of selfishness within each person. Let alone a thousand more differences between the extent of selfishness between a commoner and a Sage.

太少陰陽之短長變化는 一同之中에 有四偏하니 聖人도 所以希天也오 鄙
薄貪懦之淸濁闊狹은 萬殊之中에 有一同하니 衆人이 所以希聖也니라.

The four constitutions respond to change similarly in some ways but have four different inclinations in others. Each constitution type wishes to be closer to the heavens, as does the Sage. Yet each constitution displays different levels of ruthlessness, self-adornment, greediness, and laziness. The extent, clarity, and turbidity of these tendencies differ according to the person. Yet [regardless of the varying degrees of turbidity and clarity] all people strive to attain the wisdom of a Sage.[6]

聖人之臟도 四端也오 衆人之臟도 亦四端也니 以聖人一四端之臟으로 處
於衆人萬四端之中하니 聖人者는 衆人之所樂也오 聖人之心은 無慾也오
衆人之心은 有慾也니 以聖人一無慾之心으로 處於衆人萬有慾之中하니
衆人者는 聖人之所憂也니라.

The *Zhang* organs of both the Sage and the commoner encompass the *Sa Dan*[7] (Four Basic Characteristics). The *Sa Dan* of the Sage is unified but the *Sa Dan* of the commoner is scattered about in a thousand ways. This is why the commoner finds pleasure in attaining the wisdom of a Sage. The focused and resolute Sage doesn't have the seed of selfishness in his heart, but the commoner does. The Sage is

---

6   A Sage is one who is born with the mission to teach and enlighten others. The mind of the Sage is focused with no inclination towards selfishness or temptation. The Sage and the commoner both desire to reach closer to heaven. However, it is the Sage who doesn't sway off the path.

7   The *Sa Dan* (四端, The Four Basic Characteristics) were first mentioned in *Mencius*, credited as the work of Mengzi, a Confucian scholar who lived in the 4th century BC. In this text, Mengzi describes the four *Sa Dan* as follows: *First Sa Dan* (惻隱之心, *Ce Yin Zhi Xin*): To feel compassion and sorrow for those less fortunate; *Second Sa Dan* (羞惡之心, *Xiu Wu Zhi Xin*): To restrain from one's own unjust tendencies and to dislike malevolence; *Third Sa Dan* (辭讓之心, *Ci Rang Zhi Xin*): To humble oneself and yield to others; *Fourth Sa Dan* (是非之心, *Shi Fei Zhi Xin*): To differentiate between right and wrong.

always concerned about the fate of the commoner, whose mind is scattered in a thousand ways.[8]

然則天下衆人之臟理 亦皆聖人之臟理而才能이 亦皆聖人之才能也라 以肺脾肝腎 聖人之才能而自言曰我無才能云者 豈才能之罪哉리오 心之罪也니라

The same principles of organ function apply to both the commoner and the Sage alike. The talent and skill of the commoner are also the same as the Sage's. The lungs, spleen, liver, and kidneys all have the skills of a Sage. How can anyone say that they do not have any skill despite this fact? To say so is making a serious mistake.[9]

然之氣는 出於肺脾肝腎也오 浩然之理는 出於心也니
仁義禮智四端之氣를 擴而充之則浩然之氣 出於此也오
鄙薄貪懦一心之慾을 明而辨之則浩然之理 出於此也니라.

The lungs, spleen, liver, and kidneys give rise to *Hoyon Ji Gi*[10] (accumulated and widespread flow). The heart brings about *Hoyon Ji Ri*[11] (accumulated and widespread principle). *Hoyon Ji Ri* arises from the Four Virtues of love, humility, righteousness, and wisdom within the four organs. Ruthlessness, self-adornment, greediness, and laziness arise solely from the selfishness of the heart. *Hoyon Ji Ri* arises from the decision to recognize and overcome selfishness.[12]

聖人之心無慾云者는 非淸淨寂滅如老佛之無慾也라
聖人之心이 深憂天下之不治故로 非但無慾也라
亦未暇及於一己之慾也니 深憂天下之不治而未暇及於一己之慾者 必學不厭而敎不倦也니 學不厭而敎不倦者 卽聖人之無慾也라 毫有一己之慾則非堯舜之心也오 暫無天下之憂則非孔孟之心也니라.

The Sage's lack of selfishness cannot be compared to that of Lao Tsu or Buddha, who aimed to purify themselves and enter into Nirvana. A Sage is deeply concerned when the Emperor leads the kingdom astray. Not only do they lack selfishness, but they do not even have a second to spare in order to think about their own personal

---

8   Sages are also classified according to the four major body types and succumb to the same emotions as a commoner. Yet the Sage's emotions are balanced and expressed appropriately. The anxiety of the Sage, for example, is centered on their concern for humanity rather than his/her own selfish desires.

9   The ability to manifest our abilities and Sage-like nature starts from self-worth and self-confidence. Without believing in our potential, it would be impossible to achieve anything. Believing in the fact that we share these properties with a Sage helps us manifest them.

10   *Hoyon Ji Gi* (浩然之氣) literally translates as the *Qi* (life-force, flow) that spreads light far and wide. In this context, Lee Je-ma refers to the expression and wide distribution/movement of one's virtue.

11   *Hoyon Ji Ri* (浩然之理) literally translates as the principle that spreads light far and wide. In this context, Lee Je-ma refers to the principle upon which virtue spreads far and wide.

12   The *Gi* (氣, life-force, energy) of *Hoyon Ji Gi* and the *Ri* (理, principle) of *Hoyon Ji Ri* share a *Che* (internal) and *Yong* (external) relationship. *Ri* (virtuous principle) comes from the heart, while the organs give rise to *Gi* (life-force/movement). *Ri* is the *Che* (internal aspect), or basis of *Gi*, while *Gi* is the *Yong* (manifestation) of *Ri*. Virtuous action cannot be implemented without virtuous principle, and vice versa.

achievements. The person who is deeply concerned when the Emperor leads the kingdom astray and never has time to entertain selfish thoughts is also one who never gets tired of studying or bored of teaching. The ceaseless desire to study and teach is what is meant by the Sage's lack of selfish desire. Even the slightest bit of selfish desire sets the commoner apart from Emperors Yao and Shun. Even if for the slightest moment one loses concern for humanity, he/she cannot be compared to the stature of Confucius or Mencius.[13]

太陽人은 哀性이 遠散而怒情이 促急하니 哀性이 遠散則氣注肺而肺益 盛이오

怒情이 促急則氣激肝而肝益削하나니 太陽之臟局이 所以成形於肺大肝小 也오

少陽人은 怒性이 宏抱而哀情이 促急하니 怒性이 宏抱則氣注脾而脾益 盛이오

哀情이 促急則氣激腎而腎益削하나니 少陽之臟局이 所以成形於脾大腎小 也오

The *Song*[14] nature of the Tae Yang Individual is sorrow, which is far reaching and dispersed. The *Jung*[15] emotion of the Tae Yang Individual is anger, which is abrupt and urgent. The far-reaching and dispersed nature of sorrow gathers and increases the energy of the lungs. The abrupt and urgent emotion of their anger strikes at and severs the energy of the liver.[16] This is how the Tae Yang Individual is born with stronger lungs and a weaker liver.[17]

---

13 Lee Je-ma distinguishes a Sage from Buddha and Lao Tsu by stating that the former is ceaselessly concerned with Human Affairs and the latter with purification and Nirvana. His reference to "the ceaseless desire to study and teach" was taken directly from the Confucian *Analects*. This phrase was also quoted in the *Book of Mencius*. Lee Je-ma regarded Confucius and Mencius as Sages.

14 The *Song* (性) nature, also referred to in this situation as "predominant temperament," is an inborn, heavenly endowed characteristic that feeds the larger organ of each Sasang constitution. As a predominant temperament, the *Song* nature is a characteristic that continuously affects decision and action. Sadness, for example, plays a role in every aspect of the Tae Yang Individual's affairs. When the *Song* nature is balanced, the larger organ of each constitution remains or returns to optimum health. A balanced *Song* nature is also the vehicle that brings forth Virtue. When the *Song* nature is imbalanced, but not out of control, the individual will become vulnerable to External illness. When the *Song* nature is out of control, it morphs into the *Jung* emotion, which causes Internal illness.

15 The *Jung* (情) emotion bursts forth when an imbalance of the *Song* nature gets out of control, injuring the weaker organ of each Sasang constitution and causing Internally induced illness. Together the characters for *Song* and *Jung* form the word "*Song Jung*" (性情), a common term that translates as "nature," "disposition," or "character."

16 The *Song* nature of sorrow sends energy to and fortifies the lungs. It provides the Tae Yang Individual with the ability to express the inner Virtue of love and show compassion towards others. If this emotion is taken too far, then the *Jung* emotion of anger will burst forth, and directly injure the liver, the Tae Yang Individual's weaker organ. The inborn inclination towards uncontrolled anger is the reason why he/she has a weaker liver.

17 Lee Je-ma describes how emotional inclination, determined before birth, dictates which organs are stronger and weaker. Hence, the establishment of each body type is determined by these innate emotional inclinations, or temperaments. Each emotion, when expressed harmoniously, actually supports the health of its correlating organ. Any emotion, when taken to the extreme, will cause serious injury to its correlating organ.

The *Song* nature of the So Yang Individual is anger, which is broad and embracing. The *Jung* emotion of the So Yang Individual is sorrow, which is abrupt and urgent. The broad and embracing nature of anger gathers and increases the energy of the spleen. The abrupt and urgent emotion of their sorrow strikes at and severs the energy of the kidneys. This is how the So Yang Individual is born with a stronger spleen and a weaker kidney.

太陰人은 喜性이 廣張而樂情이 促急하니 喜性이 廣張則氣注肝而肝益盛이오

樂情이 促急則氣激肺而肺益削하나니 太陰之臟局이 所以成形於肝大肺小也오

少陰人은 樂性이 深確而喜情이 促急하니 樂性이 深確則氣注腎而腎益盛이오

喜情이 促急則氣激脾而脾益削하나니 少陰之臟局이 所以成形於腎大脾小也니라.

The *Song* nature of the Tae Eum Individual is joy, which is wide and vast. The *Jung* emotion of the Tae Eum Individual is laziness, which is abrupt and urgent. The wide and vast nature of joy gathers and increases the energy of the liver. The abrupt and urgent emotion of their laziness strikes at and severs the energy of the lungs. This is how the Tae Eum Individual is born with a stronger liver and a weaker lung.

Calmness,[18] which is deep and hard, is the *Song* nature of the So Eum individual. The *Jung* emotion of the So Eum Individual is joy, which is abrupt and urgent. The deep and hard nature of calmness gathers and increases the energy of the kidneys. The abrupt and urgent emotion of their joy strikes at and severs the energy of the spleen. This is how the So Eum Individual is born with stronger kidneys and a weaker spleen.

---

18  Every character in the Chinese language has numerous meanings that may have a positive or negative tone depending on the context in which it is used. The tone of an English word, for the most part, doesn't change depending on context. The word *calmness*, for example, has a positive tone, and may be equated with *peacefulness*. The word *laziness*, on the contrary, has a negative tone and isn't equated with calmness. The Chinese character *rak* (樂) may be interpreted as "calmness" or "laziness" depending on the situation. When not in balance, *rak* may be defined as laziness, but when balanced, calmness. Lee Je-ma emphasizes how, even though the So Eum Individual has a calm nature, he/she is also prone to being lazy and uncaring. Hence, the So Eum Individual may live a calm life or, on the contrary, be prone to external illness due to indifference. Health is therefore dependent upon how the So Eum Individual expresses this nature.

肺氣는 直而伸이오 脾氣는 栗而包오
肝氣는 寬而緩이오 腎氣는 溫而畜이니라.

The lung energy stretches directly outwards. The spleen energy is firm, and embracing. The liver energy is broad and slow. The kidney energy is Warm and nurturing.[19]

肺以呼하며 肝以吸하나니 肝肺者는 呼吸氣液之門戶也오
脾以納하며 腎以出하나니 腎脾者는 出納水穀之府庫也니라.

The lungs control inhalation while the liver controls exhalation. The inhalation and exhalation of the lungs and liver serve as a door allowing *Qi* and bodily fluids in and out of the body. The spleen absorbs while the kidney excretes. The kidney and spleen's excretion and absorption act as a warehouse that stores and distributes liquid and food throughout the body.

哀氣는 直升이오 怒氣는 橫升이오 喜氣는 放降이오 樂氣는 陷降이니라.

Sadness travels straight upwards. Anger travels diagonally upwards. Joy spreads outwards and descends. Calmness sinks directly downwards.[20]

---

19   In this section, Lee Je-ma compares organ energy with the Four Phases of Existence (元亨利貞: *Yuan, Heng, Li, Zhen*) discussed in the *I Ching*, in which King Wen assigns one or more of these attributes to each of the 64 hexagrams. The Four Phases of Existence have numerous correlations and are said to be the four basic components of all phenomena. Lee Je-ma correlates the lungs with the *Yuan* phase, which signifies upward growth, the spleen with the *Heng* phase, firm and embracing, the liver with the *Li* phase, broad and slow, and the kidneys with the *Zhen* phase, which is warm and nurturing. The four phases also correlate with the seasons: *Yuan* correlates with Spring, the Wood element, Eastern direction, and the Virtue of love. *Hyung* correlates with Summer, the Fire element, Southern direction, and the Virtue of humility. *Li* correlates with the Fall, the Metal element, Western direction, and the Virtue of righteousness. *Zhen* correlates with Winter, the Water element, Northern direction, and the Virtue of wisdom.

20   The above emotions correlate with the Four Major *Zhang* Organs, where sadness correlates with the lungs, anger correlates with the spleen, joy correlates with the liver, and calmness correlates with the kidneys. Each of the four emotions also has its energetic pathway, correlating with each of the Four Major *Zhang* Organs.

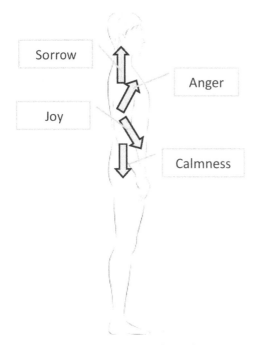

*Figure 2.1: The directional flow of emotions*

哀怒之氣는 上升이오 喜樂之氣는 下降이니 上升之氣 過多則下焦 傷이오 下降之氣 過多則上焦 傷이니라.

Since sorrow and anger flow upwards, and joy and calmness flow downwards, excessive upward flow causes injury to the Lower *Jiao*,[21] and excessive downward flow causes injury to the Upper *Jiao*.[22]

**Table 2.2: The four *Jiao* in Sasang medicine and their counterparts**

| *Jiao* | *Zhang* organ correlate | *Fu* organ correlate |
|---|---|---|
| Upper | Lungs | Esophagus |
| Mid-Upper | Spleen | Stomach |
| Mid-Lower | Liver | Small intestine |
| Lower | Kidneys | Large intestine |

---

21 "Excessive upward flow" refers to the rising of Yang from the Yang *Zhang* organs, the lungs and spleen. Excessive upward flow of Yang from the upper half of the body, or Upper *Jiao*, causes energy to circulate away from the lower half of the body, or Lower *Jiao*. In Sasang medicine, the body is divided into four *Jiao*; the Upper *Jiao*, Mid-Upper *Jiao*, Mid-Lower *Jiao*, and the Lower *Jiao*. (See Table 2.2.)

22 "Excessive downward flow" refers to the descent of Yin from the Yin *Zhang* organs, the liver and kidneys. Excessive downward flow of Yin from the lower half of the body, or Lower *Jiao*, causes energy to circulate away from the upper half of the body, or Upper *Jiao*.

哀怒之氣 順動則發越而上騰하고 喜樂之氣 順動則緩安而下墜하나니
哀怒之氣는 陽也라 順動則順而上升하고 喜樂之氣는 陰也라 順動則順而
下降이니라

When sorrow and anger flow smoothly,[23] they enhance the smooth upward flow of energy. When joy and calmness flow smoothly, they relax and calm the downward flow of energy. Sorrow and joy are Yang energies that flow smoothly upwards when balanced. Joy and calmness are Yin energies that flow smoothly downwards when in balance.

哀怒之氣 逆動則爆發而竝於上也오 喜樂之氣 逆動則浪發而竝於下也니
上升之氣 逆動而竝於上則肝腎이 傷하고 下降之氣 逆動而竝於下則脾肺
傷이니라.

When the ascent of sorrow and anger stagnates[24] and explodes upwards,[25] it will result in upper body accumulation. When the descent of joy and calmness stagnates and sinks downwards,[26] then it will result in lower body accumulation. If the upward flow of energy stagnates and accumulates, then the liver and kidneys in the lower body will be affected. If the downward flow of energy stagnates and accumulates, the spleen and lungs in the upper body will be affected.

---

23   Lee Je-ma refers to the harmonious flow of organ and emotional energy as *Sun Dong* (順動), in which sorrow and joy flow smoothly upwards and joy and leisure flow smoothly downwards. The opposite situation, referred to as *Yuk Dong* (逆動) in Korean, describes the situation in which sorrow and anger rebel/burst upwards and joy and leisure sink downwards.

24   The word "stagnation," in this case, refers to *Yuk Dong* (逆動), the opposite of *Sun Dong* (順動), harmonious flow. Lee Je-ma utilizes this term to describe imbalanced or disharmonious flow of organ energy. The excessive flow of lung energy upwards, or the excessive flow of kidney energy downwards, is referred to as *Yuk Dong* (逆動). The character for *Yuk* (逆) is also translated as "reversal" or "rebellion." In this text, Lee Je-ma also refers to *Yuk* (逆) when describing imbalanced organ flow. Hence the ascent of kidney energy, which naturally flows downward, or the descent of lung energy, which naturally flows upward, is also referred to as *Yuk Dong* (逆動), an unnatural flow that gives rise to illness.

25   The expression "explodes upwards" refers to *Pok Bal* (爆發), the opposite of *Ryang Bal* (浪發), which means to "sink downwards." It occurs when the Tae Yang Individual loses control of their *Song* nature of sorrow, or if the So Yang Individual loses control of their *Song* nature of anger. In both cases, the *Song* nature will morph into a *Jung* emotion, bursting upwards and causing injury to the largest organ of each of the above Sasang constitutions. When the Tae Yang Individual loses control of their sorrow, it will "explode upwards" in the form of anger. When the So Yang Individual loses control of their anger, it will also "explode upwards" in the form of sorrow.

26   The expression "sinks downwards" refers to *Ryang Bal* (浪發), the opposite of *Pok Bal* (爆發), which means to "explode upwards." It occurs when the Tae Eum Individual loses control of their *Song* nature of joy, or if the So Eum Individual loses control of their *Song* nature of calmness. In both cases, the *Song* nature will morph into a *Jung* emotion, sinking downwards and causing injury to the largest organ of each of the above Sasang constitutions. When the Tae Eum Individual loses control of his/her joy, it will "sink downwards" in the form of laziness or complacency. When the So Eum Individual loses control of their calmness, it will also "sink downwards" in the form of manic joy.

頻起怒而頻伏怒則腰脇이 頻迫而頻蕩也니 腰脇者는 肝之所住着處也니
腰脇이 迫蕩不定則肝其不傷乎아
乍發喜而乍收喜則胸腋이 乍闊而乍狹也니 胸腋者는 脾之所住着處也니
胸腋이 闊狹不定則脾其不傷乎아

Frequent and/or suppressed anger[27] causes repeated stress and agitation of the lumbar area and hips, which correlate with the liver. If the hips and lumbar area are constantly stressed and agitated, then how can the liver escape injury?

Fleeting moments of joy and loss of joy[28] cause the thoracic/armpit area, correlated with the spleen, to expand and contract excessively. If the chest and armpits are constantly forced to expand and contract in excess, then how can the spleen escape injury?

忽動哀而忽止哀則脊曲이 忽屈而忽伸也니 脊曲者는 腎之所住着處也니
脊曲이 屈伸不定則腎其不傷乎아
屢得樂而屢失樂則背佳頁 暴揚而暴抑也니 背佳頁者는 肺之所住着處也니
背佳頁 抑揚不定則肺其不傷乎아

Sudden bouts of sadness followed by sudden termination of sadness[29] causes the sacral area, which correlates with the kidneys, to bend forward and pull backward excessively. If the sacrum is constantly bending forward and excessively pulling backward, then how can the kidneys escape injury?

Going from long periods of calmness to long periods without feeling calm[30] causes the cervical spine,[31] correlated with the lungs, to extend backwards and flex forwards.[32] If the back of the neck is constantly extending and flexing, then how can the lungs escape injury?[33]

---

27  Frequent and suppressed anger refers to the Tae Yang Individual's *Jung* emotion.

28  Fleeting moments of joy and loss of joy refer to the So Eum Individual's *Jung* emotion.

29  Sudden bouts of sadness followed by sudden termination of sadness refers to the So Yang Individual's *Jung* emotion.

30  Going from long periods of calmness to long periods without feeling calm refers to the Tae Eum Individual's *Jung* emotion.

31  The spine is what keeps the body erect and fends off external invasion. Imbalanced emotions directly affect the spine, resulting in a lack of ability to stay upright and resist external invasion. If an area of the spine is deficient it will move excessively to compensate.

32  Excessive and imbalanced sadness, joy, calmness, and anger directly affect movement of the four major posterior areas of the body: lumbar, thoracic, sacral, and cervical spinal areas. Each of these areas also corresponds to the Four Major Organs: liver, spleen, kidneys, and lungs, respectively. Imbalanced emotion results in exceedingly repetitive movement of the weakest organ and its correlating location along the spine.

33  As mentioned above, the "explosion upwards" of the upper body *Yang Zhang* organs (lungs and spleen) results in deficiency of the lower body *Yin Zhang* organs (liver and kidneys). Hence imbalance of sorrow and anger from the lungs and spleen will cause deficiency of the liver and kidneys. Moreover, "sinking downwards" of the *Yin Zhang* organs results in deficiency of the *Yang Zhang* organs, where imbalance of joy results in deficiency of the lungs and spleen. Hence these organs cannot escape deficiency when the *Jung* emotions are imbalanced.

**Table 2.3: The effect of imbalanced *Jung* emotion on the organs and body functions**

| *Jung* emotion | Affiliated Sasang constitution | Direct organ affiliation | Explosion upwards or sinking downwards affects the… | Affected body location when imbalanced |
|---|---|---|---|---|
| Anger | Tae Yang | Spleen | Liver | Lumbar spine |
| Joy | So Eum | Liver | Spleen | Thoracic spine |
| Sadness | So Yang | Lungs | Kidneys | Sacrum |
| Calmness | Tae Eum | Kidneys | Lungs | Cervical spine |

太陽人이 有暴怒深哀하니 不可不戒오 少陽人이 有暴哀深怒하니 不可不
戒오
太陰人이 有浪樂深喜하니 不可不戒오 少陰人이 有浪喜深樂하니 不可不
戒니라.

The Tae Yang Individual should always be vigilant against their harsh and explosive anger[34] and deep-rooted sorrow.[35] The sorrow of the So Yang Individual is harsh and explosive,[36] while their anger is deep rooted.[37] These are emotions to always be cautioned against. The laziness of the Tae Eum Individual is harsh and explosive[38] and their joy[39] is deep rooted.[40] These are emotions that always need to be cautioned against. The joy of the So Eum Individual is harsh and explosive.[41] Their calmness[42] is deep rooted.[43] These are emotions that always need to be treated with caution.

---

34  Anger is the *Jung* emotion of the Tae Yang Individual, which manifests as a result of the uncontrolled *Song* nature of sorrow. Hence the Tae Yang Individual has the tendency towards harsh and explosive anger.

35  Sorrow is the *Song* nature of the Tae Yang Individual, an emotion that constantly underlies their thoughts and actions. Hence the Tae Yang Individual's sorrow is deep rooted and potentially severe.

36  Sorrow is the *Jung* emotion of the So Yang Individual, which manifests as a result of their uncontrolled *Song* nature of anger. Hence the So Yang Individual radiates towards harsh and explosive sadness.

37  Anger is the *Song* nature of the So Yang Individual, an emotion that is constantly underlying their thoughts and actions. Hence the So Yang Individual's anger is deep rooted and potentially harmful.

38  Laziness (calmness taken to the extreme) is the *Jung* emotion of the Tae Eum Individual and manifests as a result of their uncontrolled *Song* nature of joy. Hence the Tae Eum Individual has the tendency towards harsh and explosive laziness.

39  It is hard to imagine what "severe" joy means, since, in English, it has a positive connotation. As we have mentioned earlier, all emotions, when taken to the extreme, result in imbalance. When joy is extreme, it results in a craving for happiness and contentment. When this need isn't fulfilled or sustained, the So Eum Individual disdains others who are happier than them and/or retreats into their own world of unrealistic joy.

40  Joy is the *Song* nature of the Tae Eum Individual, an emotion that constantly underlies their thoughts and actions. Hence the Tae Yang Individual's joy is deep rooted and potentially severe.

41  Joy is the *Jung* emotion of the So Eum Individual, which manifests as a result of their uncontrolled *Song* nature of calmness. Hence the So Eum Individual has the tendency towards harsh and explosive joy.

42  It is hard to imagine what "severe" calmness means, since it is has a positive connotation in English. When calmness is taken to the extreme, however, it morphs into laziness and idleness.

43  Calmness is the *Song* nature of the So Eum Individual, an emotion constantly underlying their thoughts and actions. Thus the So Eum Individual's calmness is deep rooted and potentially harmful.

皐陶曰都라 在知人하며 在安民하니이다. 禹曰吁라 咸若時홀든 惟帝도
其難之러시니 知人則哲이라 能官人이며 安民則惠라 黎民이 懷之하리니
能哲而惠면 何傷乎驩兜며 何遷乎有苗며 何畏乎巧言令色孔壬이리오.

Gao Yao, the political advisor of Emperor Yu,[44] stated: "To know the common people
is to bring peace to them." Emperor Yu responded: "It is precisely as you stated.
An emperor must know the people." This was a challenge even for the powerful
Emperors Yao and Shun. Only through understanding the needs of the people can
they be governed. Kindness and respect are essential in order to establish a peaceful
society. The common people cherish the kindness and respect of their leader. How
could such a leader be worried about the actions of Huan Dou?[45] How could they
be afraid of the cunning and clever actions of You Miao?[46] A gentle and kind leader
is naturally concerned about the negative actions of such individuals for the sake of
the people [but doesn't feel anxious about or fear them].

三復大禹之訓而欽仰之曰帝堯之喜怒哀樂이 每每中節者는 以其難於知人
也오 大禹之喜怒哀樂이 每每中節者는 以其不敢輕易於知人也라 天下喜
怒哀樂之暴動浪動者 都出於行身不誠而知人不明也니 知人은 帝堯之所
難而大禹之所吁也則其誰沾沾自喜乎아 蓋亦益反其誠而必不可輕易取捨
人也니라.

Emperor Yu continued the teachings of Emperors Yao and Shun. Perhaps worthy
of the greatest respect was his ability to balance the emotions of joy, anger, sadness,
and calmness. This was because he knew how difficult it was to understand the
complexity of human nature. His ability to balance joy, anger, sadness, and laziness
was also thanks to his lack of hastiness in human affairs. Insincerity results in the
sudden and careless movement of joy, anger, sadness, and laziness. Unbalanced
emotion[47] makes it impossible to take action, practice sincerity, become wise, and
understand the complexity of human nature. If even Emperors Yu and Yao thought it
was so challenging to comprehend human nature, then how can we be satisfied with
our understanding of it? The more we cultivate our true nature through sincerity,
the easier it is to help others and not ignore their needs.

---

44  Emperor Yu, also known as Yu the Great, succeeded Emperor Shun, who granted him the throne after he
    succeeded in preventing the Yang Tse River from flooding. His father was also appointed by Emperor Shun
    to address the situation, but he didn't succeed, for which he was executed. Rather than build trenches, Yu the
    Great built a canal to divert the river's flow, hence "balancing" the Yang Tse, rather than "blocking" it.

45  Along with Gon Gong (共工), Huan Dou (驩兜), a minister of the virtuous Emperor Yao, made a failed
    attempt to oust him from power. In response, Emperor Yao exiled him to the remote area of Mt. Chongshan
    (崇山).

46  You Miao (有苗), also referred to as San Miao (三苗), was a powerful leader who controlled the southern part
    of China before Emperor Shun ascended to the throne and conquered his territory. After 70 days of retreat,
    You Miao surrendered and pledged allegiance to Emperor Shun.

47  In this sentence, Lee Je-ma refers to unbalanced emotions as the "exploding upwards" and the "sinking
    downwards" of the Jung emotions.

雖好善之心이나 偏急而好善則好善이 必不明也오 雖惡惡之心이나 偏急
而惡惡則惡惡이 必不周也라 天下事는 宜與好人做也니 不與好人做則
喜樂이 必煩也오 天下事는 不宜與不好人做也니 與不好人做則哀怒益煩
也니라.

Even though a person may wish to be benevolent,[48] if they take this desire to the extreme and act in haste, they will never bring out their benevolence. Even if one dislikes malevolence,[49] if they act hastily against it, then they will lack fairness. Those who are concerned with the affairs of the world must associate with others who follow the same path. If not, then they will feel envious of others who are happy or joyous. Those who have no interest in the affairs of the world must be careful about associating with others who follow the same path. If they associate with those who have no interest in world affairs, then they will get offended when others are sad or angry.[50]

哀怒 相成하며 喜樂이 相資하나니 哀性이 極則怒情이 動하고 怒性이 極
則哀情이 動하고 樂性이 極則喜情이 動하고 喜性이 極則樂情이 動이니
太陽人이 哀極不濟則忿怒 激外하고 少陽人이 怒極不勝則悲哀 動中하고
少陰人이 樂極不成則喜好 不定하고 太陰人이 喜極不服則侈樂이 無
厭하나니 如此而動者는 無異於以刀割臟이라 一次大動이면 十年難復이니
此는 死生壽夭之機關也니 不可不知也니라.

While sadness and anger bolster one another, joy and calmness also share the same relationship. The *Song* nature of sadness at its extreme morphs into the *Jung* emotion of anger, while the *Song* nature of anger at its extreme morphs into the *Jung* emotion of sadness. Moreover, the *Song* nature of joy at its extreme morphs into the *Jung* emotion of complacency, while the *Song* nature of calmness at its extreme leads to the *Jung* emotion of imbalanced and crooked joy. If the Tae Yang Individual doesn't control sadness, he or she will outwardly express violent anger. If the So Yang Individual doesn't overcome their anger, he or she will be plagued inwardly with profound sadness. If the So Eum Individual doesn't control calmness, he or she will drown themselves with joy from [selfish] pleasure. If the

---

48    Lee Je-ma equates "benevolence" with the manifestation of one's virtue, or highest level of potential. The "desire for benevolence" is rooted in the four senses: ears, eyes, nose, and mouth.

49    The "dislike of malevolence" is rooted in the four organs: lungs, spleen, liver, and kidneys.

50    Those who follow the way of heaven rejoice when others are joyful or calm and feel regret when they are angry or sad. Keep in mind that "joy" and "calm" are the *Song* natures of the Tae Eum and the So Eum Individual respectively. "Anger" and "sadness" are the *Song* natures of the Tae Yang and So Yang Individual respectively. Hence, it is difficult to understand the nature of others if one doesn't follow the Way of heaven. Since humans are social beings, they are strongly affected by interacting with others. Virtuous acquaintances will enhance one's virtue, and malevolent acquaintances will enhance one's negativity.

Tae Eum Individual doesn't control joy, then indulgence and laziness[51] will be boundless. There is no difference between stabbing one's own *Zhang*[52] organs and giving way to such emotions. If these emotions are expressed to the extreme, even ten years would not be enough to overcome them.[53] The imbalance and balance of the *Song* nature and *Jung* emotion is what makes the difference between premature death and longevity, dying and living. Therefore, we should never underestimate its importance.

太少陰陽之臟局短長은 陰陽之變化也라
天稟之已定은 固無可論이어니와 天稟已定之外에 又有短長而不全其天稟
者則人事之修不修而命之傾也니 不可不愼也니라.

The relative organ size[54] of each Sasang constitution depends on the [prenatal] transformation of Yin and Yang. It goes without saying that one's heavenly nature, or *Song*, is also predetermined. While all people have a heavenly nature, the relative size of their organs restricts its ability to manifest completely on its own.[55] Without taking action, [the beauty of] our heavenly nature lies dormant within. The ability to carry out *Myung* (life's path) is dependent upon whether or not one's actions are grounded in sincerity and self-cultivation. Since this process doesn't manifest of its own accord, one must always be self-aware![56]

---

51  Calmness, indulgence, and laziness are all translations of a single character, *rak* (樂). When *rak* is balanced, it manifests as calmness; when imbalanced, it manifests as indulgence and laziness. It is easier for the So Eum Individual to balance *rak* than it is for the Tae Eum, because it is the *Song* nature of the former and the *Jung* emotion of the latter Sasang constitution.

52  As mentioned before, the *Zhang* organs in Sasang medicine are the lungs, spleen, liver, and kidneys.

53  In this sentence, Lee Je-ma proclaims that once the *Jung* emotion is manifested, it is very difficult to conceal it. Once the Tae Yang Individual experiences a bout of rage, for example, he or she has the tendency to resort to this emotion continuously when under stress. Lee Je-ma equates such extreme emotional manifestation with the act of stabbing oneself, or committing emotional suicide.

54  Since Sasang medicine is based on the principle of metaphysics, Lee Je-ma isn't referring to the actual size of each organ, but rather their energetic function. "Larger" organs are considered energetically stronger and are prone to congestion and stagnation, whereas the "smaller" organs are considered energetically weaker and are prone to deficiency.

55  The difference in organ "size" has two major effects on the individual. The first is the circulation of energy and blood from the larger to the smaller organs. The second is the loss of one's pure and unfettered association with heaven, since the difference of organ size itself may be considered an imperfection. If the organs were all the same "size" and Yin and Yang within the body were completely balanced, there would be no flow. Hence, by definition, flow within the body is dependent on an imbalance of Yin and Yang, whereas perfect balance exists only within the realm of heaven itself. The discovery of, and action based on, one's *Myung* is what brings them closer to heaven and, in the process, optimizes a smooth flow from the stronger to the weaker organs.

56  In this paragraph, Lee Je-ma refers to the difference between *Chon Song* (天性) and *Chon Myung* (天命). The former, which translates as "heavenly nature," is bestowed equally within the heart of all humanity, while the latter, which means "heavenly endowed path," requires the discovery of one's "heavenly nature" and sincerity in one's affairs.

太陽人怒는 以一人之怒而怒千萬人하나니 其怒 無術於千萬人則必難堪
千萬人也오

少陰人喜는 以一人之喜而喜千萬人하나니 其喜 無術於千萬人則必難堪千
萬人也오

少陽人哀는 以一人之哀而哀千萬人하나니 其哀 無術於千萬人則必難堪千
萬人也오

太陰人樂은 以一人之樂而樂千萬人하나니 其樂이 無術於千萬人則必難堪
千萬人也니라

The *Jung* emotion of anger expressed by a single Tae Yang Individual can cause anger among ten million[57] others. If they do not find a way to control this anger, then it would assuredly be challenging for ten million others to endure it.

The *Jung* emotion of joy expressed by a single So Eum Individual can cause joy among ten million others. If they do not find a way to control this joy [and give way to selfish pleasure], then ten million others would assuredly find it challenging to bear.

The *Jung* emotion of sorrow expressed by a single So Yang Individual can cause sorrow among ten million others. If they do not find a way to overcome this sorrow, then it would assuredly pose a challenge for ten million others to endure it.

The *Jung* emotion of complacency expressed by a single Tae Eum Individual can cause complacency among ten million others. If they do not find a way to control their extremely complacent nature, then it would certainly be a challenge for ten million others to bear it.

太陽少陽人이 但恒戒哀怒之過度而不可强做喜樂하야 虛動不及也
若强做喜樂而煩數之則喜樂이 不出於眞情而哀怒 益偏也오
太陰少陰人이 但恒戒喜樂之過度而不可强做哀怒하야 虛動不及也니
若强做哀怒而煩數之則哀怒 不出於眞情而喜樂이 益偏也니라.

The two Yang constitutions (Tae Yang and So Yang) must always be vigilant of their tendency towards feeling sad and/or angered, a tendency that makes it difficult to be truly joyful or calm. Excessive effort to become joyous and calm will only be in vain. The Tae Yang and So Yang Individual cannot feel true joy or calmness by force or excessive effort. The forceful attempt to become joyful and/or calm will only result in further damage from sadness and anger.[58]

---

57  The term "ten million" is another expression for "infinity." In this context it is used to describe an infinite number of people. Hence the Tae Yang Individual's *Jung* emotion of anger affects everyone they come in contact with directly or indirectly.

58  Balancing the tendency towards excessive anger and sorrow is the only way for the Tae Yang and So Yang Individual to accomplish joy and relaxation. By nature Tae Eum and So Eum Individuals are more joyous and calm compared to the Tae Yang and So Yang Individual. Jealous of these Yin traits, the Tae Yang and So Yang Individual may attempt to achieve joy and relaxation through artificial or hasty means, which will result in further affliction of anger and sorrow.

The two Yin constitutions (Tae Eum and So Eum) must always practice caution against their tendency towards feeling too joyous and/or complacent. This tendency makes it difficult for them to be truly sorrowful or angry. Excessive effort to become sorrowful or angry will only be in vain. The Tae Eum and So Eum Individual cannot feel true sorrow or anger by force or excessive effort. The forceful attempt to become sorrowful and/or angry will only result in further damage from excess joy and/or complacency.[59]

喜怒哀樂之未發을 謂之中이오 發而皆中節을 謂之和니
喜怒哀樂未發而恒戒者 此非漸近於中者乎아
喜怒哀樂已發而自反者 此非漸近於節者乎아.

When joy, anger, sadness, and calmness are dormant, they are referred to as the emotions of the "center." When these emotions are expressed appropriately,[60] they are referred to as "harmonious." Wouldn't the act of keeping a vigilant eye on one's joy, anger, sadness, and complacency bring them closer to their center? Once the emotions of joy, anger, sadness, and complacency are expressed, wouldn't the practice of self-reflection eventually lead to harmony?

---

59  Balancing the tendency towards excessive joy and complacency is the only way for the Tae Eum and So Eum Individual to accomplish joy and relaxation. By nature, the Tae Yang and So Yang assert themselves more strongly (through anger and sorrow) when compared to the Tae Eum and So Eum constitutions. Jealous of these Yang traits, the Tae Eum and So Eum Individual may attempt to be more assertive through artificial or hasty means, resulting in further affliction from imbalanced joy and complacency.

60  The character *jul* (節) has several meanings and is translated in this sentence as "expressed appropriately." It is also the title of the 60th hexagram of the *I Ching* and signifies the "correct time and place" for action. *Jul* is also translated as "season," and in ancient times, man lived in accordance with the seasons by consuming seasonal foods and adjusting activity levels. In the Korean language, the term "*jul yi durosumnida*" contains the character for *jul*, and is often used to describe a child or adult who has modified their behavior and become morally inclined.

# Expanding and Fulfilling[1]

擴
充
論

太陽人은 哀性이 遠散而怒情이 促急하나니 哀性이 遠散者는 太陽之耳
察於天時而哀衆人之相欺也니 哀性이 非他라 聽也오 怒情이 促急者는
太陽之脾 行於交遇而怒別人之侮己也니 怒情이 非他라 怒也니라

The Tae Yang Individual's sorrow is widely dispersed and their anger is urgent and sudden.[2] Sorrow is the Tae Yang Individual's *Song* nature while anger is their *Jung* emotion. Widely dispersed sadness is the result of their ability to hear *Chon Shi*, the voice of heaven.[3] This ability makes them aware of when people are keeping secrets, or do not *listen* to each other. The ability to "hear" when others are not truthful saddens the Tae Yang Individual. Hence the nature of sadness comes from hearing. The *Jung* emotion of anger bursts forth when the Tae Yang Individual's spleen[4] engages in *Kyo Uh*, associating with others one on one, with a feeling of being looked down upon.[5] The *Jung* emotion of anger is nothing but pure anger itself.

---

1   The title of this chapter comprises the two characters *hwak* (擴: To expand, amplify, distribute) and *chung* (充: To fill, close up). Together these characters mean "expanding and fulfilling" one's *Myung*, or life's path. The term *hwak chung* was originally cited in Mengzi's *Mencius*: "Those who expand (擴) the Four Virtues within themselves and fulfill their path (充) are like a raging Fire or a bubbling Spring" (凡有四端於我者 知 皆擴而充之矣 若火之始然 泉之始達).

2   "Widely dispersed" refers to the Tae Yang Individual's chronic underlying *Song* nature of sorrow. "Urgent and sudden" refers to the acute upward explosion of the Tae Yang Individual's *Jung* emotion of anger.

3   The ability to hear *Chon Shi* is a heavenly endowed ability of the Tae Yang Individual, and it activates the *Song* nature of sorrow.

4   The spleen is associated with anger, the Tae Yang Individual's *Jung* emotion, and it is also associated with the Virtue of humility.

5   *Kyo Uh* is carried out through the Virtue of humility. The act of looking down on others comes from a lack of humility. The Tae Yang Individual is sensitive to others' lack of humility, which causes their *Jung* emotion, anger, to burst forth.

少陽人은 怒性이 宏抱而哀情이 促急하나니 怒性이 宏抱者는 少陽之
目이 察於世會而怒衆人之相侮也니 怒性이 非他라 視也오 哀情이 促急
者는 少陽之肺 行於事務而哀別人之欺己也니 哀情이 非他라 哀也니라

The So Yang Individual's anger is broad and engulfing while their sorrow is urgent and sudden.[6] Anger is the So Yang Individual's *Song* nature while sadness is their *Jung* emotion. Their broad and engulfing anger is the result of the ability to "see" *Sei Wei*, social duty and humility.[7] This ability makes them *see* clearly when people look down on each other. The ability to "see" when others are looking down on one another angers the So Yang Individual. Hence the nature of anger comes from seeing. The *Jung* emotion of sadness manifests when the So Yang Individual's lungs[8] are practicing *Sa Mu*, Human Affairs, and they feel as if others are hiding something from them. The *Jung* emotion of sadness is nothing but pure sadness itself.[9]

太陰人은 喜性이 廣張而樂情이 促急하나니 喜性而廣張者는 太陰之鼻
察於人倫而喜衆人之相助也니 喜性이 非他라 嗅也오 樂情이 促急者는
太陰之腎이 行於居處而樂別人之保己也니 樂情이 非他라 樂也니라.

The Tae Eum Individual's joy is broad and expanding while their complacency is urgent and sudden.[10] Joy is the Tae Eum Individual's *Song* nature while complacency is their *Jung* emotion. The broad and expanding joy is the result of their ability to "smell" *In Ryun*, humanity.[11] This ability makes them sense when people are helping each other. The ability to "smell" when others are helping each other makes the Tae Eum Individual feel joyful. Hence the nature of joy comes from smelling. The *Jung* emotion of complacency and laziness manifests when the Tae Eum Individual's kidneys[12] are practicing *Ko Cho*, Household Affairs, and they feel as if others are protecting[13] them. The *Jung* emotion of complacency is nothing but pure complacency itself.

---

6    "Broad and engulfing" refers to the So Yang Individual's chronic underlying *Song* nature of anger. "Urgent and sudden" denotes the acute upward explosion of the So Yang Individual's *Jung* emotion of sorrow.

7    The ability to see *Sei Wei* is a heavenly endowed ability of the So Yang Individual, and it activates the *Song* nature of anger.

8    The lungs are associated with sadness, the So Yang Individual's *Jung* emotion. They are also associated with the Virtue of wisdom.

9    The Yang (Tae Yang and So Yang) constitutions are sensitive to whether or not others are looking down on them (or each other) or hiding something from them (or each other). These sensitivities will either activate their *Song* nature or explode their *Jung* emotion depending on the constitution and the situation.

10   "Broad and expanding" refers to the Tae Eum Individual's chronic underlying *Song* nature of joy. "Urgent and sudden" denotes the acute downward sinking of the Tae Eum Individual's *Jung* emotion of complacency.

11   The ability to smell *In Ryun* is a heavenly endowed ability of the Tae Eum Individual and activates the *Song* nature of joy.

12   The kidneys are associated with complacency/laziness, the Tae Eum Individual's *Jung* emotion, and are also associated with the Virtue of love.

13   "Protection" in this context is referring to the Tae Eum Individual's inclination to take the care they receive from immediate friends and family for granted, a reflection of their complacent *Jung* emotion.

少陰人은 樂性이 深確而喜情이 促急하나니 樂性이 深確者는 少陰之口
察於地方而樂衆人之相保也니 樂性이 非他라 味也오 喜情이 促急者는
少陰之肝이 行於黨與而喜別人之助己也니 喜情이 非他라 喜也니라.

The So Eum Individual's calmness is deep and hard while their joy is urgent and sudden.[14] Calmness is the So Eum Individual's *Song* nature while joy is their *Jung* emotion. The deep and hard calmness is the result of their ability to taste *Ji Bang*, the appropriate place for action.[15] This ability makes them sense when people are protecting each other. The ability to "taste" when others are protecting each other makes the So Eum Individual feel calm and relaxed. Hence the nature of calmness comes from tasting. The *Jung* emotion of joy manifests when the So Eum Individual's liver[16] is practicing *Dang Yo*, establishing relationships with like-minded people, and they feel as if others are helping them. The *Jung* emotion of joy is nothing but pure joy itself.[17]

太陽之耳는 能廣博於天時而太陽之鼻는 不能廣博於人倫이오
太陰之鼻는 能廣博於人倫而太陰之耳는 不能廣博於天時오
少陽之目은 能廣博於世會而少陽之口는 不能廣博於地方이오
少陰之口는 能廣博於地方而少陰之目은 不能廣博於世會니라.

The ears of the Tae Yang Individual are capable of spreading *Chon Shi*, the way of heaven, far and wide.[18] However, the nose of the Tae Yang is incapable of spreading *In Ryun*, humanity, far and wide.[19]

The nose of the Tae Eum Individual is capable of spreading *In Ryun* far and wide.[20] However, the ears of the Tae Eum are incapable of spreading *Chon Shi* far and wide.[21]

---

14 "Deep and hard" refers to the So Eum Individual's chronic underlying *Song* nature of calmness. "Urgent and sudden" refers to the acute downward sinking of the So Eum Individual's *Jung* emotion of excess joy.

15 The ability to taste *Ji Bang* is a heavenly endowed ability of the So Eum Individual, and it activates the *Song* nature of calmness.

16 The liver is associated with joy, the So Eum Individual's *Jung* emotion, and is also associated with the Virtue of righteousness.

17 The Yin (Tae Eum and So Eum) constitutions are sensitive to whether or not others assist them (or each other) or protect them (or each other). These sensitivities will either activate their *Song* nature or explode their *Jung* emotion depending on the constitution and the situation.

18 The capability of spreading *Chon Shi* far and wide comes from the Tae Yang Individual's strongest sense, hearing, which correlates with their strongest organ, the lungs.

19 The incapability of spreading *In Ryun* far and wide is due to its association with smell, the Tae Yang Individual's weakest sense.

20 The capacity to spread *In Ryun* far and wide comes from the Tae Eum Individual's strongest sense, smell, which correlates with their strongest organ, the liver.

21 The incapability of spreading *Chon Shi* far and wide is due to its association with hearing, the Tae Eum Individual's weakest sense. This illustrates how Tae Yang and Tae Eum Individuals have opposing strengths and weaknesses because their energies flow as opposing Yin and Yang poles.

The eyes of the So Yang Individual are capable of spreading *Sei Wei* far and wide.[22] However, the mouth of the So Yang is incapable of spreading *Ji Bang*, establishing the appropriate place for action, far and wide.[23]

The mouth of the So Eum Individual is capable of spreading *Ji Bang* far and wide.[24] But the eyes of the So Eum are incapable of spreading *Sei Wei* far and wide.[25,26]

太陽之脾는 能勇統於交遇而太陽之肝은 不能雅立於黨與오
少陰之肝은 能雅立於黨與而少陰之脾는 不能勇統於交遇오
少陽之肺는 能敏達於事務而少陽之腎은 不能恒定於居處오
太陰之腎은 能恒定於居處而太陰之肺는 不能敏達於事務니라.

The spleen of the Tae Yang Individual is capable of courageously directing *Kyo Uh*.[27] However, the liver of the Tae Yang Individual is not capable of gracefully engaging in *Dang Yo*.[28]

The liver of the So Eum Individual is capable of gracefully engaging in *Dang Yo*,[29] but the spleen of the So Eum Individual is not capable of courageously directing *Kyo Uh*.[30]

The lungs of the So Yang Individual are capable of quickly spreading *Sa Mu*.[31] However, the kidneys of the So Yang are not capable of consistently establishing *Ko Cho*.[32]

---

22  The capacity to spread *Sei Wei* far and wide comes from the So Yang Individual's strongest sense, sight, which correlates with their strongest organ, the spleen.

23  The incapability of spreading *Ji Bang* far and wide is due to its association with taste, the So Yang Individual's weakest sense.

24  The capability of spreading *Ji Bang* far and wide comes from the So Eum Individual's strongest sense, taste, which correlates with their strongest organ, the kidneys.

25  The incapability of spreading *Sei Wei* far and wide is due to its association with sight, the So Eum Individual's weakest sense.

26  This section, correlating with *Song* (Human Nature, 性), describes the influence of *Chon Ki*, Heavenly Affairs, on each of the Sasang constitutions.

27  As mentioned above, the spleen correlates with anger, which is the Tae Yang Individual's *Jung* emotion. It also correlates with *Kyo Uh*. Hence, it is challenging for the Tae Yang Individual to conduct *Kyo Uh* without expressing their *Jung* emotion of anger. However, in this sentence Lee Je-ma illustrates how, if the Tae Yang Individual controls their *Jung* emotion, he or she is capable of courageously directing *Kyo Uh*.

28  *Dang Yo* correlates with the liver, the Tae Yang Individual's weakest organ.

29  The liver correlates with joy, which is the So Eum Individual's *Jung* emotion. It also correlates with *Dang Yo*. Hence it is challenging for the So Eum Individual to conduct *Dang Yo* without expressing their *Jung* emotion of overjoy. However, in this sentence Lee Je-ma illustrates how, if the So Eum Individual controls their *Jung* emotion, he or she is capable of gracefully engaging in *Dang Yo*.

30  *Kyo Uh* correlates with the spleen, the So Eum Individual's weakest organ.

31  The lungs correlate with sorrow, which is the So Yang Individual's *Jung* emotion. They also correlate with *Sa Mu*. Hence, it is challenging for the So Yang Individual to conduct *Sa Mu* without expressing their *Jung* emotion of sorrow. In this sentence Lee Je-ma illustrates how, if the So Yang Individual controls their *Jung* emotion, he or she is capable of courageously spreading *Sa Mu*.

32  *Ko Cho* correlates with the kidneys, the So Yang Individual's weakest organ.

The kidneys of the Tae Eum Individual are capable of consistently comforting *Ko Cho*.[33] The lungs of the Tae Eum Individual are not capable, however, of quickly spreading *Sa Mu*.[34,35]

太陽之聽이 能廣博於天時故로 太陽之神이 充足於頭腦而歸肺者 大也오
太陽之嗅 不能廣博於人倫故로 太陽之血이 不充足於腰脊而歸肝者
小也니라
太陰之嗅 能廣博於人倫故로 太陰之血이 充足於腰脊而歸肝者 大也오
太陰之聽이 不能廣博於天時故로 太陰之神이 不充足於頭腦而歸肺者
小也니라
少陽之視 能廣博於世會故로 少陽之氣 充足於背膂而歸脾者 大也오
少陽之味不能廣博於地方故로 少陽之精이 不充足於膀胱而歸腎者
小也니라.
少陰之味 能廣博於地方故로 少陰之精이 充足於膀胱而歸腎者 大也오
少陰之視 不能廣博於世會故로 少陰之氣 不充足於背膂而歸脾者
小也니라.

The Tae Yang Individual's profound ability to hear spreads *Chon Shi* far and wide. This helps their spirit fill the [cervical spine and] brain and flow abundantly around the lungs. The Tae Yang Individual's lack of smell inhibits the spread of *In Ryun* far and wide, which inhibits the blood's ability to fill the lumbar spine and circulate around the liver.

The Tae Eum Individual's profound ability to smell spreads *In Ryun* far and wide, and this helps their blood fill the lumbar spine and flow around the liver. The Tae Eum Individual's lack of hearing inhibits the spread of *Chon Shi* far and wide, and inhibits the ability of the spirit to fill the [cervical spine and] brain and circulate around the lungs.

The So Yang Individual's profound eyesight spreads *Sei Wei* far and wide. This helps their energy fill the thoracic spine and flow around the spleen. The So Yang Individual's lack of taste inhibits the spread of *Ji Bang* far and wide, which in turn inhibits the ability of essence to fill the [sacrum and] urinary bladder and circulate around the kidneys.

The So Eum Individual's profound taste spreads *Ji Bang* far and wide. This helps their essence fill the [sacrum and] bladder and flow around the kidneys. The So Eum

---

33  The kidneys correlate with complacency, which is the Tae Eum Individual's *Jung* emotion. They also correlate with *Ko Cho*. Hence, it is challenging for the Tae Eum Individual to conduct *Ko Cho* without expressing their *Jung* emotion of complacency. In this sentence Lee Je-ma illustrates how, if the Tae Eum Individual controls their *Jung* emotion, he or she is capable of courageously establishing *Ko Cho*.

34  *Sa Mu* correlates with the lungs, the Tae Eum Individual's weakest organ.

35  This section, correlating with *Myung* (divine mission, 命), describes the influence of *In Sa*, Human Affairs, on each of the Sasang constitutions.

Individual's lack of eyesight inhibits the spread of *Sei Wei* far and wide, thus the ability of energy to fill the upper back and circulate around the spleen.

**Table 3.1: Correlation between the four *Jiao*, senses, anatomy, and generators**

| *Jiao* level | Four senses | Four generators | Anatomical correlate | Strongest constitution | Weakest constitution |
|---|---|---|---|---|---|
| Upper *Jiao* | Hearing | Spirit | Brain and cervical | Tae Yang | Tae Eum |
| Mid-Upper *Jiao* | Sight | *Qi* (life-force) | Upper back and thoracic | So Yang | So Eum |
| Mid-Lower *Jiao* | Smell | Blood | Lower back and lumbar | Tae Eum | Tae Yang |
| Lower *Jiao* | Taste | Essence | bladder and sacrum | So Eum | So Yang |

太陽之怒 能勇統於交遇故로 交遇 不侮也오
太陽之喜 不能雅立於黨與故로 黨與 侮也니
是故로 太陽之暴怒 不在於交遇而必在於黨與也니라.
少陰之喜 能雅立於黨與故로 黨與 助也오
少陰之怒 不能勇統於交遇故로 交遇 不助也니
是故로 少陰之浪喜 不在於黨與而必在於交遇也니라.

The Tae Yang Individual's anger is capable of spreading *Kyo Uh* far and wide. *Kyo Uh*[36] signifies the inability to look down on others. The Tae Yang Individual's emotion of joy is not robust enough to establish elegant *Dang Yo*, which is capable of looking down on others [who do not see things the same way].[37] The explosion of their *Jung* emotion of anger [when they feel that others look down on them] results in the inability to spread *Kyo Uh*.[38] What cannot be found in *Kyo Uh* can always be found in *Dang Yo*.[39]

The So Eum Individual's joy is capable of establishing elegant *Dang Yo*,[40] which signifies the ability to help other [like-minded] people. The So Eum Individual's emotion of anger is not robust enough to courageously direct *Kyo Uh*,[41] respecting

---

36 *Kyo Uh* correlates with the Virtue of humility, and is therefore not capable of looking down on others.

37 The Tae Yang Individual's *Jung* emotion of anger is robust, but their ability to manifest the emotion of joy, the *Jung* emotion of the Tae Eum Individual, is feeble. *Dang Yo* is carried out via the emotion of joy.

38 The *Jung* emotion isn't intrinsically negative and damaging, its strength playing a significant role in Human Affairs. If the Tae Yang Individual's strong *Jung* emotion, for example, is expressed in a balanced way, it adds to the quality of *Kyo Uh*. If they lose control of this emotion, they will fail to carry out *Kyo Uh*.

39 Because it is difficult to balance their *Jung* emotion, the Tae Yang Individual often feels angered when engaging in *Dang Yo*, which is balanced with joy, not anger. This results in the upward explosion of their angry *Jung* nature due to a loss of trust and friendship with those close to them.

40 *Dang Yo* correlates with the Virtue of righteousness. Those who are righteous feel that it is their duty to help others.

41 *Kyo Uh* is the incapacity to look down on others. This quality leads to the Virtue of humility.

others. The acute downward sinking of their *Jung* emotion of excessive joy leads to the inability to establish elegant *Dang Yo*.[42] What cannot be found in *Dang Yo* can always be found in *Kyo Uh*.[43]

少陽之哀 能敏達於事務故로 事務 不欺也오
少陽之樂이 不能恒定於居處故로 居處 欺也니
是故로 少陽之暴哀 不在於事務而必在於居處也니라.
太陰之樂이 能恒定於居處故로 居處 保也오
太陰之哀 不能敏達於事務故로 事務 不保也니
是故로 太陰之浪樂이 不在於居處而必在於事務也니라.

The So Yang Individual's sorrow is capable of sagaciously conducting *Sa Mu*,[44] which signifies the ability to partake in public affairs. The So Yang Individual's emotion of calmness is not robust enough to continuously arrange *Ko Cho*, the ability to help and aid others close to them. The So Yang Individual's upward explosion of their *Jung* emotion of sadness results in the inability to conduct *Sa Mu* and leads to the inability to help others.[45] What is not found in *Sa Mu* can always be found in *Ko Cho*.[46]

The Tae Eum Individual's calmness is capable of establishing *Ko Cho*,[47] which signifies the ability to arrange one's household affairs. The Tae Eum Individual's emotion of sorrow is not robust enough to courageously spread *Sa Mu*.[48] The acute downward sinking of their *Jung* emotion of complacency leads to the inability to engage in *Ko Cho*.[49] What cannot be found in *Ko Cho* can always be found in *Sa Mu*.

---

42 If the So Eum Individual's strong *Jung* emotion is expressed in a balanced way, it adds to the quality of *Dang Yo*. If they lose control of this emotion, however, they will fail to carry out *Dang Yo* and destroy their health.

43 Because it is difficult to balance their *Jung* emotion, the So Eum Individual is often stuck in their own world (excessive joy) when engaging in *Kyo Uh*, which is balanced with anger (at one's own and others' faults), instead of joy. This results in the downward sinking of their joyful *Jung* nature, from being estranged by others.

44 *Sa Mu* correlates with the Virtue of wisdom. In other words, *Sa Mu* relies on the Virtue of wisdom for it to spread.

45 If the So Yang Individual's strong *Jung* emotion of anger is expressed in a balanced way, it adds to the quality of *Sa Mu*. If they lose control of this emotion, however, they will fail to carry out *Sa Mu*, causing self-inflicted emotional and physical injury.

46 Because it is difficult to balance their *Jung* emotion, the So Yang Individual often feels sorrow when engaging in *Ko Cho*, which is balanced with calmness, not sorrow. This results in the upward explosion of their sorrowful *Jung* nature due to a loss of balance and harmony within the home.

47 *Ko Cho* correlates with the Virtue of love. Hence, a deep sense of love is the foundation for carrying out one's household affairs.

48 If the Tae Eum Individual's strong *Jung* emotion of complacency is expressed in a balanced way, it adds to the quality of *Ko Cho*. If they lose control of this emotion, however, they will fail to carry out *Ko Cho*, causing self-inflicted emotional and physical injury.

49 Because it is difficult to balance their *Jung* emotion, the Tae Eum Individual often feels excessively complacent when engaging in *Sa Mu*, balanced with sorrow, not calmness. This results in the downward sinking of their complacent *Jung* nature due to a lack of accomplishment in public affairs.

**Table 3.2: Emotional balance and virtue**

| Balancing the *Jung* emotion of... | When in the process of... | Leads to the manifestation of the following virtue |
|---|---|---|
| Anger | *Kyo Uh* | *Ye* (humility) |
| Sorrow | *Sa Mu* | *Ji* (wisdom) |
| Excessive joy | *Dang Yo* | *Yi* (righteousness) |
| Complacency | *Ko Cho* | *In* (love) |

太陽之交遇는 可以怒로 治之이 黨與는 不可以怒로 治之也니
若遷怒於黨與則無益於黨與而肝傷也니라
少陰之黨與는 可以喜로 治之而交遇는 不可以喜로 治之也니
若遷喜於交遇則無益於交遇而脾傷也니라
少陽之事務는 可以哀로 治之而居處는 不可以哀로 治之也니
若遷哀於居處則無益於居處而腎傷也니라
太陰之居處는 可以樂으로 治之而事務는 不可以樂으로 治之也니
若遷樂於事務則無益於事務而肺傷也니라.

The Tae Yang Individual's *Kyo Uh* can be conducted with anger. *Dang Yo,* however, cannot be conducted with anger. If the Tae Yang Individual transfers their anger towards *Dang Yo,* then not only will they fail to obtain it, but they will also injure their weakest organ, the liver.

The So Eum Individual's *Dang Yo* can be conducted with joy. *Kyo Uh,* however, cannot be controlled by joy. If the So Eum Individual transfers their joy[50] towards *Kyo Uh,* then not only will they fail to obtain it, but they will also injure their weakest organ, the spleen.

The So Yang Individual's *Sa Mu* can be controlled by sorrow. *Ko Cho,* however, cannot be controlled by sorrow. If the So Yang Individual transfers their sorrow towards *Ko Cho,* then not only will they fail to obtain it, but they will also injure their weakest organ, the kidneys.

The Tae Eum Individual's *Ko Cho* can be controlled by complacency. *Sa Mu,* however, cannot be controlled by complacency. If the Tae Eum Individual transfers their complacency towards *Sa Mu,* then not only will they fail to obtain it, but they will also injure their weakest organ, the lungs.

---

50    Anger, according to Lee Je-ma, is a Yang emotion, while joy is a Yin emotion. These emotions oppose one another. Hence, joy is needed to help others feel comfortable (*Ko Cho*), but anger is needed to sift out the respectful vs. disrespectful qualities in others (*Kyo Uh*).

太陽之性氣는 恒欲進而不欲退하고 少陽之性氣는 恒欲擧而不欲措하고
太陰之性氣는 恒欲靜而不欲動하고 少陰之性氣는 恒欲處而不欲出이니라.

The *Song* nature of the Tae Yang Individual results in the constant desire to advance and aversion to retreat.[51] The *Song* nature of the So Yang Individual results in the constant desire to grip but aversion to release.[52] The *Song* nature of the Tae Eum Individual results in the constant desire for quiet and aversion to movement.[53] The *Song* nature of the So Eum Individual results in the desire to stay at home and aversion to going out.[54]

太陽之進이 量可而進也니 自反其材而不莊이면 不能進也니라
少陽之擧 量可而擧也니 自反其力而不固면 不能擧也니라
太陰之靜이 量可而靜也니 自反其知而不周면 不能靜也니라
少陰之處 量可而處也니 自反其謀而不弘이면 不能處也니라.

The Tae Yang Individual's desire to advance can only be carried out through skill and tactics.[55] Without sufficient skill and control of sheer force, there is no advancement.

The So Yang Individual's desire to grasp can only be carried out through sincere effort[56] and refraining from obstinacy. Without sincere effort and refraining from obstinacy, it will be impossible to maintain their grasp.

The Tae Eum Individual's desire for peace and quiet can only be carried out through wisdom[57] and control of selfish desire. Without sufficient wisdom and control of selfish desire, there is no peace and quiet.

The So Eum Individual's desire to dwell in a familiar setting[58] can only be carried out through consideration and planning. Without fulfilling their plan, the So Eum Individual cannot remain in a peaceful dwelling.

---

51  The *Song* nature of sorrow correlates with the Virtue of wisdom. Hence, the Tae Yang Individual constantly desires to advance and superimpose their knowledge when partaking in *Dang Yo*. While their diligence is noteworthy, there is always a time to advance and a time to retreat in *Dang Yo*.

52  The *Song* nature of anger correlates with the Virtue of humility. Hence, the So Yang Individual constantly desires to hold on to their image of humility when engaging in *Ko Cho*. They have trouble releasing this image despite the fact that security and comfort, rather than humility, is the basis for *Ko Cho*.

53  The *Song* nature of joy results in the constant desire for peace and quiet. Hence, the Tae Eum Individual always desires to carry out *Sa Mu* quietly and with the least action. While there is a place for quiet *Sa Mu*, there is also the need for activity and reform.

54  The *Song* nature of calmness results in the So Eum Individual's constant desire to remain in the comfort of home.

55  Skill and tactics correlate with *Jae Gan* (manners and skills), which, as mentioned in Chapter 1, resides in the lower back. Since the lower back is governed by the liver, the Tae Yang Individual's weakest organ, this ability does not come naturally.

56  This refers to the So Yang Individual's "effort" to remain calm by controlling their *Song* nature of anger when engaging in *Ko Cho*. The ability to remain calm correlates with *Bang Ryak* (strategic planning and tactics), which resides in the buttocks. Since the buttocks are governed by the kidneys, the So Yang Individual's weakest organ, this ability does not come naturally.

57  The reference to "wisdom" in this sentence is associated with the Tae Yang, rather than Tae Eum, constitution.

58  The desire to "dwell in a familiar setting" refers to the So Eum Individual's *Ko Cho* (knowing the appropriate place to reside) and correlates with *Bang Ryak* (strategic planning).

太陽之情氣는 恒欲爲雄而不欲爲雌하고 少陰之情氣는 恒欲爲雌而不欲
爲雄하고 少陽之情氣는 恒欲外勝而不欲內守하고 太陰之情氣는 恒欲內
守而不欲外勝이니라.

The Tae Yang Individual's *Jung* emotion is associated with the desire to be manly like a bull, and the dislike of being womanly like a doe.[59] The So Eum Individual's *Jung* emotion is associated with the desire to be womanly like a doe, and the dislike of being manly like a bull.[60]

The So Yang Individual's *Jung* emotion is associated with the desire to prevail outwardly and the dislike of focusing and cultivating themselves inwardly.[61] The Tae Eum Individual's *Jung* nature is associated with the desire to focus inwards, and the dislike of prevailing outwardly.[62]

太陽之人이 雖好爲雄이나 亦或宜雌니 若全好爲雄則放縱之心이 必過
也니라 少陰之人이 雖好爲雌나 亦或宜雄이니 若全好爲雌則偸逸之心이
必過也니라 少陽之人이 雖好外勝이나 亦宜內守니 若全好外勝則偏私之
心이 必過也니라 太陰之人이 雖好內守나 亦宜外勝이니 若全好內守則物
欲之心이 必過也니라.

Even though the Tae Yang Individual desires to be manly, they may occasionally desire to be womanly. If they desire only to be manly,[63] it would be impossible to control their desolate inclinations.

Even though the So Eum Individual desires to be womanly, they may occasionally desire to be manly. If they desire only to be womanly,[64] then it would be impossible to control their tendency to isolate themselves from others.

Even though the So Yang Individual desires to prevail outwardly, they may occasionally desire to cultivate themselves inwardly. If they desire only to prevail outwardly,[65] then it would be impossible to control their narrow-minded and conceited nature.

Even though the Tae Eum Individual desires focus inwards and to protect themselves, they may occasionally desire to prevail outwardly. If they desire only to

---

59  When sadness, the *Jung* emotion of the Tae Yang Individual, leads to sympathy and compassion, it enhances their health. If it results in anger, like that of a bull, it destroys their health.

60  When joy, the *Jung* emotion of the So Eum Individual, leads to social activity, it enhances their health. If it results in isolation and fear, like that of a doe, it destroys their health.

61  When sadness, the *Jung* emotion of the So Yang Individual, causes them to reflect, it enhances their health. If sadness causes them to avoid looking inwards, it destroys their health.

62  When calmness, the *Jung* emotion of the Tae Eum Individual, leads to giving comfort to others who are facing hard times, it enhances their health. If calmness results in laziness, it destroys their health.

63  "If they desire only to be manly" refers to the constant upward explosion of the Tae Yang Individual's angry *Jung* emotion.

64  "If they desire only to be womanly" refers to the constant downward sinking of the So Eum Individual's joyous *Jung* emotion.

65  "If they desire only to prevail outwardly" refers to the constant upward explosion of the So Yang Individual's *Jung* emotion of sorrow.

protect themselves and focus inwardly,[66] then it would be impossible to control their materialistic and indulgent nature.

**Table 3.3: Selfish tendencies and associated remedies**

| Sasang constitution | Selfish tendency | Remedy |
|---|---|---|
| Tae Yang | 放縱之心<br>Desolate, unruly, violent | Cultivating their feminine nature |
| So Eum | 逸之心<br>Secretive, reclusive | Cultivating their masculine nature |
| So Yang | 偏私之心<br>One-sided, stubborn | Looking inwards, self-reflection |
| Tae Eum | 物欲之心<br>Materialistic, lavish | Considering others, generosity |

太陽人이 雖至愚나 其性이 便便然猶延納也오 雖至不肖나 人之善惡을
亦知之也니라
少陽人이 雖至愚나 其性이 恢恢然猶式度也오 雖至不肖나 人之知愚를
亦知之也니라
太陰人이 雖至愚나 其性이 卓卓然猶敎誘也오 雖至不肖나 人之勤惰를
亦知之也니라
少陰人이 雖至愚나 其性이 坦坦然猶撫循也오 雖至不肖나 人之能否를
亦知之也니라

No matter how out of touch the Tae Yang Individual may become, they will always have the seed of tolerance and acceptance.[67] Even though they themselves may lack respect and piousness, they will always be aware[68] of whether or not others are good or bad.[69]

No matter how out of touch the So Yang Individual may become, they will always have the potential to embrace others far and wide, and be culturally adept.[70]

---

66  "If they desire only to focus inwardly" refers to the constant downward sinking of the Tae Eum Individual's complacent *Jung* emotion.

67  This "seed" is derived from the Tae Yang Individual's *Song* nature of sorrow and their innate Virtue of wisdom.

68  This ability is also derived from their Virtue of wisdom, which helps determine whether or not others are virtuous.

69  Despite their own shortcomings, each Sasang constitution has the capacity to determine the extent of others' moral behavior. This awareness may act in their favor as they choose to learn from others' shortcomings and become respectful and pious themselves, or it may cause their *Jung* nature to explode (or sink) when others do not treat them with respect.

70  "Culturally adept" refers to the So Yang Individual's profound ability to adapt to the times. This skill is the product of *Sei Wei*, their *Song* nature of anger, and their innate Virtue of humility.

Even though they themselves may lack respect and piousness, they will always be able[71] to determine who is wise and who is ignorant.

No matter how out of touch the Tae Eum Individual may become, they will always have a remarkable capacity to teach and entice others.[72] Even though they themselves may be lacking respect and piousness, they will always be able[73] to determine who is lazy and who is diligent.

No matter how out of touch the So Eum Individual may become, they will always have a calm and tranquil nature, which is capable of soothing and calming the mind of others.[74] Even though they themselves may lack respect and piousness, they will always be able[75] to determine who is capable or incapable.

太陽人은 謹於交遇故로 恒有交遇生疎人慮患之怒心하나니 此心은 出於秉彝之敬心也라 莫非至善而輕於黨與故로 每爲親熟黨與人所陷而偏怒 傷臟하나니 以其擇交之心이 不廣故也니라.

The Tae Yang Individual strongly values *Kyo Uh*,[76] and is overly concerned and easily angered when he or she thinks others are taking advantage of them. This is because the Tae Yang Individual strongly believes that others will practice fairness and humility [when engaging in *Kyo Uh*], yet it is impossible for them to find a perfectly fair person. The Tae Yang Individual is so preoccupied with *Kyo Uh* that he or she carelessly engages[77] in *Dang Yo*[78] and attempts to entrap others through intimacy, which is fed by selfish anger, resulting in damage to their liver. Hence the Tae Yang Individual has trouble keeping an open mind when choosing new friends.

71  This ability is also derived from their innate Virtue of humility. According to Confucian philosophy, humility forms a *Che* (internal, latent)/*Yong* (external, manifest) relationship with wisdom. Humility is the basis of wisdom, and wisdom is the basis for humility. Accordingly, those who are incapable of being humble are also considered ignorant and unwise.

72  This capacity is derived from the Tae Eum Individual's *Song* nature of joy and their innate Virtue of righteousness. Others are attracted to their joyous nature and righteous character.

73  This capacity is also derived from the Tae Eum Individual's innate Virtue of righteousness, which gives them the ability to determine whether or not action is based in sincerity. The unrighteous Tae Eum may criticize others for being lazy despite their own laziness.

74  The So Eum Individual's tranquility is derived from the So Eum Individual's *Song* nature of calmness and their innate Virtue of love.

75  This ability is also derived from the So Eum Individual's innate Virtue of love, which gives them the ability to differentiate between actions based in sincerity vs. selfishness.

76  In this context, *Kyo Uh* may be interpreted as "mutual respect and humility."

77  The Tae Yang Individual doesn't find value in conforming to group values and norms.

78  As mentioned earlier, *Dang Yo* correlates with the liver. The Tae Yang Individual's precarious engagement in *Dang Yo* leads to a weakened liver.

少陰人은 謹於黨與故로 恒有黨與親熟人擇交之喜心하나니 此心은 出
於秉彛之敬心也라 莫非至善而輕於交遇故로 每爲生疎交遇人所誣而偏
喜 傷臟하나니 以其慮患之心이 不周故也니라.

The So Eum Individual strongly values *Dang Yo*.[79] They single out and attempt to establish close relationships with [one or two] members of a group, which results in a feeling of joy.[80] The desire for intimacy is because the So Eum Individual strongly believes that others will feel the same way and automatically respect each other when engaging in *Dang Yo*, yet it is impossible for them to find a perfectly respectful person. The So Eum Individual is so focused on *Dang Yo* that he or she carelessly engages in *Kyo Uh*[81] and attempts to shut out those within the group who they are not close to. Seeking joy in this way causes injury to their spleen. The So Eum Individual's own actions are to blame because he or she doesn't take a well-rounded approach when considering friendships.

少陽人은 重於事務故로 恒有出外興事務之哀心하나니 此心은 出於秉
彛之敬心也라 莫非至善而不謹於居處故로 每爲主內做居處人所陷而偏
哀 傷臟하나니 以其重外而輕內故也니라.

The So Yang Individual strongly values *Sa Mu*,[82] yet they always feel saddened when leaving their home to carry out a mission. This sadness is because the So Yang Individual strongly believes that others should practice fairness when engaging in *Sa Mu*, yet it is impossible for them to find a perfectly respectful person. The So Yang Individual is so preoccupied with *Sa Mu* that he or she carelessly engages in *Ko Cho*[83] by endangering and leaving behind others who dwell at home—a result of extreme sadness that affects the health of their kidneys. The So Yang Individual's own actions are to blame because they think lightly of internal/household affairs while focusing primarily on external affairs.

---

79  In this context, *Dang Yo* refers to interaction with others who have similar interests and goals in mind. Unlike the Tae Eum Individual, who often finds comfort in the group setting, the So Eum Individual has a tendency to refine their *Dang Yo*, to the point of disregarding the needs of the group.

80  This can easily become an unbalanced feeling of joy, which is a result of excessive comfort, believing that an intimate friend will always be respectful and kind to them. In this case, the So Eum Individual will be lacking in consideration of their friend's feelings and refuse to reflect on their own role in the friendship.

81  *Kyo Uh* correlates with the spleen. The Tae Yang Individual's precarious engagement in *Kyo Uh* leads to a weakened spleen.

82  *Sa Mu*, in this context, refers to public affairs, goals, and tasks.

83  *Ko Cho*, in this context, refers to household or personal affairs and correlates with the kidneys. The Tae Yang Individual's precarious engagement in *Ko Cho* leads to weakened kidneys.

太陰人은 重於居處故로 恒有主內做居處之樂心하나니 此心은 出於秉彛
之敬心也라 莫非至善而不謹於事務故로 每爲出外與事務人所誑而偏樂이
傷臟하나니 以其重內而輕外故也니라.

The Tae Eum Individual strongly values *Ko Cho* because they feel extremely relaxed and complacent when engaging in internal/household affairs. They strongly believe that others should also practice fairness when engaging in *Ko Cho*, yet it is impossible for them to find a perfectly fair person to carry out these actions. The Tae Eum Individual is so focused on *Ko Cho* that he or she doesn't value *Sa Mu*,[84] and therefore attempts to entrap those who value external affairs. Seeking complacency in this way causes injury to their lungs. The Tae Eum Individual's own actions are to blame as they think lightly of external affairs while focusing primarily on internal/household affairs.

太陰之頷은 宜戒驕心이니 太陰之頷에 若無驕心이면 絶世之籌策이 必在
此也니라. 少陰之臆은 宜戒矜心이니 少陰之臆에 若無矜心이면 絶世之經
綸이 必在此也니라.

The Tae Eum Individual must practice caution against the tendency towards *Kyo Shim*,[85] residing in their chin.[86] If they rid themselves of *Kyo Shim*, then a profound sense of *Ju Chek*[87] will always manifest.

The So Eum Individual must practice caution against the tendency towards *Gung Shim*,[88] which resides in their chest.[89] If they rid themselves of *Gung Shim*, then a profound sense of *Kyung Ryun*[90] will always manifest.

---

84 The Tae Eum Individual values internal affairs (*Ko Cho*) more than external affairs (*Sa Mu*).

85 *Kyo Shim* (驕心) may be interpreted as "arrogance," "haughtiness," or "conceitedness."

86 The chin is located in the Upper *Jiao* and receives *Qi* (energy, life-force) from the lungs. Since the lungs are the weaker organ of the Tae Eum Individual, they have difficulty regulating and controlling *Kyo Shim*.

87 By regulating *Kyo Shim*, the Tae Eum Individual strengthens their Upper *Jiao* and lungs, hence increasing flow to the chin. Since the chin is also where *Ju Chek* resides, regulation of *Kyo Shim* will enable them to strategize and calculate profit from loss (*Ju Chek*).

88 *Gung Shim* (矜心) may be interpreted as "self-praise," "boasting," and "stinginess."

89 The chest is located in the Mid-Upper *Jiao* and receives *Qi* (energy, life-force) from the spleen. Since the spleen is the smallest organ of the So Eum Individual, it has difficulty regulating and controlling *Gung Shim*.

90 By regulating *Gung Shim*, the So Eum Individual strengthens their Mid-Upper *Jiao* and spleen, hence increasing flow to the chest. Since the chest is also where *Kyung Ryun* resides, *Gung Shim* regulation enables them to govern and administrate affairs through intuition and wisdom (*Kyung Ryun*).

太陽之臍는 宜戒伐心이니 太陽之臍에 若無伐心이면 絶世之行檢이 必在
此也니라. 少陽之腹은 宜戒夸心이니 少陽之腹에 若無夸心이면 絶世之度
量이 必在此也니라.

The Tae Yang Individual must practice caution against the tendency towards *Bol Shim*,[91] which resides in the umbilicus.[92] If they rid themselves of *Bol Shim*, then a profound sense of *Heng Gom*[93] will always manifest.

The So Yang Individual must practice caution against *Gwa Shim*,[94] which resides in their lower abdomen.[95] If they rid themselves of *Gwa Shim*, then a profound sense of *Do Ryang*[96] will always manifest.

少陰之頭는 宜戒奪心이니 少陰之頭에 若無奪心이면 大人之識見이 必在
此也니라 太陰之肩은 宜戒侈心이니 太陰之肩에 若無侈心이면 大人之威
儀 必在此也니라

The So Eum Individual must practice caution against the tendency towards *Tal Shim*,[97] which resides in the head.[98] If they rid themselves of *Tal Shim*, then they are able to manifest *Shik Kyun*,[99] equivalent to that of a *Dae In*.[100]

---

91  *Bol Shim* (伐心) may be interpreted as "violence," "ruthlessness," and "cruelty."

92  The umbilicus is located in the Mid-Lower *Jiao* and receives *Qi* (energy, life-force) from the liver. Since the liver is the smallest organ of the Tae Yang Individual, it has difficulty regulating and controlling *Bol Shim*.

93  By regulating *Bol Shim*, the Tae Yang Individual strengthens their Mid-Lower *Jiao* and liver, hence increasing flow to the umbilicus. Since the umbilicus is also where *Heng Gom* resides, regulating *Bol Shim* enables them to reflect on their actions and decipher between what is morally right and wrong (*Heng Gom*).

94  *Gwa Shim* (夸心) may be interpreted as "self-conceit," "extravagance," and "rudeness."

95  The lower abdomen is located in the Lower *Jiao* and receives *Qi* (energy, life-force) from the kidneys. Since the kidneys are the weakest organ of the So Yang Individual, they have difficulty regulating and controlling *Gwa Shim*.

96  By regulating *Gwa Shim*, the So Yang Individual strengthens their Lower *Jiao* and kidneys, hence increasing flow to the lower abdomen. Since the lower abdomen is also where *Do Ryang* resides, regulating *Gwa Shim* enables them to embrace and tolerate others through the Virtue of love (*Do Ryang*).

97  *Tal Shim* (奪心), the "desire to take from others," is also referred to as *Chon Shim* (擅心), the desire to deprive others of virtue.

98  As mentioned in Chapter 1, *Chon Shim* (擅心) lurks within the head, which correlates with the Upper *Jiao* and lungs. Recall how the So Yang Individual's *Jung* emotion and the Tae Yang Individual's *Song* nature of sadness also correlate with the lungs and are hence prone to *Chon Shim*. In this section, Lee Je-ma illustrates how *Chon Shim* (expressed here as *Tal Shim*) isn't only limited to the Yang constitutions, but all other Sasang constitutions, to some degree, may be prone. Since the So Eum Individual, for example, has a weaker Upper *Jiao* and lacks in Yang energy, he/she must guard against the inclination towards *Chon Shim*. Note how both a lack of Yang energy, as in the case of the Yin constitutions, and an excess of Yang energy, as in the case of the Yang constitutions, both may lead to *Chon Shim*.

99  By regulating *Tal Shim*, the So Eum Individual strengthens their Upper *Jiao* and lungs, hence increasing flow to the head. Since the head is also where *Shik Kyun* resides, the So Eum is therefore able to maximize their ability to know the right time to take action (*Shik Kyun*).

100  The *Dae In* (大人), or "magnificent one," is a title used in Asian philosophy to describe an individual who has attained the highest level of virtue through utmost sincerity in self-cultivation.

The Tae Eum Individual must practice caution against the tendency towards *Chi Shim*,[101] residing in their shoulders.[102] If they rid themselves of *Chi Shim*, then it is possible to manifest *Wi Eui*,[103] equivalent to that of a *Dae In*.

少陽之腰는 宜戒懶心이니 少陽之腰에 若無懶心이면 大人之材幹이 必在 此也니라. 太陽之臀은 宜戒竊心이니 太陽之臀에 若無竊心이면 大人之方 略이 必在此也니라.

The So Yang Individual must practice caution against the tendency towards *Na Shim*,[104] which resides in the lower back.[105] If they rid themselves of *Na Shim*, then they are able to manifest *Jae Gan*,[106] equivalent to that of a *Dae In*.

The Tae Yang Individual must practice caution against *Jul Shim*,[107] residing in their buttocks.[108] If they rid themselves of *Jul Shim*, then it is possible to manifest *Bang Ryak*,[109] equivalent to that of a *Dae In*.

---

101  *Chi Shim* (侈心) may be interpreted as "extravagance" or "immoderation."

102  *Chi Shim* lurks within the shoulders, correlated with the Upper *Jiao* and spleen. Recall how the Tae Yang Individual's *Jung* emotion and the So Yang Individual's *Song* nature of anger also correlate with the spleen and are prone to *Chi Shim*. In this section, Lee Je-ma illustrates how *Chi Shim* isn't limited only to the Yang constitutions, but all other Sasang constitutions, to some degree, may be prone. Since the Tae Eum Individual, for example, has a weaker Upper and Mid-Upper *Jiao* and lacks in Yang energy, they must guard against the inclination towards *Chi Shim*. Note how both a lack of Yang energy, as in the case of the Yin constitutions, and an excess of Yang energy, as in the case of the Yang constitutions, both may lead to *Chi Shim*.

103  By regulating *Chi Shim*, the Tae Eum Individual strengthens their Mid-Upper *Jiao* and spleen, hence increasing flow to the shoulders. Since the chest is also where *Wi Eui* resides, the Tae Eum Individual is therefore able to maximize their ability to show respect towards others and manifest dignity (*Wi Eui*).

104  *Na Shim* (懶心) may be interpreted as "laziness," "lassitude," or "lack of volition."

105  *Na Shim* lurks within the lower back, correlated with the Mid-Lower *Jiao* and the liver. Recall how the So Eum Individual's *Jung* emotion and the Tae Eum Individual's *Song* nature of joy also correlate with the liver and are prone to *Na Shim*. In this section, Lee Je-ma illustrates how *Na Shim* isn't limited only to the Yin constitutions, but all other Sasang constitutions, to some degree, may be prone. Since the So Yang Individual has a weaker Mid-Lower *Jiao* and lacks in Yin energy, they must guard against the inclination towards *Na Shim*. Note how both a lack of Yin energy, as in the case of the So Yang Individual, and an excess of Yin energy, as in the case of the So Eum Individual, both may lead to *Na Shim*.

106  By regulating *Na Shim*, the So Yang Individual strengthens their Mid-Lower *Jiao* and liver, hence increasing flow to the lower back. Since the lower back is also where *Jae Gan* resides, the So Yang Individual is therefore able to maximize their skills and manners (*Jae Gan*).

107  *Jul Shim* (竊心) may be interpreted as "the desire to steal from others" or "selfishness."

108  *Jul Shim* lurks within the buttocks, which correlates with the Lower *Jiao* and the kidneys. Recall how the Tae Eum Individual's *Jung* emotion and the So Eum Individual's *Song* nature of complacency/calmness also correlate with the kidneys and are prone to *Jul Shim*. In this section, Lee Je-ma illustrates how *Jul Shim* isn't limited only to the Yin constitutions, but all other Sasang constitutions, to some degree, may be prone. Since the Tae Yang Individual, for example, has a weaker Lower *Jiao* and lacks in Yin energy, they must guard against the inclination towards *Jul Shim*. Note how both a lack of Yin energy, as in the case of the Yang constitutions, and an excess of Yin energy, as in the case of the Yin constitutions, may lead to *Jul Shim*.

109  By regulating *Jul Shim*, the Tae Yang Individual strengthens their Lower *Jiao* and kidneys, hence increasing flow to the buttocks. Since the buttocks are also where *Bang Ryak* resides, the Tae Yang Individual is therefore able to maximize their strategic planning and tactics (*Bang Ryak*).

Chapter 4 ——————————————————————

# The *Zhang Fu* Organs[1]

肺部位는 在頷下背上하고 胃脘部位는 在頷下胸上故로 背上胸上以上은
謂之上焦오 脾部位는 在脊하고 胃部位는 在膈故로 脊膈之間을 謂之中
上焦오 肝部位는 在腰하고 小腸部位는 在臍故로 腰臍之間을 謂之中下
焦오 腎部位는 在腰脊下하고 大腸部位는 在臍腹下故로 脊臍下以下를
謂之下焦라.

The lungs are located between the cervical spine and thoracic spine. The esophagus
is located below the chin and above the chest. The Upper *Jiao* includes everything
above the chest and mid-spine.

The spleen is located in the thoracic-spine area. The stomach is located
in the diaphragmic area. The area between the thoracic-spine and diaphragm is
called the Mid-Upper *Jiao*.

The liver is located in the lumbar-spine area and the small intestine is located in
the umbilical area. The area between the lumbar-spine and the umbilicus is referred
to as the Mid-Lower *Jiao*.

The kidneys are located in the sacral area and the large intestines are located in
the lower abdomen area (below the umbilicus). The area between the sacrum and
below the umbilicus is referred to as the Lower *Jiao*.[2]

---

1   The *Zhang* (臟) organs are associated with Yin and are referred to as solid organs. The *Fu* (腑) organs are
    associated with Yang and are referred to as hollow organs. Chinese medicine denotes a total of five Yin *Zhang*
    organs (lungs, spleen, liver, kidneys, and heart) and six Yang *Fu* organs (large intestine, stomach, Gall bladder,
    Urinary bladder, small intestine, and Triple Burner). Sasang medicine describes four Yin *Zhang* organs (lungs,
    spleen, liver, and kidneys) and four Yang *Fu* pairs (esophagus, stomach, small intestine, and large intestine).

2   In the above paragraph, Lee Je-ma describes the metaphysical location of the lungs, spleen, liver, and kidneys.
    This isn't the precise anatomical location. Instead it describes the location of each organ based on its energetic
    function.

水穀이 自胃脘而入于胃하고 自胃而入于小腸하고 自小腸而入于大
腸하고 自大腸而出于肛門者 水穀之都數 停畜於胃而薰蒸爲熱氣하고 消
導於小腸而平淡爲凉氣니熱氣之輕淸者 上升於胃脘而爲溫氣하고 凉氣之
質重者 下降於大腸而爲寒氣니라.

*Su Gok*[3] travels from the esophagus to the stomach. It then travels from the stomach to the small intestine, and then from the small intestine to the anus. From the anus it exits the body. *Su Gok* also accumulates in the stomach and undergoes fermentation, which results in heat energy. *Su Gok* is then sent to the small intestine, which guides and purifies food with its Cool nature. Lighter, clearer, and warmer energy from *Su Gok* is then sent from the small intestine upwards to the esophagus, where it is transformed into Warm energy. Heavier, turbid, and cooler *Su Gok*-related substances are sent from the small intestine to the large intestine where they transform into Cold energy.

胃脘이 通於口鼻故로 水穀之氣 上升也오 大腸이 通於肛門故로 水穀之
氣 下降也오胃之體 廣大而包容故로 水穀之氣 停畜也오
小腸之體 狹窄而屈曲故로 水穀之氣 消導也니라.

The esophagus is connected with the mouth and nose and sends the [clear] *Su Gok* energy upwards.

The large intestine is connected with the anus and sends [turbid] *Su Gok* energy downwards.

The structure of the stomach is wide and embracing, which allows for the accumulation of *Su Gok* energy.

The structure of the small intestine is narrow and curved, which helps guide *Su Gok* energy.

**Table 4.1: Relationship between the Sasang *Fu*[4] organs and *Su Gok***

| Body part | Temperature | Function | Movement |
|---|---|---|---|
| Esophagus | Warm energy | Sends heavier *Su Gok* to stomach and lighter *Su Gok* upwards | Pivotal |
| Stomach | Hot energy | Carries out fermentation and sends *Su Gok* to small intestine | Inwards and downward |
| Small intestine | Cool energy | Sends warmer/pure *Su Gok* to esophagus and cooler/turbid *Su Gok* to the large intestine | Pivotal |
| Large intestine | Cold energy | Sends *Su Gok* downward to the anus | Downward |

3    The term *Su Gok* contains the characters for water (水) and grain (穀). Lee Je-ma utilizes this as a general term to describe ingested food and drink. *Su Gok* is either emitted from the body via the anus or transformed into energy within the small intestine and rises upwards.

4    In Sasang medicine, there are four major *Fu* organs: the esophagus, stomach, small intestine, and large intestine.

水穀溫氣 自胃脘而化津하야 入于舌下하야 爲津海니 津海者는 津之所舍
也라 津海之淸氣 出于耳而爲神하고 入于頭腦而爲膩海니 膩海者는 神之
所舍也라 膩海之膩汁淸者 內歸于肺하고 濁滓 外歸于皮毛故로 胃脘與舌
耳頭腦皮毛는 皆肺之黨也니라.

Warm-natured food gets transformed into *Jin*[5] inside of the esophagus, which then enters the sublingual area to form *Jin Hei*,[6] the place where *Jin* accumulates.

The pure *Jin* fluids then travel to the ear and are transformed into *Shin*[7] (spirit), which proceed to the brain to form *Ni Hei*,[8] the place where *Shin* resides.

The pure fluids[9] of *Ni Hei* then travel to the lungs and the turbid *Ni Hei* fluids travel outwards to [nourish and produce] the skin and hair. The lung group[10] encompasses the esophagus, tongue, ears, skin, and hair.

水穀熱氣 自胃而化膏하야 入于ᄀ間兩乳하야 爲膏海니 膏海者는 膏之所
舍也라 膏海之淸氣 出于目而爲氣하고 入于背膂而爲膜海니 膜海者는 氣
之所舍也라 膜海之膜汁淸者 內歸于脾하고 濁滓 外歸于筋故로 胃與兩乳
目背膂筋은 皆脾之黨也니라.

Hot-natured food gets transformed into *Go*[11] inside of the stomach. It then enters the area between the breasts to form the *Go Hei*,[12] the place where *Go* accumulates.

The pure *Go Hei* fluids then travel to the eyes and are transformed into the *Gi*.[13] The *Gi* then travels to the upper spine to form the *Mak Hei*,[14] the place where the *Gi* resides.

The pure fluids of the *Mak Hei* then travel internally to the spleen and the turbid *Mak Hei* fluids travel outwards to the tendons. The stomach, breasts, eyes, upper spine, and tendons all correlate with the spleen group.[15]

---

5   *Jin* (津) is the term for bodily fluid produced in the Upper *Jiao*. The *Jin* fluids have a lower density than the fluids of the other *Jiao*. As energy and fluids descend within the body, they get thicker.

6   *Jin Hei* (津海) is interpreted as the "Sea of *Jin*," or the "place where *Jin* accumulates." Since Sasang medicine is based on metaphysical energetic principles, the reference to organ and fluid isn't to be correlated directly with anatomy. A loose correlation, however, can be made between each metaphysical and physical correspondence. The *Jin* fluids, for example, can be loosely correlated with saliva, since both are in charge of initiating the process of digestion in the upper body and have a lighter consistency compared to the fluids of the Mid-Upper *Jiao*, Mid-Lower *Jiao*, and Lower *Jiao*.

7   *Shin* (神) is defined as "spirit," which resides in the brain in the form of *Ni Hei*.

8   *Ni Hei* (膩海) is defined as the "Sea of *Ni*," or the "place where the spirit resides." In Sasang medicine it is equated with the human brain.

9   This is a translation of the character *Jup* (汁), which can be interpreted as "juice," "sap," "extract," or "soup." Lee Je-ma considered the brain to be of soup-like consistency.

10  The lung group or *Pei Ji Dang* (肺之黨) is another term for the Upper *Jiao*, which is controlled by the lungs.

11  *Go* (膏) is the Mid-Upper *Jiao* bodily fluid. It is thicker than *Jin* but lighter than *Yu*.

12  *Go Hei* (膏海) is interpreted as the "Sea of *Go*," or the "place where the *Go* resides." In Sasang medicine it is equated with the stomach.

13  *Gi* (氣), pronounced in Chinese as "Qi," is defined as "energy" or "life-force."

14  *Mak Hei* (膜海) is defined as the "Sea of *Mak*."

15  The spleen group or *Bi Ji Dang* (脾之黨) is another term for the Mid-Upper *Jiao*, which is controlled by the spleen.

水穀凉氣 自小腸而化油하야 入于臍하야 爲油海니 油海者는 油之所舍
也라
油海之淸氣 出于鼻而爲血하고 入于腰脊而爲血海니 血海者는
血之所舍也라 血海之血汁淸者 內歸于肝하고 濁滓 外歸于肉故로 小腸與
臍鼻腰脊肉은 皆肝之黨也니라

Cool-natured food gets transformed into *Yu*[16] inside of the small intestine. From there *Yu* enters the umbilical area to form the *Yu Hei*,[17] the place where *Yu* accumulates.

The pure *Yu Hei* fluids then travel to the nose and are transformed into the blood, which travels on to the lower spine to form the *Hyul Hei*,[18] the place where the blood resides.

The pure fluids of the *Hyul Hei* then travel internally to the liver and the turbid *Hyul Hei* fluids travel outwards to the muscles. The small intestine, umbilicus, nose, and lower back all correlate with the liver group.[19]

水穀寒氣 自大腸而化液하야 入于前陰毛際之內하야 爲液海니 液海者는
液之所舍也라 液海之淸氣 出于口而爲精하고 入于膀胱而爲精海니 精海
者는 精之所舍也라 精海之精汁淸者 內歸于腎하고 濁滓 外歸于骨故로
大腸與前陰口膀胱骨은 皆腎之黨也니라.

Cold-natured food gets transformed into *Ek*[20] inside of the large intestine. It then enters the area covered by pubic hair to form the *Ek Hei*,[21] the place where *Ek* accumulates.

The pure *Ek Hei* fluids travel on to the mouth and are transformed into the essence. The essence then travels to the bladder to form the *Jung Hei*,[22] the place where the essence resides.

The pure fluids of the *Jung Hei* then travel internally to the kidney and the turbid *Jung Hei* fluids travel outwards to the bones. The large intestine, reproductive organs, mouth, and urinary bladder all correlate with the kidney group.[23]

---

16    *Yu* (油) is the Mid-Lower *Jiao* bodily fluid. It is thicker than *Go* but lighter than *Ek*.

17    *Yu Hei* (油海) is defined as the "Sea of *Yu*," or the "place where *Yu* resides." In Sasang medicine it is equated with the small intestine.

18    *Hyul Hei* (血海) is defined as the "Sea of *Hyul*," or the "place where *blood* is stored."

19    The liver group or *Gan Ji Dang* (肝之黨) is another term for the Mid-Lower *Jiao*, which is controlled by the liver.

20    *Ek* (液) is the Lower *Jiao* bodily fluid. It is thicker than *Jin*, *Go*, and *Yu* fluids.

21    *Ek Hei* (液海) is defined as the "Sea of *Ek*," or the "place where *Ek* resides." In Sasang medicine it is equated with the large intestine.

22    *Jung Hei* (精海) is defined as the "Sea of *Jung*," or the "place where *essence* is stored." It is equated with the urinary bladder.

23    The kidney group or *Shin Ji Dang* (腎之黨) is another term for the Lower *Jiao*, which is controlled by the kidneys.

**Table 4.2: The transformation of *Su Gok***

| *Fu* organ | From *Su Gok* it produces... | Then is sent to the... | Pure energy goes to the... | Then to the... | Pure energy goes to the... | Turbid energy goes to the... |
|---|---|---|---|---|---|---|
| Esophagus | *Jin* (via Warm energy) | Sublingual area (*Jin Hei*) | Ear where it becomes *Shin* | Brain (*Ni Hei*) | Lungs | Skin, hair |
| Stomach | *Go* (via Hot energy) | Chest (*Go Hei*) | Eyes where it becomes *Gi* | Upper spine (*Mak Hei*) | Spleen | Tendons |
| Small intestine | *Yu* (via Cool energy) | Umbilicus (*Yu Hei*) | Nose where it becomes *Hyul* | Lower spine (*Hyul Hei*) | Small intestine | Muscles |
| Large intestine | *Ek* (via Cold energy) | Pubic area (*Ek Hei*) | Mouth where it becomes *Jung* | bladder (*Jung Hei*) | Large intestine | Bones |

**Table 4.3: The organ groups and their associations**

| Organ | Associated anatomy |
|---|---|
| lung group | esophagus, tongue, ears, skin, hair |
| spleen group | stomach, breasts, eyes, upper spine, tendons |
| liver group | Small intestine, umbilicus, nose, lower spine, muscles |
| kidney group | Large intestine, reproductive organs, mouth, urinary bladder |

耳는 以廣博天時之聽力으로 提出津海之淸氣하야 充滿於上焦하야
爲神而注之頭腦하야 爲膩하야 積累爲膩海하고
目은 以廣博世會之視力으로 提出膏海之淸氣하야 充滿於中上焦하야
爲氣而注之背脊하야 爲膜하야 積累爲膜海하고

The power of the ears enables us to hear the far-reaching[24] sound of *Chon Shi*. This power also encourages the release of pure *Jin Hei* energy, which fills the Upper *Jiao* and then becomes the *Shin*. The pure energy of *Shin* then pours into the brain and is transformed into *Ni*. The accumulation of *Ni* eventually becomes the *Ni Hei*.

The power of the eyes enables them to see the far-reaching sights of *Sei Wei*. This power also encourages the release of pure *Go Hei* energy, which fills the Mid-Upper *Jiao*, becoming *Gi*. The pure energy of *Gi* then flows into the upper spine and is transformed into *Mak*. The accumulation of *Mak* fluids eventually becomes the *Mak Hei*.

---

24    "Far-reaching" refers to the influence of Heavenly Affairs, or *Chon Ki*.

鼻는 以廣博人倫之嗅力으로 提出油海之淸氣하야 充滿於中下焦하야
爲血而注之腰脊하야 爲凝血하야 積累爲血海하고
口는 以廣博地方之味力으로 提出液海之淸氣하야 充滿於下焦하야
爲精而注之膀胱하야 爲凝精하야 積累爲精海니라.

The power of the nose enables it to smell the far-reaching scent of *In Ryun*. This power also encourages the release of pure *Yu Hei* energy, which fills the Mid-Lower *Jiao* and then transforms into *Hyul*. The pure energy of *Hyul* then pours into the lower spine and is further transformed into blood. The accumulation of blood eventually becomes the *Hyul Hei*.

The power of the mouth enables it to experience the far-reaching taste of *Ji Bang*. This power also encourages the release of pure *Ek Hei* energy, which fills the Lower *Jiao* and then transforms into *Jung*. The pure energy of *Jung* travels on to the urinary bladder and is further transformed into essence. The accumulation of essence eventually becomes the *Jung Hei*.

肺는 以鍊達事務之哀力으로 吸得膩海之淸汁하야 入于肺하야
以滋肺元而內以擁護津海하야 鼓動其氣하야 凝聚其津하고
脾는 以鍊達交遇之怒力으로 吸得膜海之淸汁하야 入于脾하야
以滋脾元而內以擁護膏海하야 鼓動其氣하야 凝聚其膏하고
肝은 以鍊達黨與之喜力으로 吸得血海之淸汁하야 入于肝하야
以滋肝元而內以擁護油海하야 鼓動其氣하야 凝聚其油하고
腎은 以鍊達居處之樂力으로 吸得精海之淸汁하야 入于腎하야
以滋腎元而內以擁護液海하야 鼓動其氣하야 凝聚其液이니라.

With the strength of sorrow, associated with *Sa Mu*, the lungs absorb pure fluids from *Ni Hei*. After absorption, the pure fluids from the *Ni Hei* enter the lungs, nourish their essence, and protect the *Jin Hei*. The pure *Ni Hei* fluids also condense and gather the *Jin* fluids.[25]

With the strength of anger, associated with *Kyo Uh*, the spleen absorbs pure fluids from *Mak Hei*. After absorption, the pure fluids from *Mak Hei* enter the spleen, nourish its essence, and protect the *Go Hei*. The pure *Mak Hei* fluids also condense and gather the *Go* fluids.

With the strength of joy, associated with *Dang Yo*, the liver absorbs pure fluids from *Hyul Hei*. After absorption, the pure fluids from the *Hyul Hei* enter the liver, nourish its essence, and protect the *Yu Hei*. The pure *Hyul Hei* fluids also condense and gather the *Yu* fluids.

With the strength of calmness, associated with *Ko Cho*, the kidneys absorb pure fluids from the *Jung Hei*. After absorption, the pure fluids from the *Jung Hei* enter

---

25   Notice how in the previous section *Jin* becomes *Ni*. In this section, *Ni* condenses, gathers, and protects *Jin*. Hence, *Jin* and *Ni* have a reciprocal, mutually supportive, relationship. This relationship is also carried out between *Go* and *Mak*, *Yu* and *Hyul*, and *Ek* and *Jung*.

the kidneys, nourish their essence, and protect the *Ek Hei*. The pure *Jung Hei* fluids also condense and gather the *Ek* fluids.

**Table 4.4: The influence of Human Affairs on the bodily fluids**

| These organs… | Utilize these temperaments… | Associated with this Human Affair… | To absorb pure fluids from… | In order to nourish their essence and protect… |
|---|---|---|---|---|
| Lungs | Sorrow | *Sa Mu* | *Ni Hei* | *Jin Hei* |
| Spleen | Anger | *Kyo Uh* | *Mak Hei* | *Go Hei* |
| Liver | Joy | *Dang Yo* | *Hyul Hei* | *Yu Hei* |
| Kidneys | Calmness | *Ko Cho* | *Jung Hei* | *Ek Hei* |

津海之濁滓則胃脘이 以上升之力으로 取其濁滓而以補益胃脘하고
膏海之濁滓則胃 以停畜之力으로 取其濁滓而以補益胃하고
油海之濁滓則小腸이 以消導之力으로 取其濁滓而以補益小腸하고
液海之濁滓則大腸이 以下降之力으로 取其濁滓而以補益大腸이니라.

The energy of the esophagus rises upwards to acquire the leftover turbid *Jin* fluids. Once acquired, these fluids serve to protect the esophagus.

The energy of the stomach stores and accumulates the leftover turbid *Go* fluids. Once acquired, these fluids serve to protect the stomach.

The energy of the small intestine directs and guides the leftover turbid *Yu* fluids. Once acquired, these fluids serve to protect the small intestine.

The energy of the large intestine descends and releases the leftover turbid *Ek* fluids. Once acquired, these fluids serve to protect the large intestine.

膩海之濁滓則頭 以直伸之力으로 鍛鍊之而成皮毛하고
膜海之濁滓則手 以能收之力으로 鍛鍊之而成筋하고
血海之濁滓則腰 以寬放之力으로 鍛鍊之而成肉하고
精海之濁滓則足 以屈强之力으로 鍛鍊之而成骨이니라.

The head has a natural ability to stay upright and stretched outwards. This ability facilitates the transformation of turbid *Ni Hei* fluids into skin and hair.

The hands have the natural ability to gather and collect. This ability facilitates the transformation of turbid *Mak Hei* fluids into the tendons.

The lower back has the natural ability to stretch and release. This ability is what facilitates the transformation of turbid *Hyul Hei* fluids into the muscles.

The legs have the natural ability to extend and flex. This ability facilitates the transformation of turbid *Jung Hei* fluids into the bones.

是故로 耳必遠聽하며 目必大視하며 鼻必廣嗅하며 口必深味니
耳目鼻口之用이 深遠廣大則精神氣血이 生也오 淺近狹小則精神氣血이
耗也니라. 肺必善學하고 脾必善問하고 肝必善思하고 腎必善辨이니
肺脾肝腎之用이 正直中和則津液膏油 充也오 偏倚過不及則津液膏油 爍
也니라.

Accordingly, it is necessary for the ears to hear sounds from afar, the eyes to see from a distance, the nose to be sensitive to distant scents, and the mouth to have an acute sense of taste. The acute ability to hear, see, smell, and taste gives rise to the *Jung*, *Shin*, *Gi*, and *Hyul*. If the above senses lose this capability, then *Jung*, *Shin*, *Gi*, and *Hyul* will dissipate and waste away. It is also necessary for the lungs to contribute to studying, the spleen to contribute to inquiry, the liver to contribute to deep thought, and the kidneys to help with distinction. If the lungs, spleen, liver, and kidneys function in harmony, then the *Jin*, *Ek*, *Go*, and *Yu* fluids will flourish. If the above organs become biased, deficient, or excessive, then the *Jin*, *Ek*, *Go*, and *Yu* fluids will perish.[26]

**Table 4.5: Sense and organ influence on the bodily fluids**

| Acuity of this sense | Gives rise to and preserves… | Organ | Natural ability… | Gives rise to and preserves… |
|---|---|---|---|---|
| Hearing | *Shin* | lungs | Study | *Jin* |
| Sight | *Gi* | spleen | Inquiry | *Go* |
| Smell | *Hyul* | liver | Deep thought | *Yu* |
| Taste | *Jung* | kidney | Distinction | *Ek* |

膩海여 藏神하고 膜海여 藏靈하고 血海여 藏魂하고 精海여 藏魄이니라.
津海여 藏意하고 膏海여 藏慮하고 油海여 藏操하고 液海여 藏志니라.

The *Sea of Ni* stores the *Shin* (consciousness), the *Sea of Mak* stores the *Yong* (subconscious), the *Sea of Hyul* stores the *Hun* (ethereal aspect of the mind), the *Sea of Jung* stores the *Baek* (material aspect of the mind).

---

26 Recall how the senses are the closest connection with heaven. If these senses are impaired, then the connection with heaven will also weaken, resulting in the wasting away of *Jung*, *Shin*, *Gi*, and *Hyul*. Also, note that the organs are the closest connection in the body to the senses. If the organ energy is impure, then the connection with heaven through the senses also gets muddied, further impairing the *Fu* organ (esophagus, stomach, small intestine, large intestine) function of producing *Jin*, *Ek*, *Go*, and *Yu*.

The *Sea of Jin* gives rise to *Yi* (justification), the *Sea of Go* gives rise to *Ryuh* (consideration), the *Sea of Yu* gives rise to *Jo* (conduct), the *Sea of Ek* gives rise to *Ji* (willpower).[27]

**Table 4.6: The eight components of the mind**

| Component | Chinese character | Definition |
|---|---|---|
| *Shin* | 神 | Conscious, inspiration, emotion, insight |
| *Yong* | 靈 | Subconscious, deep-seated emotion |
| *Hon* | 魂 | Immaterial, spiritual, vision, creativity |
| *Baek* | 魄 | Material, focus, concrete, physical |
| *Yi* | 意 | Intention, distinction, integrity, righteousness |
| *Ryuh* | 慮 | Consideration, thinking, study, modesty |
| *Jo* | 操 | Conduct, control, gather, handle |
| *Ji* | 志 | Willpower, drive, meaning, memory |

頭腦之膩海는 肺之根本也오 背膂之膜海는 脾之根本也오
腰脊之血海는 肝之根本也오 膀胱之精海는 腎之根本也니라.

The *Sea of Ni*, located within the brain, forms the lungs. The *Sea of Mak*, located within the upper spine, forms the spleen. The *Sea of Hyul*, located within the lower back, forms the liver. The *Sea of Jung*, located within the urinary bladder, forms the kidneys.

舌之津海는 耳之根本也오 乳之膏海는 目之根本也오
臍之油海는 鼻之根本也오 前陰之液海는 口之根本也니라.

The *Sea of Jin*, located under the tongue, forms the ears. The *Sea of Go*, located within the chest, forms the eyes. The *Sea of Yu*, which surrounds the umbilical area, forms the nose. The *Sea of Ek*, located within the reproductive area, forms the mouth.

---

27   Each component of the mind is intricately connected, forming a *Che* (internal)/*Yong* (external) relationship. The *Shin* (神) refers primarily to present emotional and conscious feelings, while the *Yong* (靈) is associated with deep underlying, often non-expressed, emotions. The *Yong* (靈), in this case, is *Che* (internal), while the *Shin* is the *Yong* (external) aspect. The *Baek* (魄) is associated with the material aspect of the body, and is the *Yong* (external) aspect of the *Hon* (魂), which is associated with the immaterial aspect of the body. The *Baek* is bound by concrete possession and accomplishment, while the *Hon* is constantly trying to free itself from the material. The *Hon* is activated when we are asleep to promote the process of dreaming, whereas the *Baek* is activated when we are conscious and awake. Upon death, the *Baek* returns to the earth, while the *Hon* dissipates upwards towards the heavens. The *Baek* is also referred to as the "material spirit," while the *Hon* is also referred to as the "ethereal/immaterial spirit." The *Yi* and *Ryuh* components also form a *Che*/*Yong* relationship. The virtuous "intention" of *Yi* forms the foundation (*Che*) of *Ryuh* "consideration," its outward manifestation, or *Yong*. Finally, it is necessary to "gather" and "collect" one's energy via the *Jo* component in order to manifest the "willpower" and "drive" of the *Ji* spirit. Hence, *Jo* is considered the *Che* aspect of *Ji*.

心이 爲一身之主宰하야 負隅背心하고 正向┌中하야 光明瑩澈하야
耳目鼻口 無所不察하며 肺脾肝腎이 無所不忖하며 頷臆臍腹이 無所不
誠하며 頭手腰足이 無所不敬이니라.

The heart is located in the center of the chest directly between both breasts. From such a prominent location, it shines clearly and brightly, presiding over the entire body. It provides the four senses with the boundless ability to govern; the Four *Zhang* Organs with the unlimited ability to calculate and decipher; the chin, chest, umbilical area, and lower abdomen with immeasurable sincerity; and the head, hands, lower back, and feet with infinite respect and reverence.

## Chapter 5

# The Basic Principles of Medicine[1]

醫
源
論

書에 曰若藥이 不瞑眩이면 厥疾이 不瘳라하니 商高宗時에 已有瞑眩藥
驗而高宗이 至於稱歎則醫藥經驗이 其來已久於神農黃帝之時라하니 其
說은 可信於眞也而本草 素問이 出於神農黃帝之手라하니 其說은 不可信
於眞也라. 何以言之오 神農黃帝時에는 文字가 應無하야 後世文字로 澆
漓例法故也니라.

It was once written that if the consumption of medicine doesn't result in dizziness
or cause loss of consciousness, then it cannot cure illness. During the Shang
Dynasty there were numerous herbs that could elicit this effect in patients, and
doctors valued this quality. Since this theory goes back further than the *Shennong
Bencaojing*[2] and *Huang Di Neijing*,[3] the average person accepts it without question.
However, it is difficult to subscribe to the *Ben Cao Lun* and *Su Wen*-based idea that
the above theory was inscribed directly from Shen Nong and Huang Di. This is
because written language was not yet developed during the age of Shen Nong and
Huang Di. It wasn't until much later that a simple form of undeveloped written
language was utilized.

---

1   The title of this chapter is a combination of the character *Eui* (醫), which translates as medicine, doctor, and
    healing, and *Won* (源), which means basis, principle, and foundation.

2   The *Shennong Bencaojing* (神農本草經), or *The Classic of Herbal Medicine*, is credited with the work of
    Shennong, translated as the "God of Agriculture," who supposedly lived around 2800 BC. While the original
    text doesn't exist, it was said to consist of three volumes with 365 herbal remedies and their specific functions.
    It is likely that this text was a compilation of medical knowledge from approximately 300 BC to 200 AD.

3   The *Huang Di Neijing* (黃帝內經), or *Yellow Emperor's Inner Canon*, consists of a question-and-answer
    conversation between the legendary Emperor Huang Di and his minister, pen named Qi Bo. This text, which
    is said to have been written over 2000 years ago, is the compilation of two parts, the *Su Wen* (素問, *Simple
    Questions*) and the *Ling Shu* (靈樞, *Spiritual Pivot*), each containing 81 chapters.

衰周秦漢以來로 扁鵲이 有名而張仲景이 具備得之하야 始爲成家著
書하니 醫道가 始興하고 張仲景以後에 南北朝隋唐醫가 繼之而至于
宋하야 朱肱이 具備得之하야 著活人書하니 醫道中興하니 朱肱以後에
元醫李杲 王好古 朱震亨 危亦林이 繼之하고 而至于明하야 李梴 龔信이
具備得之하고 許浚이 具備傳之하야 著東醫寶鑑하니 醫道復興하니라.

The book entitled *Bian Que Nan Jing*[4] was well known from the last part of the Zhou Dynasty through the Qin and Han Dynasties. This book was discovered by Zhang Zhongjing,[5] a distinguished physician and medical author who played a significant role in developing [Eastern] medicine. After he passed away, doctors of the Southern and Northern (420–581), Sui (581–618), and Tang (618–907) Dynasties followed in his footsteps. Zhu Gong[6] of the Song Dynasty (960–1279) expanded on previous teachings in his text entitled *Huoren Shu*. During the Yuan Dynasty (1279–1369) Doctors Li Gao,[7] Wang Hao Gu,[8] Zhu Zhenheng,[9] and Wei Yilin[10] also followed

---

4     The *Bian Que Nan Jing* (扁┌難經) was written by the earliest known physician in China, Bian Que (died in 310 BC). He was said to have started out as a hostel staff member who received supernatural powers as a gift from an elderly man in return for his kind attendance. Bian Que eventually became well known throughout China after warning the Emperor of his eminent disease. The Emperor didn't heed his warning and died soon afterwards.

5     Zhang Zhongjing (150–219 AD) authored the *Shang Han Lun* (傷寒論), a text that Lee Je-ma refers to throughout the remainder of this book. In this treatise, he classified illness into six stages of pathogenic influence: Tai Yang, Yang Ming, Shao Yang, Tai Yin, Shao Yin, and Jue Yin. The title and compilation of this treatise was provided by his disciple Wang Shu He, who divided the original *Shang Han Lun* into two books: *Shang Han Lun* and *Jin Gui Yao Lue* (金匱要略). The *Jin Gui Yao Lue*, also authored by Zhang Zhongjing, covers diseases not mentioned in the *Shang Han Lun*, such as lung diseases, edema, diabetes, *Bi* syndrome, Summer Heat, stroke, and gynecological issues. The above title was given by his disciple Wang Shu He.

6     Zhu Gong was a famous physician and scholar of the *Shang Han Lun* School. His treatise entitled *Huoren Shu* (活人書, *Revive the People*), written in 1112 AD, contains 100 questions and answers regarding the contents of the *Shang Han Lun*. His purpose was to offer a practical approach to utilizing the principles of the *Shang Han Lun*. Zhu Gong believed that it was necessary to immerse oneself in the study of channel theory in order to understand the pathogenesis of disease.

7     Li Gao (1279–1368), also known as Li Dongyuan, author of the *Pi Wei Lun* (脾胃論, *Treatise on the stomach and spleen*), claimed that all illness is derived from imbalances of the stomach and spleen. The formula entitled *Bu Zhong Yi Qi Yang* is just one example of several well-known prescriptions born from this treatise. Li Gao introduced the concept of *Yin Fire*, which results from spleen deficiency and its inability to ascend clear fluids and descend turbid fluids. The accumulation of fluids in the lower body causes heat rebellion in the upper body, leading to *Yin Fire*.

8     Wang Hao Gu (1200–1264), a disciple of Li Gao, was known for his view on Yin patterns, that they are much more challenging to diagnosis and treatment compared to Yang patterns.

9     Zhu Zhenheng (1281–1358), also known as Master Zhu Danxi, is known for his emphasis on balancing *Minister Fire*, or vital force originating from within the kidneys, by preserving the body's Yin component and preventing the tendency towards excessive Yang accumulation, which results from inappropriate diet and overindulgence of sexual intercourse. He authored the text entitled *Bencao Yanyi Buyi* (本草衍義補遺, *Supplement and Expansion of Materia Medica*).

10     Although Lee Je-ma equates Wei Yilin (1277–1347) with the *Shang Han Lun* School, he is perhaps best known for authoring the text entitled *Shiyi Dexiaofang* (世醫得效方), in which he described treatments for bone fractures and introduced joint-adjustment techniques. He was also known to use herbal anesthetics during his orthopedic surgical procedures.

this legacy. Doctors Li Chan[11] and Gong Xin[12] of the Ming Dynasty (1368–1644) also expanded on previous teachings. Afterwards, medicine continued to advance with the help of Heo Jun[13] and the *Dongeui Bogam*.[14]

蓋自神農黃帝以後 秦漢以前은 病證藥理를 張仲景이 傳之하고
魏晋以後 隋唐以前은 病證藥理를 朱肱이 傳之하고
宋元以後 明以前은 病證藥理를 李梴 龔信 許浚이 傳之하니
若以醫家의 勤勞功業을 論之則當以張仲景 朱肱 許浚으로 爲首而李梴 龔
信이 次之니라.

Zhang Zhongjing was the most influential doctor from the time of Shen Nong and Huang Di to the dynasties of Qin and Han in regard to his knowledge of disease and herbal treatment. Zhu Gong was the most influential doctor from the Wei and Qin to the Sui and Tang Dynasties in regard to his knowledge of disease and herbal treatment. Li Chan, Gong Xin, and Hou Jun were the most influential doctors from the Song and Yuan to the Ming Dynasties for their knowledge of disease and herbal treatment. If we were to weigh the merit of their contribution to medicine, doctors Zhang Zhongjing, Zhu Gong, and Hou Jun would stand out above the rest, with the work of doctors Li Chan and Gong Xin immediately following in order of reverence.

本草는 自神農黃帝以來로 數千年世間流來經驗而神農時에 有本草하고
殷時에 有湯液本草하고 唐時에 有孟詵食療本草 陳藏器本草拾遺하고
宋時에 有龐安常本草補遺와 日華子本草하고 元時에 有王好古湯液本
草니라.

The *Shennong Bencaojing* and *Huang Di Neijing* were the product of accumulated experience from thousands of years since the time of Shen Nong. The *Tangye*

---

11  Li Chan was a doctor of the Ming Dynasty who wrote the *Yixue Rumen* (醫學入門, *Introduction to Medicine*). He strongly believed that a deep understanding of medicine could only be achieved after a thorough study of Confucian teachings. This unprecedented perspective was later shared by Lee Je-ma, who broke away from the common belief that Daoist, rather than Confucian, principles are of primary significance in Oriental medicine.

12  Gong Xin, author of *Gujin Yijian* (古今醫鑑, *Newly Amended Mirror of Ancient and Modern Medicine*), was a famous doctor of the Ming Dynasty who with his son, Gong Tingxian, served as a physician in the Imperial Medical Academy. His son wrote other well-known texts such as the *Manbing Huichun* (萬病回春, *Restoration of Health from Myriad Diseases*).

13  Heo Jun (1539–1615) was a Korean medical doctor and author of the *Dongeui Bogam* (東醫寶鑑). He was born the son of a mistress who was destined to be nothing other than a societal outcast. Yet his incredible sincerity and interest in medicine led him to eventually become the king's personal physician.

14  The *Dongeui Bogam* (東醫寶鑑), or *Mirror of Eastern Medicine*, authored by Heo Jun (1539–1615), consists of five chapters, which describe the physiology, etiology, and treatment strategy for numerous diseases, based on both Korean and Chinese medical teachings. (See the Introduction for more information about the *Dongeui Bogam*.)

*Bencao*[15] was made available during the Yin Dynasty. During the Tang Dynasty, Meng Shen (621–713 AD) authored the book entitled *Cang Liao Ben Cao*,[16] and Chen Zhang Qi (687–757 AD) wrote the *Supplementation to the Ben Cao Shi Yi*.[17] During the Song Dynasty, Pang An Jiao (1042–1099 AD) composed the *Ben Cao Bu Yi*[18] and Ri Hua Zi authored the *Ri Hua Zi Ben Cao*.[19] During the Yuan Dynasty, Wang Hao Gu composed a revised version of the *Tangye Bencao*, and entitled it *Wang Hao Gu Tangye Bencao*.[20]

少陰人病證藥理를 張仲景이 庶幾乎昭詳發明而宋元明諸醫家 盡乎昭詳
發明하고 少陽人病證藥理를 張仲景이 半乎昭詳發明而宋元明諸醫家 庶
幾乎昭詳發明하고 太陰人病證藥理를 張仲景이 略得影子而宋元明諸
醫家 太半乎昭詳發明하고 太陽人病證藥理를 朱震亨이 略得影子而本
草에 略有藥理니라

Most of the treatment methods and medicinal principles of the So Eum Individual were covered in detail by Zhang Zhongjing. The remaining methods and principles were introduced during the Song and Yuan Dynasties.

Only half of the treatment methods and medicinal principles of the So Yang Individual were covered in detail by Zhang Zhongjing. The other half was introduced during the Song and Yuan Dynasties.

15    The original *Tangye Bencao* (湯液本草), or *Materia Medica of Decoctions*, was written during the Shang Dynasty (1766–1122 BC; also known as the Yin Dynasty). There are no surviving records of this text.

16    The *Cang Liao Ben Cao* (食療本草), or *Food-Based Materia Medica*, is a two-volume text written by Meng Shen of the Tang Dynasty. This book focuses on the use of common foods for treating illness. The original text has been lost with the exception of two remaining sections contained in the *Leizheng Bencao* (類證本草), or *Materia Medica of Combined Syndromes*.

17    The *Ben Cao Shi Yi* (本草拾遺), or *Supplementation to the Materia Medica*, written by Chen Zhang Qi of the Tang Dynasty, includes several herbal ingredients that were left out of previous medical texts and ten major formulae, each containing two herbs, which he researched during his clinical practice. Remedies include the use of Tong Cao (*Medulla Tetrapanacis*) and Fang Ji (*Radix Aristolochia*) for moving stagnant *Qi*, cow meat and Ren Shen (*Radix Ginseng*) for *Qi* deficiency, and Ma Huang (*Herba Ephedrae*) and Ge Gen (*Radix Puerariae*) for channel excess.

18    The text entitled *Ben Cao Bu Yi* (本草補遺), or *Additional Supplementation to the Materia Medica*, was written by Pang An Jiao of the Song Dynasty. It contains herbal prescriptions for tumors, Cold-induced toxins, and seasonally related Warm Febrile disease.

19    The text entitled *Ri Hua Zi Ben Cao* (日華子本草), or *Ri Hua Zi's Materia Medica*, contains in 20 chapters detailed descriptions, classification, and practical application of 600 different herbs. Most of this book has not survived the test of time.

20    The text entitled *Wang Hao Gu Tangye Bencao* (王好古湯液本草), or *Wang Hao Gu's Materia Medica of Decoctions*, written by Wang Hao Gu in 1298, is a revised version of the Shang Dynasty's *Tangye Bencao*, and is commonly referred to by the same title. In this text, he emphasizes the use of tonic herbs instead of purgatives during the later stage of febrile disease. His focus was on supporting the body rather than harshly attacking disease.

The Tae Eum Individual's treatment methods and medicinal principles were only roughly delineated by Zhang Zhongjing. During the Song and Yuan Dynasties these became far more advanced.

The Tae Yang Individual's treatment methods and medicinal principles were only briefly contained in Zhu Zhenheng's text entitled *Bencao Yanyi Buyi*.

余가 生於醫藥經驗이 五千載後하야 因前人之述하야 偶得四象人臟腑性理하야 著得一書하니 名曰壽世保元이라 原書中에 張仲景所論太陽病少陽病陽明病太陰病少陰病厥陰病은 以病證名目而論之오 余가 所論太陽人少陽人太陰人少陰人은 以人物名目而論之也니 二者를 不可混看이오 又不可厭煩然後에 可以探其根株而採其枝葉也라 若夫脈法者는 執證之一端也니 其理는 在於浮沈遲數而不必究其奇妙之致也오 三陰三陽者는 辨證之同異也니 其理는 在於腹背表裏而不必究其經絡之變也니라.

It was through immense fortune that after 5–6000 years of medical history, and the knowledge brought to us from doctors of the past, that I was able to decipher the physiology and organ-based principles of Sasang Constitutional Medicine. [In honor of this discovery] I decided to write the current text entitled *Dongeui Susei Bowon*.

It was the writings of Zhang Zhongjing that brought to life the terms Tai Yang, Shao Yang, Yang Ming, Tai Yin, Shao Yin, and Jue Yin in relation to the progression of illness. I was the first to associate Tai Yang, Shao Yang, Tai Yin, and Shao Yin[21] with the four constitution types. It is important not to confuse the above two approaches [even though they utilize the same titles]. Only after a thorough investigation can they be clearly differentiated. This distinction can be compared to differentiating the leaves from the branches of a tree.

As far as pulse diagnosis is concerned, it is only necessary to focus on superficial, deep, slow, and fast rates. It is not necessary to delve into the other obscure pulse patterns. The use of the Three Yin and Three Yang method[22] is a way to differentiate between the various types of illness. Yet when it comes to the location of illness, it is not necessary to decipher which channel is affected, but instead, where it is

---

21   The terms Tai Yang, Shao Yang, Tai Yin, and Shao Yin (in Chinese) are pronounced Tae Yang, So Yang, Tae Eum, and So Eum, respectively, in the Korean language. Lee Je-ma refers to the latter pronunciation elsewhere in this text.

22   In this sentence, Lee Je-ma refers to the Six Stages of Illness outlined in the *Shang Han Lun*: Tai Yang, Shao Yang, Yang Ming, Tai Yin, Shao Yin, and Jue Yin. The Six Stages of Illness also correlate with the Six *Zhang* (the Five Major *Zhang* with Pericardium added) and Six *Fu* Organs and their respective meridians, whereas Tai Yang correlates with the small intestine and Urinary bladder, Shao Yang with the Triple Burner and the Gall bladder, Yang Ming with the large intestine and stomach, Tai Yin with the lungs and spleen, Shao Yin with the heart and kidneys, and Jue Yin with the Pericardium and liver.

presented along four major aspects of the body: the abdomen, spine,[23] exterior, and interior.[24]

古人이 以六經陰陽으로 論病인 故로 張仲景이 著傷寒論에 亦以六經陰
陽으로 該證證而 以頭痛 身疼 發熱 惡寒 脈浮者로 謂之太陽病證이라
하고 以口苦 咽乾 目眩 耳聾 胸脇滿 寒熱往來 頭痛 發熱 脈弦細者로 謂
之少陽病證이라 하고 以不惡寒 反惡熱 汗自出 大便秘者로謂之陽明病
證이라 하고 以腹滿 時痛 口不燥 心不煩而自利者로謂之太陰病證이라
하고 以脈微細 但欲寐 口燥 心煩而自利者로 謂之少陰病證이라 하고 以
初無腹痛 自利等證而傷寒六七日 脈微緩 手足厥冷 舌卷 囊縮者로 謂之
厥陰病證이라 하니

In ancient times, doctors utilized the Six Channel and Yin/Yang theories to classify illness. Zhang Zhongjing also used this approach in his book, the *Shang Han Lun*, which correlates Tai Yang illness with the occurrence of head and body aches, chills and fever, and a superficial pulse. It also associates Shao Yang illness with a bitter taste, thirst, dryness of the throat, dizziness, tinnitus, flank pain, alternate fever and chills, and a wiry and narrow pulse. Yang Ming illness is characterized by no occurrence of chills but an increase in fever, spontaneous sweating, and dry stools. Fullness of the stomach with occasional abdominal pain, no occurrence of thirst or unsettled feeling in the chest, and uncontrollable diarrhea is referred to as Tai Yin illness. Shao Yin illness is associated with a minute pulse, fatigue, a constant desire to sleep, an unsettled/anxious feeling in the chest, thirst, and uncontrollable diarrhea. The absence of stomach pain and uncontrollable diarrhea after six to seven days of Shang Han illness with a slow and minute pulse, cold extremities, and stiffness of the tongue and contraction of the scrotum is referred to as a Jue Yin illness.

---

23 The *Bok* (腹), or abdomen, and *Bei* (背), or spine, correlate with the anterior and posterior aspects of the body. As mentioned in Chapter 1, the four major aspects of the anterior body are the chin, chest, umbilicus, and abdomen. Lee Je-ma collectively describes them here as *Bok*. The four major posterior aspects of the body are the cervical, thoracic, lumbar, and sacral spine, collectively referred to as *Bei*. Each of the four major anterior and posterior aspects correlate with the Four Temperaments of sorrow, anger, joy, and calmness. Hence the anterior/posterior location of imbalance within the body will depend on the manifestation of the Four Temperaments. Recall that each constitution will have different temperamental inclinations, causing various levels of imbalance in each of the above areas of the body.

24 External (表) and internal (裏) illness manifest differently according to the constitution type. As mentioned in Chapter 2, each body type has a different *Song* (性) nature and *Jung* (情) emotion. Imbalance of the *Song* nature will lead to external disorders, and imbalance of the *Jung* emotion will lead to internal disorders. Heat and Cold also affect each constitution differently. External disorders of the Tae Yang and So Eum Individuals correlate with Heat-induced syndromes, and internal disorders correlate with Cold-induced syndromes. External disorders of the Tae Eum and So Yang Individuals correlate with Cold-induced syndromes, and internal disorders with Heat-induced syndromes.

六條病證中에 三陰病證은 皆少陰人病證也오 少陽病證은 即少陽人病證也오 太陽病證과 陽明病證은 則少陽人少陰人太陰人 病證에 均有之而少陰人病證에 居多也니라.古昔以來로 醫藥法方이 流行世間하야 經歷累驗者를 仲景이 採撫而著述之하니 蓋古之醫師가 不知心之愛惡所欲과 喜怒哀樂偏着者爲病而但知 脾胃水穀 風寒暑濕 觸犯者爲病인 故로 其論病論藥全局이 都自少陰人 脾胃水穀中出來而少陽人 胃熱證藥이 間成有焉하고 至於太陰人太陽人病情則全昧也니라.

Out of the above six types of sickness, the three Yin stages are associated with the So Eum constitution. The Shao Yang illness only applies to the So Yang constitution. For the most part, the Tai Yang and Yang Ming sicknesses apply evenly to the So Yang, So Eum, and Tae Eum constitutions. However, the So Eum constitution is affected by these disorders slightly more often than the other types.

The *Shang Han Lun* is the product of accumulated experience from ancient Oriental medical doctors, and is a modification of the well-read ancient text entitled *Yi Yao Fa Fang*.[25] Most doctors of the past didn't consider that when emotions such as love, hate, selfishness, joy, anger, sadness, and cheerfulness are over-expressed, they could contribute to the onset of illness. On the contrary, they assumed that the onset of illness was due to digestive disorders, Wind, Cold, Heat, and/or Dampness. Therefore, most of the ancient medical discoveries were based on the deficient spleen and stomach of the So Eum constitution and the occasional formula to treat stomach Heat of the So Yang constitution. There is no trace of treatment theory for the Tae Eum and Tae Yang Individuals' illness.

岐伯이 曰傷寒一日에 巨陽이 受之인 故로 頭項痛 腰脊强이오 二日에 陽明이 受之하니 陽明은 主肉이라 其脈이 挾鼻絡於目인 故로 身熱 目疼而鼻乾 不得臥也오 三日에 少陽이 受之하니 少陽은 主膽이라 其脈이 循脇絡於耳인 故로 胸脇痛而耳聾하나니 三陽經絡이 皆受其病而未入於臟인 故로 可汗而已오 四日에 太陰이 受之하니 太陰脈은 布胃中絡於嗌인 故로 腹滿而嗌乾이오 五日에 少陰이 受之하니 少陰脈은 貫腎絡於肺 繫舌本인 故로 口燥 舌乾而渴이오 六日에 厥陰이 受之하니 厥陰脈은 循陰器而絡於肝인 故로 煩滿而囊縮하나니 三陰三陽 五臟六腑가 皆受病하야 榮衛不行하며 五臟이 不通則死矣니라.

Qi Bo stated that the first stage of Shang Han influence is referred to as Tai Yang, marked by a sore throat, headache, and achiness of the lower back and spine. The second stage of Shang Han influence is referred to as Yang Ming, which primarily

---

25   The *Yi Yao Fa Fang* (醫藥法方) is a text that supposedly formed the basis of Zhang Zhongjing's Shang Han theory and the medicinal principles of ancient China. There are no surviving records of its content or scope.

affects the skin and muscles. The Yang Ming meridian[26] flows from the sides of the nose to the eyes. Hence this stage is marked by fever, eye pain, dryness of the nasal passages, and insomnia. The third stage of Shang Han illness is referred to as Shao Yang. This stage of illness primarily affects the Gall bladder. The Shao Yang meridian[27] flows from the flanks to the ears. Hence this stage is marked by chest/flank pain and tinnitus. Even if all of the three Yang channels are affected, the illness is still considered to be external and not affecting the internal organs. In the Yang stages, the body will sweat in order to release the illness.

The fourth stage of Shang Han influence is referred to as Tai Yin. The Tai Yin meridian[28] travels from the stomach to the throat. Hence this stage is marked by stomach fullness and a dry throat. The fifth stage of Shang Han influence is referred to as Shao Yin. The Shao Yin meridian[29] travels from the kidney to the lungs, and then to the tongue. This stage is marked by dryness of the tongue and mouth with thirst. The sixth stage of Shang Han influence is referred to as Jue Yin. The Jue Yin meridian[30] travels from the reproductive organs to the liver. This stage is thus marked by an unsettled and anxious feeling in the chest and contraction of the scrotum. If the *Three Yin* and *Three Yang*[31] are all influenced by Shang Han, then the blood will have trouble circulating and the organs will lack communication, leading to imminent death.

---

26 The Yang Ming meridian refers to the path of energy, or *Qi* (氣), that begins from the large intestine, travels through the neck, and to the face. It is also referred to as the Hand Yang Ming meridian. The Foot Yang Ming meridian starts from the stomach, flows down the lateral anterior leg, and to the second toe.

27 The Shao Yang meridian refers to the path of energy, or *Qi* (氣), that begins from the Gall bladder, travels through the flank, and to the ears. It is also referred to as the Foot Shao Yang meridian. The Hand Shao Yang meridian correlates with the *San Jiao* (Triple Burner). It starts from the lateral aspect of the fourth finger, flows up the posterior aspect of the arm, and to the ear.

28 The Tai Yin meridian refers to the path of energy, or *Qi* (氣), that begins from the spleen, travels through the medial aspect of the leg, and to the first toe. It is also referred to as the Foot Tai Yin meridian. The Hand Tai Yin meridian starts from the lungs, travels through the medial aspect of the arm, and to the thumb.

29 The Shao Yin meridian refers to the path of energy, or *Qi* (氣), that begins from the kidney, travels through the medial aspect of the leg, and to the center of the sole. It is also referred to as the Foot Shao Yin meridian. The Hand Shao Yin meridian starts from the heart, travels through the axillary, down the medial aspect of the arm, and to the fifth finger.

30 The Jue Yin meridian refers to the path of energy, or *Qi* (氣), that begins from the liver, travels through the medial aspect of the leg, and to the first toe. It is also referred to as the Foot Jue Yin meridian. The Hand Jue Yin meridian starts from the pericardium, travels down the medial aspect of the arm, and to the third finger.

31 The *Three Yin* and the *Three Yang* refer to the six stages of Shang Han illness: Tai Yang, Yang Ming, Shao Yang, Tai Yin, Shao Yin, and Jue Yin.

兩感於寒者는 必不免於死니 兩感寒者는 一日에 巨陽과 少陽이 俱病
則頭痛 口乾而煩滿하고 二日에 陽明과 太陰이 俱病則腹滿 身熱 不飮
食 譫語하고 三日에 少陽과 厥陰이 俱病則耳聾 囊縮而厥하고 水漿不入
口하며 不知人하며 六日에 死니 其死는 皆以六七日之間이오 其愈는 皆
以十日已上이니라.

If all of the Yin and Yang channels are affected by Shang Han illness, then the possibility of death cannot be escaped. In this case, both the Tai Yang and the Shao Yin stages will be affected on the first day of Shang Han attack. This situation is marked by headaches, thirst, and an unsettled and anxious feeling in the chest. The second day of onset is marked by the concurrence of the Yang Ming and Tai Yin stages. This situation will be marked by fullness of the stomach, fever, inability to ingest food, and incoherent speech. The third day of onset is marked by the concurrence of the Shao Yang and Jue Yin stages. This situation is marked by deafness, contraction of the scrotum, coldness of the hands and feet, the inability to drink plain water or rice milk, and loss of consciousness. Death will likely occur after six days in this situation. [In general, if all six stages are affected, then] it will take six to seven days to die. Recovery will take ten or more days.

論曰靈樞素問에 假托黃帝하야 異怪幻惑하니 無足稱道나 方術好事者之
言이 容或如是니 不必深責也니라 然이나 此書에 亦是古人之經驗而五臟
六腑와 經絡鍼法과 病證修養之辨이 多有所啓發則實是醫家格致之宗主
而苗脈之所自出也니 不可全數其虛誕之罪而廢其啓發之功也니라 蓋此
書는 亦古之聰慧博物之言과 方士淵源修養之述也니 其理를 有可考而其
說을 不可盡信이니라.

In my opinion, the *Ling Shu*[32] and *Su Wen*[33] were falsely credited with the words of Emperor Huang Di. Yet just because it is not his writing doesn't automatically refute its authenticity.[34] The *Ling Shu* and *Su Wen* are products of our ancestors' accumulated knowledge regarding the Five *Zhang* and the Six *Fu* Organs, channel theory, acupuncture, disease pathology, and self-cultivation, and reopened the door to extensive ancient wisdom. The *Ling Shu* and *Su Wen* are rooted in the common knowledge of ages past and the teaching of shamans [who inscribe fortune tablets,

---

32  The *Ling Shu* (靈樞), also known as the *Spiritual Pivot* or *Divine Pivot*, along with the *Su Wen*, are credited with being the most ancient, and often most revered, texts in Oriental medicine, which date back to the first century BC. The *Ling Shu* and *Su Wen* each consist of 12 scrolls and 81 chapters in a question-and-answer format, based on a conversation between Emperor Huang Di and his personal physician/minister Qi Bo. The contents of the *Ling Shu* have a spiritual and esoteric focus, and the *Su Wen* contains precise acupuncture prescriptions for particular diseases based on Yin Yang and Five Elemental Theory.

33  The *Su Wen* (素問) is also known as *The Yellow Emperor's Classic*, or *Huang Di Neijing* (黃帝內經).

34  Lee Je-ma, along with most other modern historians and scholars, hold that the *Ling Shu* and *Su Wen* are works of numerous authors who credited their authorship with Emperor Huang Di. This perspective reflects the idea that doctors and scholars of ancient China were more interested in contributing their knowledge than receiving individual recognition.

incantations, and herbs in the treatment of illness]. With this in mind, it is not necessary to over-criticize or take for granted these teachings. In fact, the *Ling Shu* and *Su Wen* can be likened to a bud from which the core of Oriental medical study emerged [throughout the ages]. With this in mind, I do not find it appropriate to cold-heartedly deny the merit of the above teachings.

岐伯所論에 巨陽가 少陽과 少陰經病은 皆少陽人病也오 陽明과 太陰經病은 皆太陰人病也오 厥陰經病은 少陰人病이니라.

The Tai Yang, Shao Yang, and Shao Yin stages described by Qi Bo correlate with illness of the So Yang constitution. The Yang Ming and Tai Yin stages correlate with the illness of the Tae Eum Individual, and the Jue Yin stage with the illness of the So Eum Individual.

# Part II

# CLINICAL APPLICATION

Chapter 6 ————————————

# The So Eum Individual's Illness

少
陰
人
論

## Section 1
## The So Eum Individual's Kidney Heat Causing Exterior Heat Syndrome[1]
## 少陰人腎受熱表熱病

張仲景 傷寒論에 曰發熱 惡寒 脈浮者는 屬表하니 卽太陽證也ㅣ니라.
太陽傷風은 脈이 陽浮而陰弱하니 陽浮者는 熱自發이오 陰弱者는 汗自
出이니 嗇嗇惡寒하며 淅淅惡風하다가 翕翕發熱하며 鼻鳴乾嘔하니
桂枝湯을 主之니라.

According to Zhang Zhongjing, chills, fever, and a superficial radial pulse indicate Tai Yang stage illness. The superficial pulse of Tai Yang *Shang Feng* syndrome indicates floating Yang and deficient Yin. Floating Yang will lead to symptoms of fever, while Yin weakness results in spontaneous sweating. If there are frequent chills, an aversion to Cold and/or Wind, hot flashes, audible nasal breathing, and dry heaves, then *Gui Zhi Tang* (Cinnamon Twig Decoction) should be prescribed.

---

1    The Exterior syndrome of each of the four Sasang constitutions isn't to be correlated directly with Exterior disorders mentioned in the *Shang Han Lun*, such as Tai Yang illness. Rather, the So Eum Individual has four major stages of Exterior illness: (a) Tai Yang, (b) Tai Yang/Jue Yin, (c) Yang Ming, and (d) Jue Yin. Keep in mind that external disorders of the So Eum Individual originate from the inability to regulate and harmonize their *Song* nature of calmness and The desire to protect/comfort nobody other than oneself, which affects the flow of kidney energy and causes external vulnerability. Internal disorders, on the contrary, originate from the sinking of the So Eum Individual's *Jung* nature of joy, affecting the stomach and causing internal weakness. Also worthy of note is that Exterior syndromes are not necessarily less threatening than Interior syndromes, as suggested in the *Shang Han Lun*. The onset of sweating during the common cold of a Tai Yang stage illness of the So Eum Individual, for example, is already the first stage of *Mang Yang* syndrome, a life-threatening situation involving Yang depletion.

危亦林 得效方에 曰四時瘟疫에는 當用香蘇散이니라. 龔信 醫鑑에 曰傷
寒 頭痛 身疼 不分表裏證에는 當用藿香正氣散이니라.

In the *De Xiao Fang*,[2] Wei Yilin mentions the use of *Xiang Su San* (Cyperus and Perilla Leaf Powder) for four seasonal epidemic disorders. In the *Gujin Yijian*,[3] Gong Xin states that *Huo Xiang Zheng Qi San* (Agastache Powder to Rectify the Qi) can be used for Shang Han disorders, which are difficult to classify as Interior or Exterior, and are marked by headaches and aching of the entire body.

論曰張仲景所論에 太陽傷風에 發熱惡寒者는 即少陰人 腎受熱 表熱病
也니 此證에 發熱 惡寒而無汗者는 當用桂枝湯 川芎桂枝湯 香蘇散 芎歸
香蘇散 藿香正氣散이오 發熱惡寒而有汗者는 此는 亡陽初證也니 必不可
輕易視之하고 先用黃芪桂枝湯 補中益氣湯 升陽益氣湯 三日連服而汗不
止 病不愈則當用桂枝附子湯

From my perspective, the Tai Yang *Shang Feng* syndrome described by Zhang Zhongjing, marked by spontaneous fever and chills, is nothing other than the So Eum Individual's *kidney Heat causing Exterior Heat* syndrome. In this case, if there is no sweating then *Gui Zhi Tang* (Cinnamon Twig Decoction), *Cheongung Gyeji Tang* (Lee Je-ma's Lovage Root and Cinnamon Twig Decoction), *Xiang Su San* (Cyperus and Perilla Leaf Powder), *Gunggwi Hyangsu San* (Lee Je-ma's Cyperus and Perilla Leaf Powder with Lovage and Angelica Root), and *Gwakhyang Jeonggi San* (Lee Je-ma's Agastache Powder to Rectify the Qi) can be used. If sweating is present in the above situation, caution should be practiced since it indicates the first stage of *Mang Yang* (Yang Collapse). In this case, *Huanggi Gyeji Tang* (Lee Je-ma's Cinnamon Twig Astralagus and Aconite Decoction), *Bochung Ikgi Tang* (Lee Je-ma's Tonify the Middle and Augment the Qi Decoction), or *Seungyang Ikgi Tang* (Lee Je-ma's Raise the Yang and Benefit the Qi Decoction) can be prescribed. If after taking these formulae sweating is still present and the other symptoms do not improve, then *Gyeji Buja Tang* (Lee Je-ma's Cinnamon Twig and Prepared Aconite Decoction), *In Sam Gyeji Buja Tang* (Lee Je-ma's Ginseng, Cinnamon Twig, and Aconite Decoction), and *Seungyang Ikgi Buja Tang* (Lee Je-ma's Raise the Yang and Benefit the Qi Decoction with Aconite) can be prescribed.

---

2   The *De Xiao Fang* (得效方, *Efficacious Remedies of the Physicians*), also referred to as *Shi Yi De Xiao Fang*, was written by Wei Yilin and published in 1337, during the Yuan Dynasty.

3   The *Gujin Yijian* (古今醫鑑, *Newly Amended Mirror of Ancient and Modern Medicine*), written by Gong Xin, consists of eight volumes, covering pulse diagnosis, disease etiology, herbal function, and a discourse on the flow of bodily *Qi* according to the seasons. He also elaborated on internal, gynecological, pediatric, and ears/nose/throat disorders.

**Table 6.1: The So Eum Individual's kidney Heat causing Exterior Heat syndrome[4]**

| Method of action | Situation addressed | Lee Je-Ma's adopted and modified formulae |
|---|---|---|
| Release Exterior Cold pathogen by ascending kidney and promoting light sweating | Initial stage Tai Yang illness with no sweating, indicating the absence of *Mang Yang* syndrome and focus on releasing the Exterior pathogen with Warm, Yang-natured acrid herbs | *Gui Zhi Tang* (Adopted) (Cinnamon Twig Decoction) |
| | | *Cheongung Gyeji Tang* (Lee Je-ma's Lovage Root and Cinnamon Twig Decoction) |
| | | *Xiang Su San* (Adopted) (Cyperus and Perilla Leaf Powder) |
| | | *Gunggwi Hyangsu San* (Lee Je-ma's Cyperus and Perilla Leaf Powder with Lovage and Angelica Root) |
| | | *Gwakhyang Jeonggi San* (Lee Je-ma's Agastache Powder to Rectify the Qi) |
| Release Exterior Cold pathogen by raising kidney and spleen Yang, preserve weakened spleen Yang, and avoid further sweating | Tai Yang stage illness with onset of excessive sweating, indicating early stage *Mang Yang* syndrome. Treatment focuses on supporting Yang and releasing Exterior | *Huanggi Gyeji Tang* (Lee Je-ma's Cinnamon Twig Astralagus and Aconite Decoction) |
| | | *Bochung Ikgi Tang* (Lee Je-ma's Tonify the Middle and Augment the Qi Decoction) |
| | | *Seungyang Ikgi Tang* (Lee Je-ma's Raise the Yang and Benefit the Qi Decoction) |
| Release Exterior Cold pathogen by raising kidney and spleen Yang, strongly preserve weakened spleen Yang, and avoid further sweating | Tai Yang stage illness with consistent excessive sweating due to significant Yang deficiency with middle to later stage *Mang Yang* syndrome | *Gyeji Buja Tang* (Lee Je-ma's Cinnamon Twig and Prepared Aconite Decoction) |
| | | *In Sam Gyeji Buja Tang* (Lee Je-ma's Ginseng, Cinnamon Twig, and Aconite Decoction) |
| | | *Seungyang Ikgi Buja Tang* (Lee Je-ma's Raise the Yang and Benefit the Qi Decoction with Aconite) |

---

4    The above reference to "adopted" indicates *Shang Han Lun*-based formulae that consist entirely of herbal ingredients that correlate directly with the So Eum constitution. "Modified" refers to other *Shan Han Lun*-based formulae with added ingredients to enhance their effect, or omitted ingredients, which are not suitable for the So Eum constitution. Please refer to the last section of this chapter for a concise list of ingredients and modification details.

張仲景이 曰太陽病에 脈浮緊하며 發熱無汗而衄者는 自愈也ㅣ니라.

According to Zhang Zhongjing, if the pulse is superficial and rapid, with no sweating during Tai Yang stage illness, then the patient will recover on their own.

太陽病 六七日에 表證이 因在하고 脈微而沈하며 反不結胸하고 其人如 狂者는 以熱在下焦니 小腹이 當滿이오 小便이 自利者는 下血하면 乃 愈하니 抵當湯을 主之니라.

[According to Zhang Zhongjing,] if after five to six days [of Tai Yang illness] there is no improvement and the patient experiences the onset of *Ul Kwang*[5] syndrome with no signs of insanity, accompanied by a minute pulse, Heat in the Lower *Jiao*, fullness and hardness in the lower abdomen, but no urination issues, then blood simply needs to flow downwards. In this case *Di Dang Tang* (Rhubarb and Leech Decoction) can be prescribed.

太陽證에 身黃發狂하고 小腹이 硬滿하며 小便이 自利者는 血證이니 宜 抵當湯이오 傷寒에 小腹이 滿하면 應小便不利어늘 今反利者는 以有血 也ㅣ니라.

[According to Zhang Zhongjing,] during an episode of Tai Yang illness there may be symptoms of jaundice, psychosis, tightness, and fullness of the lower abdomen without any urinary issues. These symptoms indicate that the pathogen has entered the blood level,[6] for which the prescription of *Di Dang Tang* is suitable. In most cases of Shang Han illness, if there is fullness of the lower abdomen, then urination will become an issue. In this particular case, however, urinary output will still be sufficient and smooth because there is no deficiency of blood.[7]

太陽病이 不解하고 熱結膀胱하야 其人이 如狂하며 血自下者는 自愈오 但小腹이 急結者는 宜攻之니 宜桃仁承氣湯이니라.

[According to Zhang Zhongjing,] there may be difficulty overcoming a Tai Yang illness with signs of Heat building up in the urinary bladder and concurrent symptoms of psychosis. This can naturally be resolved if the blood is able to flow

---

5    *Ul Kwang* syndrome is the result of an Exterior pathogenic influence causing chills and fever, accumulation of phlegm in the Upper *Jiao*, and inability to sweat. It is often accompanied by psychosis and madness.

6    According to the *Shang Han Lun*, when a pathogen enters the blood level there may be symptoms such as high fever, severe irritability, jaundice, tightness and fullness in the lower abdomen, psychosis, skin maculae, hematemesis, epistaxis, hematuria, hematochezia, and/or convulsions.

7    Difficult urination during the other stages of Shang Han illness may indicate blood deficiency since blood and urine share the same source, the *Jin Ye* bodily fluids.

downwards.[8] However, if the lower abdomen hardens [due to a lack of blood supply] then *Tao Ren Cheng Qi Tang*[9] (Peach Pit Decoction to Order the Qi) is called for.

太陽病外證이 未除而數下之면 遂下利不止하고 心下痞硬하야 表裏不解니 人蔘桂枝湯을 主之니라.

[According to Zhang Zhongjing,] if diarrhea is promoted before the resolution of a Tai Yang illness, causing uncontrollable bowel flow and epigastric *Bi Ying* syndrome,[10] and the spontaneous occurrence of Exterior and Interior symptoms, then it is necessary to prescribe *Ren Shen Gui Zhi Tang* (Cinnamon Twig Decoction with Ginseng).[11]

論曰此證에 其人如狂者는 腎陽이 困熱也오 小腹이 硬滿者는 大腸이 怕寒也라 二證이 俱見이어든 當先其急이니 腎陽이 困熱則當用川芎桂枝湯 黃芪桂枝湯 八物君子湯하야 升補之하며 大腸이 怕寒則當用藿香正氣散 香砂養胃湯하야 和解之하되 若外熱이 包裡冷而毒氣重 結於內하야 或將有養虎遺患之弊 則當用巴豆丹하야 下利一二度하고 因以藿香正氣散 八物君子湯으로 和解而峻補之니라.

From my perspective, symptoms of psychosis, present along with Tai Yang illness, are due to the stagnation of kidney Yang, causing Heat accumulation.[12] Tightness and fullness in the lower abdomen are due to the influence of Cold on the large intestine.[13] If both of these symptoms occur simultaneously then we must address the stagnant Yang Heat within the kidneys with *Cheongung Gyeji Tang* (Lee Je-ma's Lovage Root and Cinnamon Twig Decoction), *Huanggi Gyeji Tang* (Lee Je-ma's Cinnamon Twig Astralagus and Aconite Decoction), *Palmul*

---

8     Psychosis, in this situation, is due to Tai Yang stage pathogenic influence causing uproot/rebellion of blood and *Qi*.

9     *Tao Ren Cheng Qi Tang* (Peach Pit Decoction to Order the Qi) is mentioned in Zhang Zhongjing's *Shang Han Lun*. It consists of Tao Ren (*Semen Pruni Persicae*) 12–15g, Da Huang (*Radix et Rhizoma Rhei*) 12g, Gui Zhi (*Ramulus Cinnamomi Cassiae*) 6g, Mang Xiao (*Natrii Sulfas*) 6g, and Zhi Gan Cao (*Radix Glycyrrhizae*) 6g.

10    "Epigastric *Bi Ying* syndrome," or *Xin Xia Bi Ying* (心下痞硬), is one indication of acute Tai Yin stage syndrome, marked by tightness, fullness, (subjective) hardness, and stagnation of the epigastric area. It is the result of weakness of the stomach and accumulation of Cold toxin in the epigastric area. Please note that Lee Je-ma differentiates between the *Bi Ying* syndrome of the So Eum Individual and that of the So Yang Individual. In the So Eum Individual's case, the epigastrium feels hard to the patient but is actually soft to the touch, and in the So Yang Individual's case, the epigastrium doesn't only feel hard to the patient, but is also hard to the touch. The former situation is due to weakness of stomach *Qi* and accumulation of Cold toxin, whereas the latter situation is due to build-up of fluids in the chest during a Tai Yang stage illness.

11    The standard dose of 4g of Ren Shen (*Radix Ginseng*) is added to *Gui Zhi Tang* in this formula. The precise dosage of Ren Shen may change according to the patient and his or her presentation.

12    Displaced Heat is due to the entrapment of Yang within the kidneys, accumulating pressure over time, and eventually rebelling upwards. The upwards rebellion of Yang and Heat may result in psychosis. This condition, also known as *Ulchuk Panggwang* (鬱縮膀胱—see also following footnote), is addressed through the administration of herbs that encourage the ascent of kidney Yang.

13    This syndrome is referred to as *Daejang Pahan* (大腸怕寒), or "influence of Cold on the large intestine." It occurs as a result of a Cold pathogenic influence causing tightness, fullness, constipation, and a Cold sensation above the lower abdomen upon palpation.

*Gunja Tang* (Lee Je-ma's Eight Ingredient Gentlemen Decoction), and the like. These formulae support the ascent of, and tonify, Yang energy. If there are only symptoms related to the Cold influence of the large intestine, the prescription of *Hyangsa Yangwi Tang* (Lee Je-ma's Cyperus and Hawthorn Enliven the stomach Decoction) can be used to harmonize the interior and disperse External Heat. If Heat continuously surrounds the Cold within the body, it will repeatedly trap Cold toxin. This can be compared to raising a tiger that eventually attacks its owner. In this case, *Padu Dan* (Lee Je-ma's Croton Seed Pill) should be prescribed to promote bowel movement until there are one to two bouts of diarrhea. Immediately afterwards, formulae such as *Gwakhyang Jeonggi San* (Lee Je-ma's Agastache Powder to Rectify the Qi) and *Palmul Gunja Tang* (Lee Je-ma's Eight Ingredient Gentlemen Decoction) can be prescribed to reestablish harmony and follow up with the intense tonification of Yang.

**Table 6.2: *Daejang Pahan* and *Ulchuk Panggwang* syndromes**

| Method of action | Situation addressed | Formula name |
|---|---|---|
| Ascend trapped Yang within the kidneys | Tai Yang stage illness with Cold influence of the large intestine (*Daejang Pahan* syndrome) causing Cold and hardness sensation (to touch) of the lower abdomen without psychosis (less severe) | *Hyangsa Yangwi Tang* (Lee Je-ma's Cyperus and Hawthorn Enliven the stomach Decoction) |
| | Tai Yang stage illness with displaced Yang causing psychosis (*Ulchuk Panggwang* syndrome) and Cold influence of the large intestine (*Daejang Pahan* syndrome) causing Cold and hardness sensation (to touch) of the lower abdomen (more severe) | *Cheongung Gyeji Tang* (Lee Je-ma's Lovage Root and Cinnamon Twig Decoction) *Huanggi Gyeji Tang* (Lee Je-ma's Cinnamon Twig Astralagus and Aconite Decoction) *Palmul Gunja Tang* (Lee Je-ma's Eight Ingredient Gentlemen Decoction) |
| Evacuate Cold toxin by promoting diarrhea | Significantly displaced Yang (*Ulchuk Panggwang* syndrome) with significant Cold influence of the large intestine (*Daejang Pahan* syndrome) leading to constipation (Yang Ming syndrome) and accumulation of Cold toxins (most severe) | *Padu Dan* (Lee Je-ma's Croton Seed Pill) |
| Extinguish remaining Yang Ming stage illness, harmonize the Interior, and tonify Yang | Prescribed after promoting flow of bowel with Ba Dou (*Semen Crotonis*) to support Yang and extinguish remaining traces of pathogen | *Gwakhyang Jeonggi San* (Lee Je-ma's Agastache Powder to Rectify the Qi) *Palmul Gunja Tang* (Lee Je-ma's Eight Ingredient Gentlemen Decoction) |

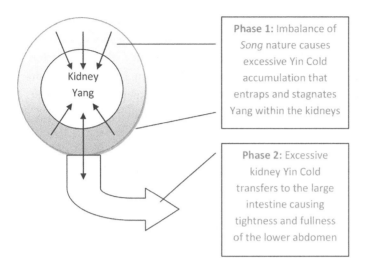

*Figure 6.1: The Daejang Pahan syndrome of the So Eum Individual*

張仲景所論에 下焦血證은 卽少陰人 脾局陽氣가 爲寒邪所掩抑 而腎局陽
氣가 爲邪所拒하야 不能直升連接於脾局하야 鬱縮膀胱之證也니 其人如
狂者는 其人이 亂言也오 如見鬼狀者는 怳惚譫語也니라.

What Zhang Zhongjing refers to as a Lower *Jiao* blood-level disorder is, in my opinion, actually the influence of Cold invasion leading to blockage of spleen Yang of the So Eum Individual. This will eventually cause restraint of the kidney Yang energy. The invasion of Cold impedes the ability of the kidney energy to connect with the spleen. This results in the accumulation of [turbid] energy in the urinary bladder.[14] Zhang Zhongjing's reference to "psychosis" [during the less critical stage of this disease] involves the mumbling of incoherent speech. His reference to "hallucination" [during the critically acute stage of this disease] describes this incoherent mumbling and fading consciousness.

---

14  This syndrome is referred to as *Ulchuk Panggwang* (鬱縮膀胱), or stagnation of urinary bladder energy due to the inability of Yang ascent from the kidney to the spleen group. As mentioned in the previous chapter, the urinary bladder is a component of the kidney group, or *Shin Ji Dang* (腎之黨). ence, kidney Yang deficiency and Yang stagnation within the kidneys will eventually lead to urinary bladder heat stagnation and dysuria.

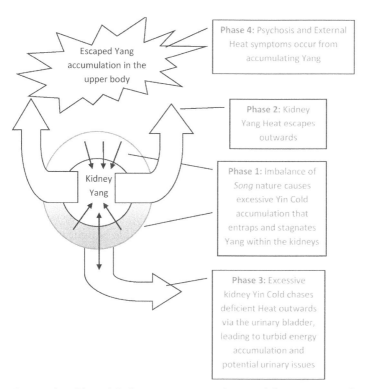

Phase 4: Psychosis and External Heat symptoms occur from accumulating Yang

Escaped Yang accumulation in the upper body

Phase 2: Kidney Yang Heat escapes outwards

Kidney Yang

Phase 1: Imbalance of *Song* nature causes excessive Yin Cold accumulation that entraps and stagnates Yang within the kidneys

Phase 3: Excessive kidney Yin Cold chases deficient Heat outwards via the urinary bladder, leading to turbid energy accumulation and potential urinary issues

*Figure 6.2: The Ulchuk Panggwang syndrome of the So Eum Individual*

太陽病 表證因在者는 身熱煩腦而惡寒之證이 間有之也오 太陽病 外證이 除者는 身熱煩腦而惡寒之證이 都無之也니 此證에 益氣而升陽則得其上策也어니와 破血而解熱則出於下計也니라.

The lingering Tai Yang illness is characterized by the affliction of Heat with occasional chills. The absence of chills with Heat affliction is a sign that the exterior influence has been removed. Here it is necessary to preserve the body's energy by promoting the ascent of [kidney] Yang.[15] It would be foolish to promote blood movement and clear Heat [as described in the *Shang Han Lun*] in such a situation.

---

15   This is done initially by promoting the ascent of spleen Yang.

太陽病 外證이 未除而數下之면 遂下利不止云云者는 亦可見古人之於此 證에 用承氣湯則下利不止인 故로 遂變其方而用抵當桃仁湯耳니라. 太 陽病 外證이 未除則陽氣其力이 雖有鬱抑이나 猶能振寒而與寒邪相爭於 表也어니와 若外證이 盡除則陽氣其力이 不能振寒而遂爲窮困縮伏之 勢 也니 攻下之藥이 何甚好藥而必待陽氣窮困縮伏 之時而應用耶아 人蔘桂 枝湯이 不亦晚乎아

The ancient doctors were aware that severe diarrhea will result if it is mistakenly promoted before the resolution of a Tai Yang illness. The precaution was mentioned as a result of prescribing *Cheng Qi Tang* (Order the Qi Decoction) during Tai Yang illness, which resulted in incessant diarrhea. *Di Dang Tang* (Rhubarb and Leech Decoction) was prescribed as an antidote. When a Tai Yang illness lingers, it is a sign that Yang had been suppressed but is still intact and capable of fighting against the exterior pathogenic Cold. When the symptoms of Tai Yang illness disappear [without other signs of improvement] it is a sign that Yang can no longer push away the Exterior Cold and is in a desperate state of oppression. Why would anyone want to promote diarrhea in this situation and cause further exhaustion of Yang? Wouldn't it be too late to prescribe [a tonic such as] *Ren Shen Gui Zhi Tang* (Cinnamon Twig Decoction with Ginseng) to remedy the situation?

張仲景이 曰婦人이 傷寒에 發熱하고 經水가 適來適斷하며 畫日明 了하고 夜則譫語하야 如見鬼狀은 此爲熱入血室이니 無犯胃氣及上二 焦면 必自愈니라. 陽明病에 口燥嗽水하고 不欲嚥은 此는 必衄이니 不可 下니라.

Zhang Zhongjing stated that if a female contracts a Shang Han illness marked by fever and chills, irregular menses, psychosis, and hallucinations only at night, then she is suffering from Uterine Heat, and that as long as Uterine Heat doesn't travel to the stomach and penetrate the Middle and Upper *Jiao*, the illness will resolve naturally. If during Yang Ming illness the patient is thirsty but unable to swallow, then she will definitely experience nosebleeds.[16] In this case it is necessary to refrain from promoting diarrhea.

---

16  Nose bleeding with thirst and the inability to swallow fluids is due to the occurrence of Yang Ming stage illness, in which stomach Heat causes thirst, but parched dryness leads to the inability to swallow and absorb fluids.

陽明病 不能食에 攻其熱하면 必「이니 傷寒에 嘔多하면 雖有陽明
病이라도 不可攻이오 胃家實 不大便과 若表未解及有半表者는 先以桂枝
柴胡하야 和解라사 乃可下也니라.

[According to Zhang Zhongjing,] if during a Yang Ming stage illness appetite is
lacking and the Heat Clearing Method[17] is used, dry heaves will occur indefinitely.
If dry heaves occur during the occurrence of Shang Han illness, even in the situation
of Yang Ming, Heat should not be cleared. If during the occurrence of *Wei Jia
Shi*[18] there is constipation and a lingering exterior pathogen, it is indicative of a
half-exterior and half-interior syndrome, and is necessary to first employ the exterior-
releasing properties of Gui Zhi (*Ramulus Cinnamomi Cassiae*) and Chai Hu (*Radix
Bupleuri*)[19] and only afterwards promote bowel movement.[20]

論曰右諸證에 當用藿香正氣散 香砂養胃湯 八物君子湯이니라.

From my perspective, the above situations call for the use of *Gwakhyang Jeonggi San*
(Lee Je-ma's Agastache Powder to Rectify the Qi), *Hyangsa Yangwi Tang* (Lee Je-ma's
Cyperus and Hawthorn Enliven the stomach Decoction), and *Palmul Gunja Tang*
(Lee Je-ma's Eight Ingredient Gentlemen Decoction).

**Table 6.3: Tai Yang/Yang Ming syndrome**

| Indications | Lee Je-ma's modified formulae |
|---|---|
| Tai Yang illness which transfers into Yang Ming stage illness with *Wei Jia Shi* syndrome (constipation, displaced Heat in the stomach, tidal fever) | *Gwakhyang Jeonggi San* (Lee Je-ma's Agastache Powder to Rectify the Qi) |
| | *Hyangsa Yangwi Tang* (Lee Je-ma's Cyperus and Hawthorn Enliven the stomach Decoction) |
| | *Palmul Gunja Tang* (Lee Je-ma's Eight Ingredient Gentlemen Decoction) |

17  The "Heat Clearing Method" refers to the use of Cold-natured purgatives.

18  *Wei Jia Shi* (胃家實), translated as "excess in the stomach house," refers to displaced Heat accumulation and
dryness of the stomach, leading to constipation, tidal fever, incoherent speech, and excessive sweating of the
hands and feet, a hallmark syndrome of Yang Ming stage illness. Yet elsewhere in this chapter, Lee Je-ma also
refers to *Wei Jia Shi* occurrence during a Tai Yang or Tai Yin stage illness. In such cases, he simply denotes
the occurrence of constipation along with other Tai Yang or Tai Yin symptoms, without significant Heat and
dryness of the stomach. The *Wei Jia Shi* of the Yang Ming stage involves significant Heat accumulation leading
to stomach dryness and constipation.

19  The suggestion to administer Chai Hu (*Radix Bupleuri*) was made by Zhang Zhongjing. Lee Je-ma associates
this herb with the So Yang rather than So Eum Individual.

20  Releasing Heat through the bowel results in diarrhea.

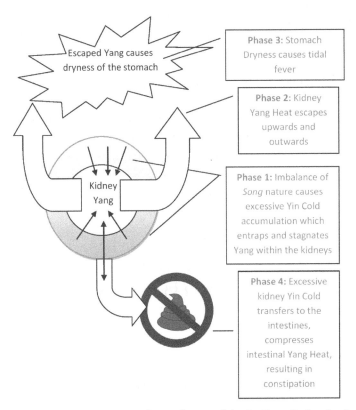

*Figure 6.3: The Wei Jia Shi syndrome of the So Eum Individual*

張仲景이 曰陽明之爲病은 胃家實也니라. 問曰緣何得陽明病고 答曰太陽病에 發汗 若下 若利小便者는 此는 亡津液하야 胃中이 乾燥하나니 因轉屬陽明하야 不更衣 內實大便難者는 此名陽明病也니라. 傷寒에 轉屬陽明하면 其人이 「然微汗出也니라.

According to Zhang Zhongjing, *Wei Jia Shi* is the hallmark syndrome of Yang Ming stage illness. In the *Shang Han Lun*, he posed the question, "Why does Yang Ming occur?" and answered that it occurs if too much sweating, diarrhea, or urination is promoted during the Tai Yang illness. Inappropriate treatment in the Tai Yang stage will cause the *Jin Ye* fluids to dry up, leading to general body dryness. This dryness then causes the transformation of illness from the Tai Yang to the Yang Ming stage, marked by constipation or abdominal fullness with difficult bowel movement. He stated further that if an illness transfers to the Yang Ming stage there will be a mild, clammy sweat.

傷寒에 若吐 若下後에 不解하야 不大便 五六日至十餘日하며 日哺에
所發潮熱이며 不惡寒하고 狂言하며 如見鬼狀하야 若劇者는 發則不識
人하며 循衣 摸床하고 惕而不安하며 微喘直視하나니 脈弦者는 生하고
脈濇者는 死니라.

[According to Zhang Zhongjing,] if after vomiting or diarrhea, the Shang Han illness has not resolved, and there are five to six or ten days of constipation, late afternoon (3–5pm) tidal fever without chills, incoherent speech, hallucinations with possible fits, aggressive behavior, and/or seizures with the inability to recognize others, fear of the unknown, anxiety, shortness of breath, and/or staring into space, then there will be one of two outcomes. If these symptoms occur with a wiry pulse, there is a good prognosis. If the pulse has a coarse or rough texture, then death is imminent.

論曰秦漢時 醫方治法에 大便秘燥者를 有大黃治法하고 無巴豆治法인
故로 張仲景이 亦用大黃大承氣湯하야 治少陰人 太陽病이 轉屬陽明
病하야 其人┌然微汗出하고 胃中이 燥煩實하야 不大便五六日至十餘
日하며 日哺에 發潮熱하고 不惡寒 狂言하며 如見鬼狀之時而用之則神
效라하고 若劇者는 發則不識人하고 循衣摸床하며 惕而不安하고 微喘直
視하니 用之於此則脈弦者는 生이오 脈濇者는 死라하니 蓋此方은 治少
陰人 太陽病이 轉屬陽明하야 不大便五六日하고 日哺에 發潮熱者에 可
用而其他則不可用也

In my experience, during the Jin and Han Dynasties Da Huang (*Radix et Rhizoma Rhei*) was mentioned as a remedy for constipation and dry stools, but there has been no mention of using Ba Dou (*Semen Crotonis Pulveratum*) for the same reason. Zhang Zhongjing was able to produce miraculous results using Da Huang by prescribing *Da Cheng Qi Tang* (Major Order the Qi Decoction) to treat a So Eum Individual suffering from a Tai Yang stage illness that transferred into a Yang Ming stage illness. This individual experienced clammy sweating, stomach dryness with discomfort and fullness, five to ten days of constipation, tidal fever,[21] a lack of chills,[22] incoherent speech, and hallucinations. In an extreme case he treated an individual with the inability to recognize others, fits and aggressive behavior, fear of the unknown, anxiety, shortness of breath, and staring into space. Zhang Zhongjing said that if the above formula is used and the pulse is wiry, there will be a good prognosis. If the pulse is rough and coarse, then death is imminent. The use of *Da Cheng Qi Tang* for the So Eum Individual is restricted to situations in which a Tai Yang illness transforms into the Yang Ming level with the occurrence of tidal fever and no bowel movement for five to six days.

---

21  Tidal fever, a hallmark symptom of Yang Ming stage illness, is a cyclical fever that occurs from 3pm to 5pm.

22  A "lack of chills" in this situation indicates that the pathogen has entered the Yang Ming stage of illness.

仲景이 知此方有可用不可用之時候인 故로 亦能昭詳 少陰人太陽陽明病
證 候也라 蓋仲景一心精力이 都在於探得大承氣湯可用時候인 故로 不可
用之時候를 亦昭詳知之也니라.

Zhang Zhongjing was aware of the appropriate use of *Da Cheng Qi Tang* (Major Order the Qi Decoction) and its use in cases involving the pathogenic transfer from Tai Yang to Yang Ming syndrome of the So Eum Individual. His wholehearted efforts combined with the accumulated knowledge of his predecessors led to the appropriate application of *Da Cheng Qi Tang*.

仲景의 太陽陽明病 藥方中에 惟桂枝湯 人蔘桂枝湯이 得其彷彿而大承氣
湯則置人死生於茫無津涯之中하니 必求大承氣湯可用時候而待其不大便
五六日하고 日哺發潮熱 狂言時하면 是이 豈美法也哉아 蓋少陰人病候는
自汗不出則脾不弱也오 大便이 秘燥則胃實也니라. 少陰人 太陽陽明病에
自汗不出하고 脾不弱者는 輕病也니 大便雖硬이라도 用藥하면 易愈也

Zhang Zhongjing included the primary use of *Gui Zhi Tang* (Cinnamon Twig Decoction) and *Ren Shen Gui Zhi Tang* (Cinnamon Twig Decoction with Ginseng) for when Tai Yang stage illness transfers into Yang Ming syndrome. If the use of *Da Cheng Qi Tang* (Major Order the Qi Decoction) can only be prescribed after five to six days of constipation, tidal fever, and incoherent speech, how can it be an appropriate treatment method for the So Eum Individual?[23] In such situations, life, itself, is at risk.[24] The Tai Yang/Yang Ming stage syndrome of the So Eum Individual [without the loss of Yang] occurs when there is constipation without sweating. A lack of sweat during the Tai Yang and Yang Ming stages indicates the absence of *Bi Yao*[25] syndrome, which can be overcome easily with the use of the above herbal combinations. Even with constipation in such situations, herbal therapy can easily lead to recovery.

---

23  In this sentence Lee Je-ma argues that no matter how effective a formula may be in a single situation, it isn't necessarily the only one to be used. *Da Cheng Qi Tang* is a formula prescribed for the Tae Eum Individual, not the So Eum Individual. Even though it has a remarkable effect in this situation, other formulae prescribed for the So Eum are equally if not more effective. Moreover, the use of Da Huang (*Radix et Rhizoma Rhei*) in this situation may eventually make matters worse since it has a Cool nature, which can lead to further Yang deficiency.

24  The occurrence of tidal fever and sweating for five or more days is a sign of severe Heat blockage in the stomach and weakness of spleen energy. Excessive spontaneous sweating is a direct indication of spleen deficiency and loss of Yang.

25  *Bi Yao* (脾約), or spleen weakness, is a condition resulting from excessive sweating due to inappropriate diaphoretic treatment or a preexisting lack of Yang energy. The latter occurs as a result of Tai Yang illness with spontaneous Yang deficiency leading to the escape of Yang energy through the skin pores. This is also referred to as the first stage of *Mang Yang* syndrome.

故로 大黃 枳實 厚朴 芒硝之藥도 亦能成功於此時而劇者는 猶有半生半
死하나니 若用八物君子湯 升陽益氣湯 與巴豆丹則雖劇者라도 亦無 脈弦
者는 生하고 脈濇者는 死之理也니라. 又太陽病 表證因在時에 何不早用
溫補升陽之藥 與巴豆하야 預圖其病而必待陽明病 日晡發潮熱 狂言時에
用承氣湯하야 使人半生半死耶아.

The use of Da Huang (*Radix et Rhizoma Rhei*), Zhi Shi (*Fructus Aurantii Immaturus*), Hou Po (*Mangnolia Officinalis*), and Mang Xiao (*Natrii Sulfas*) are suitable for the Tai Yang/Yang Ming syndrome of the So Eum Individual without *Bi Yao* syndrome. However, in severe situations, only 50 percent of those inflicted will survive. The odds of survival are increased by employing the use of *Palmul Gunja Tang* (Lee Je-ma's Eight Ingredient Gentlemen Decoction), *Seungyang Ikgi Tang* (Lee Je-ma's Raise the Yang and Benefit the Qi Decoction), and *Badu Dan* (Lee Je-ma's Croton Seed Pill). In such situations if the pulse is palpable, the patient will survive. If it is not palpable, death is imminent. I cannot understand why the methods of warming, tonifying, and ascending Yang were not traditionally used during the Tai Yang stage to prevent the onset of Yang Ming stage illness [of the So Eum Individual]. Wouldn't this be more efficient than waiting until the onset of tidal fever and incoherent speech, with the survival rate decreasing to only 50 percent?

許叔微本事方에 曰一人이 病傷寒하야 大便不利하며 日晡에 發潮
熱하며 手循衣縫하고 兩手撮空하며 直視喘急이어늘 諸醫가 皆走하니
此誠惡候라 仲景이 雖有證而無法하고 但云脈弦者는 生하고 脈濇者는
死라함을 護且救之하야 與小承氣湯 一服하니 而大便利하고 諸疾이 漸
退하며 脈且微弦하더니 半月에 愈하니라.

In the *Puji Ben Shi Fang*[26] (*Practical Formulae for Universal Benefit*), Xu Shu-wei wrote that he once treated a patient who was suffering from a life-threatening Shang Han illness marked by constipation, tidal fever,[27] uncontrolled waving movement of the arms, shortness of breath, and staring into space. Most attending physicians had given up and avoided further treatment due to the condition's gravity. Zhang Zhongjing described this situation without providing a remedy, simply stating that if the pulse is wiry, there is a chance of survival. Yet, if it is choppy,[28] death is imminent. Xu Shu-wei treated this patient with *Xiao Cheng Qi Tang* (Minor

---

26  The *Puji Ben Shi Fang* (本事方, *Practical Formulae for Universal Benefit*) was written in 1132 by Xu Shu-wei, a scholar of the *Shang Han Lun* school of thought. In this text, he includes 300 herbal remedies and numerous acupuncture protocols for 20 categories of illness, including Stroke, liver, Gall bladder, lung, kidney, heart, small intestine, spleen Disorders, Headache, and Dizziness. Xu Shu-wei also emphasized the importance of preserving and cultivating pre-natal Qi, or the Fire of the kidneys.

27  Tidal fever (潮熱) refers to the sudden onset of fever occurring between 3pm and 5pm.

28  A choppy pulse (濇脈), also referred to as a rough pulse, is slow, weak, and may skip beat(s) but then recover its normal rhythm. It feels uneven, like a knife scraping bamboo, and indicates blood deficiency with damaged *Jin Ye* fluids or inadequate blood flow due to obstruction (Huynh, H. (1981) *Pulse Diagnosis*: Paradigm Publications).

Order the Qi Decoction), and after just one pack (two doses of herbs) his bowel movement was regulated. His symptoms continued to fade, and in fifteen days, his pulse became wiry [indicating recovery].

王好古海藏書에 曰一人이 傷寒에 發狂欲走하며 脈虛數이어늘 用柴胡湯하니 反劇하야 以蔘 芪 歸 朮 陳皮 甘草로 煎湯一服하니 狂定하고 再服하니 安睡而愈니라.

In the *Haizang Shu*[29] (*Hai Zang's Collection of Work*) Xu Shu-wei stated that he once treated an individual who went mad and ran away. His pulse was deficient and rapid, and his symptoms became worse after Xu Shu-wei prescribed Chai Hu Tang (*Bupleurum Decoction*). For this he prescribed a formula containing Ren Shen (*Radix Ginseng*), Dang Gui (*Radix Angelicae Sinensis*), Bai Zhu (*Radix Atractylodis Macrocephalae*), Chen Pi (*Pericarpium Citri Reticulatae*), and Gan Cao (*Radix Glycyrrhizae*). After a single dose, his patient began to calm down, and he slept peacefully that same evening following the second dose.

醫學綱目에 曰嘗治循衣摸床者 數人할새 皆用大補氣血之劑하니 惟一人이 兼厂振脈代어늘 逐於補劑中에 略加桂하니 亦振止하고 脈和하야 而愈니라.

In the *Yixue Gangmu*[30] (*Compendium of Medicine*) Lou Ying recalled treating several patients who nervously fidgeted with their clothes by prescribing a formula to tonify both *Qi* and blood. One of his patients started to experience muscle twitching and an intermittent pulse,[31] but improved steadily after he added Rou Gui (*Cortex Cinnamomi*) to the above tonics.

成無己 明理論에 曰潮熱은 屬陽明하니 必於日晡時發者는 乃爲潮熱也라. 陽明之爲病은 胃家實이니 胃實則譫語하며 手足에 厂然汗出者는 此는 大便已硬也니 譫語有潮熱하면 承氣湯으로 下之하고 熱不潮者는 勿服이니라.

Cheng Wuji stated in his book *Mingli Lun* (*Expounding on the Treatise*)[32] that tidal fever occurring only at dawn is a reflection of Yang Ming illness. This can also be referred to as *Wei Jia Shi*, which is accompanied by incoherent speech and excessive

---

29 The *Haizang Shu* (海藏書) is written by Wang Hao Gu (1200–1264), a disciple of Li Gao, who was known for his view on Yin patterns, stating that they are much more challenging to diagnose and treat compared to Yang patterns. "Hai Zang" is another name given to Wang Hao Gu.

30 The *Yixue Gangmu* (醫學綱目), written by Lou Ying (1332–1402), is a 40-volume text that categorizes diseases into two categories: Yin and Yang.

31 An intermittent pulse (脈代) is slow and weak, and pauses at regular intervals. It indicates the decline of *Zhang* organ energy (Huynh, H. (1981) *Pulse Diagnosis*: Paradigm Publications).

32 The *Mingli Lun* (明理論), also referred to as the *Shanghan Mingli Lun*, written by Cheng Wuji (1063–1156), is a four-volume commentary on the *Shang Han Lun* often read as an introduction to the teachings of Zhang Zhongjing.

sweating of the hands and feet. These are signs that the bowels have already started to harden. *Cheng Qi Tang* (Order the Qi Decoction) can be prescribed only for those who have tidal fever and delirium. It should be avoided in the absence of tidal fever.

朱震亨 丹溪心法에 曰傷寒壞證에 昏沈垂死는 一切危急之證이니 好人蔘 一兩을 水煎하야 一服而盡하니 汗이 自鼻梁上出하야 涓涓如水하니라.

In Zhu Zhenheng's book entitled *Danxi Xinfa* (*The Teachings of Danxi*), he recalled an individual who was suffering from a debilitating Shang Han illness and was on the verge of death. Zhu Zhenheng immediately prescribed 37.5g of high-quality Ren Shen (*Radix Ginseng*) boiled in water. His patient consumed the formula in one dose and immediately started to drip sweat from the base of his nose.

論曰右論은 皆以張仲景 大承氣湯으로 始作俑而可用不可用之候를 難 知인 故로 紛紜多惑而始知張仲景之不可信也니라. 張仲景大承氣湯은 元 是殺人之藥而非活人之藥則大承氣湯은 不必擧論이라. 此胃家實病에 不 更衣發狂證에는 當用巴豆全粒하거나 或用獨蔘八物君子湯하며 或先用 巴豆하고 後用八物君子湯하야 以壓之니라.

In my opinion, the advice provided by the above doctors was modeled directly after Zhang Zhongjing's *Da Cheng Qi Tang* (Major Order the Qi Decoction). They do not offer enough detail regarding when to employ or avoid the use of this formula. Their advice also contains a certain amount of superstition, making it difficult for doctors of later ages to accept the teachings of Zhang Zhongjing. The use of *Da Cheng Qi Tang* can destroy the health of a patient rather than restore it. If *Wei Jia Shi* occurs with symptoms of madness and uncontrollable fidgeting,[33] I recommend prescribing one seed [without removal of the husk][34] of Ba Dou (*Semen Crotonis*) or *Doksam Palmul Tang* (Lee Je-ma's Added Ginseng Eight Ingredient Gentlemen Decoction), instead of *Da Cheng Qi Tang* (Major Order the Qi Decoction). These symptoms can also be overcome with the initial use of Ba Dou (*Semen Crotonis*) [to promote bowel movement] followed by *Palmul Gunja Tang* (Lee Je-ma's Eight Ingredient Gentlemen Decoction).

張仲景이 曰陽明病은 外證이 身熱 汗自出 不惡寒反惡熱이니라. 傷寒陽 明病에 自汗出하며 小便數則液이 內竭하야 大便이 必難이오 其脾가 爲 約이니 麻仁丸을 主之니라.

Zhang Zhongjing stated that the Exterior-related symptoms associated with Yang Ming illness are fever, spontaneous sweating, increased aversion to Heat, and absence of chills. He also mentioned that if, in the course of a Yang Ming stage illness there

---

33 "Fidgeting" is a translation of *Bu Geng Yi* (不更衣), nervously fiddling with the button or the lapel of one's clothes.

34 When prescribing Ba Dou (*Semen Crotonis*) in Sasang medicine, the husk is not removed from the seeds.

is spontaneous sweating and frequent urination, then fluid deficiency will result, causing the difficult passage of stool. This is a sign of *Bi Yao* and should be treated with *Ma Ren Wan* (Hemp Seed Formula).

陽明病에 自汗出하며 小便이 自利者는 此爲津液內竭이니 大便이 雖 硬이나 不可攻之오 宜用蜜導法하야 通之니라. 陽明病에 發熱 汗多者는 急下之니 宜大承氣湯이니라.

[According to Zhang Zhongjing,] if in the course of a Yang Ming stage illness spontaneous sweating and urinary incontinence occur, fluid loss will eventually lead to the difficult passage of stool. In this case, laxatives are not to be administered, but instead, honey as an enema [can help the passage of stools]. If a Yang Ming illness includes fever and excessive sweating, *Da Cheng Qi Tang* (Major Order the Qi Decoction) should be administered immediately.

李「醫學入門에 汗多不止를 謂之亡陽이니 如心痞 胸煩하고 面靑하며 膚「者는 難治오 色黃하며 手足溫者는 可治니라. 凡汗漏不止하야 眞 陽이 脫亡인 故로 謂之亡陽이니 其身이 必冷하고 多成痺寒하며 四肢拘 急하나니 桂枝附子湯을 主之니라.

In Li Chan's *Yixue Rumen*[35] (*Introduction to Medicine*), he states: "*Mang Yang* (Yang Collapse) is a condition marked by uncontrollable sweating. If *Mang Yang* is accompanied by vexation and fullness in the chest (a condition known as heart *Bi* syndrome), bluish-pale complexion, and muscle twitching, it will be difficult to overcome. The condition is treatable if the complexion is yellowish and the hands/feet are Warm. Uncontrollable sweating is a sign of Yang essence (眞陽) escaping from the body. During an episode of *Mang Yang*, the body will always feel cold, leading to numbness and contraction of the extremities (a condition referred to as Cold *Bi* syndrome), for which *Gui Zhi Fu Zi Tang* (Cinnamon Twig and Aconite Decoction) is appropriate."

嘗治少陰人 十一歲兒의 汗多亡陽病할새 此兒가 勞心焦思하야 素證이 有時以泄瀉爲憂而每飯時에 汗流滿面矣라. 忽一日에 頭痛, 發熱, 汗自 出하며 大便秘燥하니 以此兒素證이 泄瀉爲憂인 故로 頭痛, 身熱, 便秘, 汗出之熱證을 以其反於泄瀉寒證而曾不關心하고 尋常治之하야 以黃芪 桂枝 白芍藥等屬으로 發表矣하니 至于四五日에 頭痛發熱이 不愈니라.

I once treated an 11-year-old So Eum child with *Mang Yang* syndrome who had a history of anxiety, which caused him occasional diarrhea and excessive facial sweating

---

35 The *Yixue Rumen* (醫學入門, *Introduction to Medicine*) was written by Li Chan in 1575. It consists of nine chapters, four of which are devoted to the discussion of internal disorders and five to external disorders. It contains over 30,000 topics related to the Six Pathogenic Influences of the mind, *Qi*, and spirit. Areas of medicine include gynecology, pediatrics, surgery, internal medicine, etc.

when he ate. On one occasion, he suddenly experienced a headache with excessive sweating [throughout his body] and constipation. As I was particularly concerned about his ongoing bouts of diarrhea [and not his constipation], focus was placed on his dispelling the Exterior with Huang Qi (*Radix Astragali Membranacei*), Gui Zhi (*Ramulus Cinnamomi Cassiae*), and Bai Shao Yao (*Radix Paeoniae Lactiflorae*) rather than addressing his Heat-related symptoms that caused headaches, fever, constipation, and excessive sweating. Four to five days later, his headaches and fever didn't resolve.

六日平明에 察其證候則大便燥結이 已四五日이오 小便이 赤澁二三匙而 一晝夜間에 小便度數가 不過二三次오 不惡寒而發熱하며 汗出度數則一 晝夜間에 二三四次不均而人中則或有時有汗하고 或有時無汗하며 汗流 滿面體하니 其證이 可惡이라. 始覺汗多亡陽證候하니 眞是危證也라. 急 用巴豆一粒하고 仍煎黃芪桂枝附子湯에 用附子一錢하야 連服二貼하야 以壓之하니 至于末刻하야 大便이 通하고 小便이 稍淸而梢多라.

On the sixth day I observed his situation around midnight and noticed that he had not had a bowel movement for four to five days. His urine was a reddish color and difficult to pass, producing only two to three spoonfuls two to three times within a 48-hour period. There was also no sign of chills, but a feverish sensation with two to three bouts of excessive sweating. Even though sweating sporadically occurred underneath his nose,[36] at other times it would simply drip like a faucet from his entire body. It was so difficult to witness such a deplorable situation! Only after it became significantly worse did I realize that it was an acute case of *Mang Yang* syndrome, so I immediately administered one seed of Ba Dou (*Semen Crotonis*) followed by two packets of *Huanggi Gyeji Buja Tang* (Lee Je-ma's Cinnamon Twig Astralagus and Aconite Decoction) with 3.75g of Fu Zi (*Radix Aconiti*). Finally at 2pm the following day, he had a bowel movement and his urine output increased, becoming slightly clearer.

其翌日은 卽得病七日也로 以小兒로 附子太過之慮인 故로 以黃芪桂枝附 子湯 一貼으로 分兩日服矣하니 兩日後에 其兒亡陽證이 又作하야 不惡 寒, 發熱, 汗多而小便이 赤澁하며 大便이 秘結如前하고 面色이 帶靑하며 間有乾咳하니 病勢가 比前하면 太甚이라. 其日은 卽得病九日也로 時則 已時末刻也라 急用巴豆一粒하고 仍煎人蔘桂枝附子湯 用人蔘五錢 附子 二錢하야 連二貼으로 以壓之하니

On the second day of treatment, and seven days after the start of illness, I started to worry about prescribing too much Fu Zi (*Radix Aconiti*) to a young child, so

---

36  According to Lee Je-ma, sweating under the nose is a sign of recovery from illness for the So Eum Individual. In this case, as the body feebly attempted to overcome illness, there was merely occasional sweating under the nose only to be followed by *Mang Yang* sweating, which flows from the entire body.

I reduced the dosage of *Huanggi Gyeji Buja Tang* (Lee Je-ma's Cinnamon Twig Astralagus and Aconite Decoction) to one pack for two days. After only two days, *Mang Yang* returned as he started to show signs of fever without chills, excessive sweating, reddish and difficult urination, hard stools, bluish complexion, and dry cough. These symptoms appeared worse than his first bout of *Mang Yang*, so I immediately prescribed one seed of Ba Dou (*Semen Crotonis*)[37] with *Insam Gyeji Buja Tang* (Lee Je-ma's Ginseng Cinnamon Twig and Aconite Decoction) with 18.75g of Ren Shen (*Radix Ginseng*) and 7.5g of Fu Zi (*Radix Aconiti*) continuously for two days straight.

至于日晡하야 大便이 始通하나 小便이 稍多而色赤則一也어늘 又用人蔘桂枝附子湯 用人蔘五錢 附子二錢하야 一貼服矣하니 至于二更夜에 其兒가 側臥而頭不能擧하고 自吐痰一二匙而乾咳仍止라
其翌日에 又用人蔘桂枝附子湯 人蔘五錢 附子二錢 三貼하니 食粥二三匙하고 每用藥後則身淸凉無汗하고 小便이 稍多而大便必通이라.

By sunset, even though his urine was still reddish, his bowel and urine output increased. At midnight, after another pack of the above formula, he lay down without being able to lift his head. Shortly afterwards, he suddenly coughed up two to three spoonfuls of phlegm and his spell of dry coughing stopped. After another two days and three packs of *In Sam Gyeji Buja Tang* (Lee Je-ma's Ginseng Cinnamon Twig and Aconite Decoction) with 18.75g of Ren Shen (*Radix Ginseng*) and 7.5g of Fu Zi (*Radix Aconiti*), he was finally able to ingest two to three spoonfuls of rice gruel. He felt more comfort with every consecutive dose of herbs. His sweating ceased, bowels began to flow better, and urine became clearer.

又翌日에 用此方二貼하니 食粥半碗하고 又翌日에 用此方二貼하니 食粥半碗有餘하고 身淸凉하야 自起坐房室中하니 此日은 卽得病十二日也라
此三日內에 身淸凉하고 無汗하며 大便通하고 小便淸而多者는 連用附子二錢하야 日二三貼之故也라.

After two more days with two further packs of herbs, he was able to eat close to a half bowl of rice gruel, and after another two days with two more packs of herbs, he was able to completely finish a half bowl of rice gruel. By the 12th day, he felt a stronger sense of relief and could sit upright by himself. Within another three days he experienced even more relief, without any further sweating, constipation, or unclear and inconsistent urine flow thanks to the two to three herbal packs containing 7.5g of Fu Zi (*Radix Aconiti*) every day that I prescribed.

---

37   Lee Je-ma utilized Ba Dou here to eliminate Cold toxin accumulation of the spleen by strongly descending spleen Yin and ascending kidney Yang.

至于十三日하니 又起步門庭而擧頭하나 不能仰面이어늘 懲前小兒附子
太過之慮하야 用黃芪桂枝附子湯에 用附子一錢하야 每日二貼服하니 至
于七八日하야 頭面은 稍得仰擧而面部에 浮腫이라. 又每日二貼服하야 至
于七八日하니 頭面을 又得仰擧而面部浮腫도 亦減하니라. 其後에 用此
方하야 每日二貼服하니 自得病初로 至於病解가 前後一月餘에 用附子가
凡八兩矣니라.

On the 13th day, he was able to walk in his garden, but could not hold his head up
straight or take his gaze away from the ground. I started to worry about prescribing
too much Fu Zi (*Radix Aconiti*) to a young child, so I reduced its dosage to 3.75g
and continued to administer two packs a day of *Huanggi Gyeji Buja Tang* (Lee Je-
ma's Cinnamon Twig Astralagus and Aconite Decoction). After seven to eight days,
he was able to raise his head slightly. I noticed that his face also started to swell
due to water retention. After continuing the above dosage for seven more days, he
was able to lift his head completely with ease, and his facial edema disappeared. I
continued with this dose of herbs for another month until he completely overcame
his illness, providing him with a grand total of 300g of Fu Zi (*Radix Aconiti*).

張仲景이 曰陽明病이 有三病하니 太陽陽明者는 脾約이 是也오
正陽陽明者는 胃家實이 是也오 少陽陽明者는 發汗하고 利小便하나 胃
中이 燥煩實하고 大便難이 是也니라.

Zhang Zhongjing mentioned that there are three types of Yang Ming illness. The
Tai Yang/Yang Ming syndrome, which is also referred to as *Bi Yao*, the Zhong Yang/
Yang Ming illness, also called *Wei Jia Shi*, and the Shao Yang/Yang Ming illness,
which is induced by excessive use of diaphoretics or promotion of urine, and is
marked by excessive dryness and vexation felt in the stomach area, accompanied by
constipation.

論曰張仲景所論 陽明三病에 一曰脾約者는 自汗出 小便利之證也오
二曰胃家實者는 不更衣 大便難之證也오 三曰發汗 利小便 胃中燥煩實
者는 此亦胃家實也니其實은 非三病也오 二病而已니라. 仲景意 脾約云
者는 津液이 漸竭하야 脾之潤氣가 漸約之謂也오胃家實云者는 津液이 已
竭하야 胃之全局이 燥實之謂也니라.

From my perspective, the three levels associated with Zhang Zhongjing's Yang Ming syndrome are (a) *Bi Yao* syndrome, which is marked by spontaneous sweating,[38,39] (b) *Wei Jia Shi* (Type A), marked by uncontrolled fidgeting and constipation, and (c) *Wei Jia Shi* (Type B), caused by excessive diaphoresis or promotion of urine, leading to severe dryness of the stomach. Since two of the above stages can be classified as *Wei Jia Shi*, there are actually only two stages of Yang Ming rather than three. The *Bi Yao* syndrome that Zhang Zhongjing mentions is due to the drying up of *Jin Ye* fluids, which eventually leads to the weakening of the spleen energy. *Wei Jia Shi* [of the Yang Ming stage] refers to the situation in which the fluids have already dried up considerably, leading to acute dryness of the entire stomach area.

中古戰國秦漢之時에 醫家單方經驗이 其來已久하야 汗, 吐, 下 三法이 始
爲盛行하니 太陽病表證이 因在者는 或以麻黃湯으로 發汗하고 或以猪苓
湯으로 利小便하며 或以承氣湯으로 下之러니 承氣湯으로 之則下利不止
之證이 作矣오 麻黃湯이나 猪苓湯으로 發汗하거나 利小便則胃中燥煩實
大便難之證이 作矣할새

The three methods of promoting sweat, vomit, and evacuation [of the bowels and urination] were well developed by the advent of the Warring States, Jin, and Han periods. This is why they were able to treat long-term Tai Yang illnesses with Exterior-releasing formulae such as *Ma Huang Tang* (Ephedra Decoction) to promote sweating, *Zhu Ling Tang* (Polyporus Decoction) to promote urination, and *Cheng Qi Tang* (Order the Qi Decoction) to promote diarrhea. Yet there are situations in which diarrhea doesn't cease after using *Cheng Qi Tang*. The use of *Ma Huang Tang* (Ephedra Decoction) or *Zhu Ling Tang* may also lead to severe stomach dryness and constipation.

---

38    Although it is less likely, sweating may also occur with *Wei Jia Shi* syndrome. However, *Bi Yao* sweat doesn't form drops and instead flows like a river from all parts of the body. *Wei Jia Shi* sweating drips from the forehead. Note that *Bi Yao* sweating indicates *Mang Yang* (Yang Collapse). The difference between *Bi Yao* and more acute stages of *Mang Yang* is that the former has less sweating and normal urine flow. The acute (critical) stages of *Mang Yang* syndrome have copious sweating and difficult urination.

39    There may also be minor constipation along with *Bi Yao* syndrome, but constipation is a hallmark sign of *Wei Jia Shi*.

仲景이 有見於此인 故로 以脾約之自汗出, 自利小便者로 脾之潤氣가 漸約하야 亦將爲胃燥煩實之張本矣라하나 然이나 脾約은 自脾約也오 胃家實은 自胃家實也니 寧有其病이 先自脾約而後에 至於胃家實之理耶아

When Zhang Zhongjing observed these conditions, he assumed that spontaneous sweating and frequent urination were a result of the gradual weakening of the spleen. He predicted that this was the eventual cause of stomach dryness. Actually, *Bi Yao* and *Wei Jia Shi* may occur on their own. How can we say that only after spleen deficiency can we witness stomach excess?

胃家實 脾約 二病은 如陰證之太陰少陰病하야 虛實證狀이 顯然不同하니 自太陽病表證이 因在時에 已爲兩路分岐하야 元不相合이니라. 太陽病表證이 因在而其人如狂者는 鬱狂之初證也오 陽明病 胃家實 不更衣者는 鬱狂之中證也오 陽明病에 潮熱 狂言 微喘 直視者는 鬱狂之末證也오

Both *Bi Yao* and *Wei Jia Shi* will eventually lead to Tai Yin and Shao Yin stage illnesses and their symptomatic presentation is differentiated according to excess and deficiency patterns. From the onset, Tai Yang sickness can advance in two uniquely different directions: *Ul Kwang* syndrome and *Mang Yang* syndrome. The early (lighter) stage of *Ul Kwang* syndrome is marked by emotional instability due to lingering Tai Yang illness. The middle stage of *Ul Kwang*, also referred to as Yang Ming/*Wei Jia Shi,* is marked by constipation. Lastly, the final (critical) stage of *Ul Kwang* syndrome is characterized by tidal fever, incoherent speech, shortness of breath, and stupor, or staring into space without the ability to recognize others.

太陽病에 發熱惡寒 汗自出者는 亡陽之初證也오 陽明病에 不惡寒 反惡熱 汗自出者는 亡陽之中證也오 陽明病에 發熱汗多者는 亡陽之末證也니 蓋 鬱狂證은 都是身熱自汗不出也오 亡陽證은 都是身熱自汗出也니라.

The early (lighter) stage of *Mang Yang* is marked by spontaneous sweating. The middle stage of *Mang Yang* is marked by a lack of chills and increasing feverish feeling with spontaneous sweating as seen in the beginning stages of Yang Ming illness. Lastly, the final (acute) stage of *Mang Yang* syndrome is characterized by fever and copious spontaneous sweating as in the more acute stages of Yang Ming stage illness. A major difference between *Ul Kwang* and *Mang Yang* syndromes is that, for the most part, *Ul Kwang* syndrome is marked by a lack of sweating while *Mang Yang* is accompanied by sweating. Both, however, include symptoms of fever.

陰證에 口中和而有腹痛泄瀉者는 太陰病也오 口中不和而有腹痛泄瀉
者는 少陰病也며 陽證에 自汗不出而有頭痛身熱者는 太陽陽明病 鬱狂證
也오 自汗出而有頭痛身熱者는 太陽陽明病 亡陽證也니라

Each of the Yin stage syndromes has its own unique etiology and symptomatic presentation. Tai Yin stage symptoms are characterized by a lack of thirst, indigestion, and diarrhea. Thirst [with desire to moisten the mouth rather than swallow liquids], indigestion, and diarrhea are characteristics of the Shao Yin stage.

Each of the Yang stage syndromes (Yang Ming/*Ul Kwang*, Yang Ming/*Mang Yang*) also has its own unique etiology and symptomatic presentation. The Tai Yang/ Yang Ming stage *Ul Kwang* syndrome is characterized by a lack of (spontaneous) sweating, headache, and fever. The Tai Yang/Yang Ming stage *Mang Yang* illness is characterized by excessive spontaneous sweating, headache, and fever.

陰證之太陰病과 陽證之鬱狂病은 有輕證重證也오 陰證之少陰病과 陽
證之亡陽病은 有險證危證也니 亡陽과 少陰病은 自初痛으로 已爲險
證하다가 繼而危證也니라.

The Yin symptoms[40] of the Tai Yin stage and the Yang symptoms[41] of the *Ul Kwang* syndrome both have mild or moderate health effects. The Yin symptoms of Shao Yin syndrome and the Yang symptoms[42] of the *Mang Yang* syndrome both have severe or life-threatening effects. Severe health risks are present from the onset of both Shao Yin and *Mang Yang* syndromes, as they can quickly become life threatening.

亡陽病證은 非但觀於汗也오 必觀於小便多少也니 若小便이 清利而自汗
出則脾約病也니 此는 險證也오 小便이 赤澁而自汗出則陽明病 發熱汗多
也니 此는 危證也라. 然이나 少陽人裡熱證과 太陰人表熱證에 亦有汗多
而小便赤澁者하니 宜察之오 不可誤藥이니라.

The severity of *Mang Yang* syndrome is determined by urine output. Clear and smooth urination indicates a relatively lighter form of *Bi Yao*, and is severe but not life threatening. Copious spontaneous sweating with signs of Yang Ming stage illness such as reddish and difficult urination and fever indicate a life-threatening situation. Keep in mind, however, that the So Yang Individual's Internal Heat and the Tae Eum Individual's External Heat syndromes may also be accompanied by reddish and difficult urine with excessive sweat. It is therefore crucial to practice caution[43] in order to avoid prescribing the wrong formula.

---

40    The Yin symptoms of the Tai Yin stage are diarrhea, indigestion, and lack of thirst.

41    The Yang symptoms of the *Ul Kwang* syndrome are constipation, emotional instability, and fever.

42    The Yang symptoms of *Mang Yang* refer to fever and sweating. Although these symptoms may appear to be the result of excessive Yang, they are actually signs of Yang exhaustion and its escape upwards.

43    As a precaution it is necessary in this situation to clearly distinguish the constitution of the patient by examining body-type-specific traits before administering herbs.

**Table 6.4: Comparison between False\* Heat and False Cold-related symptoms of the So Eum and So Yang Individual**

| Constitution | Strongest organ | Strongest energy | Easily misinterpreted symptoms | Addressed with |
|---|---|---|---|---|
| So Eum | Kidneys | Cold | False\* Heat symptoms due to accumulation of Cold and escape of Yang Heat | Herbs that *warm* the spleen (despite Heat-related symptoms) |
| So Yang | Spleen | Hot | False\* Cold symptoms due to accumulation of Heat and escape of Cold Yin | Herbs that *cool* the kidneys (despite Cold-related symptoms) |

*\* Here "false" refers to Heat-related symptoms that are actually due to Cold and Cold-related symptoms actually due to Heat. The former situation is a result of Cold chasing Heat out to the exterior and the latter situation is due to Heat chasing Cold out to the exterior.*

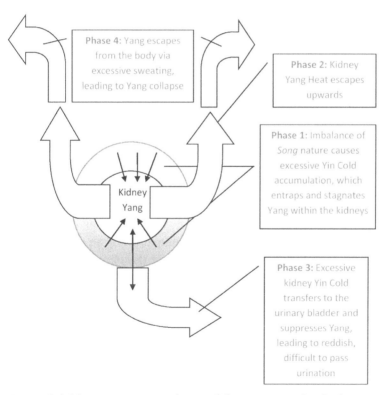

*Figure 6.4: The Mang Yang syndrome of the So Eum Individual*

胃家實病이 其始焉에는 汗不出, 不惡寒하고 但惡熱而其病이 垂危則濈然
微汗出 潮熱也니 濈然微汗出潮熱者는 表寒振發之力이 永竭故也니 胃
竭之候也오 脾約病이 其始焉에는 身熱 汗自出 不惡寒而若其病이 垂危
則發熱, 汗多而惡寒也니 發熱汗多而惡寒者는 裡熱撑支之勢가 已窮故也
│니 脾絶之候也니라.

As I mentioned before, the onset of *Wei Jia Shi* is characterized by a feverish sensation
with a lack of sweating and chills. In acute cases, a slight amount of sticky sweating
may occur with tidal fever. These symptoms occur when the ability to fight off an
External Cold-induced pathogen slowly diminishes and the stomach energy begins
to dry out.

The onset of *Bi Yao* is characterized by a feverish sensation and sweating without
the occurrence of chills. In severe cases, however, chills will accompany symptoms
of fever and excessive sweating. These symptoms occur when the ability to bear
Internal Heat has diminished and the spleen energy has considerably weakened.

張仲景이 曰厥陰證은 手足厥冷하며 小腹痛 煩滿 囊縮하며 脈微欲絶이니
宜當歸四逆湯이니라. 凡厥者는 陰陽氣가 不相順接하야 便爲厥이니 厥
者는 手足逆冷이 是也니라. 傷寒 六七日에 尺寸脈이 微緩者는 厥陰에 受
病也라 其證이 小腹煩滿而囊縮하나니 宜用承氣湯으로 下之니라. 六七
日에 脈至皆大하며 煩而口噤하여 不能言躁擾者는 必欲解也니라

According to Zhang Zhongjing, *Dang Gui Si Ni Tang* (Tangkuei Decoction for
Frigid Extremities) should be prescribed for the Jue Yin stage illness, marked by
frigid extremities, pain, fullness, and an unsettled feeling in the lower abdomen,
contraction of the scrotum, and a pulse so minute that it is almost non-existent.
As a general rule, Jue Yin-related illness results from the inability of Yin and Yang
to intermingle, causing a constant sensation of coldness in the hands and feet. A
minute and slow radial pulse after five to six days of battling a Shang Han illness is
characteristic of the Jue Yin stage, which is also accompanied by an unsettling and
full sensation of the lower abdomen and contraction of the scrotum. In this case,
*Cheng Qi Tang* (Order the Qi Decoction) should be prescribed to promote diarrhea.

He also stated that if there is a large and excessive radial pulse after six to seven
days of battling a Shang Han illness with a feverish and unsettled feeling, locking of
the jaw with inability to speak, and irritability, then it is a sign of recovery.[44]

---

44  At first glance, these acute-natured symptoms do not appear to be indicative of recovery. However, in the
case of a So Eum Individual, they represent the first stage of recovery from devastated Yang due to the onset
of a Jue Yin stage illness. The occurrence of Yang and Heat-related symptoms, such as a full pulse, lockjaw,
and irritability, have a better prognosis than the Yin and Cold-related symptoms of a minute pulse, and
contraction of the scrotum.

朱肱 活人書에 曰厥者는 手足逆冷이 是也라 手足指頭가 微寒者는 謂之 淸이니 此疾은 爲輕이오 陰厥者는 初得病에 便四肢厥冷하고 脈沈微而 不數하며 足多攣하니라. 傷寒 六七日에 煩滿, 囊縮하며 尺寸이 俱微緩 者는 足厥陰經이 受病也라 其脈이 微浮는 爲欲愈오 不浮는 爲難愈니 脈浮緩者는 必囊不縮이오 外證에 必發熱惡寒은 爲欲愈니 宜桂麻各半 湯이니라.

Zhu Gong states in his *Huoren Shu* that *Jue* (厥), characterized by frigid hands and feet, should be differentiated from a condition referred to as *Wei Han* (微寒), a minor illness in which the fingers and toes are only slightly cold to the touch. If, from the beginning stages of *Jue*, the hands and feet are ice cold and the pulse is sinking, minute, and not rapid, spasms will likely occur. If a Shang Han illness lingers for seven to eight days and is accompanied by fullness in the chest with vexation, contraction of the scrotum, and a slightly delayed pulse, then it has settled in the Foot Jue Yin channel of the liver. If the pulse is slightly superficial, there is a good chance of survival; the absence of a superficial pulse is a grave sign.

若尺寸이 俱沈短者는 必囊縮하니 毒氣入腹이라 宜承氣湯으로 下之니 速用承氣湯하면 可保五生一死니라. 六七日에 脈微浮者는 否極泰來니 水 升火降하야 寒熱이 作而大汗하야 解矣니라.

[Zhu Gong also states that] when the pulse is superficial and slightly delayed with Exterior-related signs of chills and fever, but the scrotum is not contracted, it indicates that the body is overcoming a Jue Yin stage illness, in which case it is necessary to prescribe *Gui Ma Ge Ban Tang* (Combined Cinnamon Twig and Ephedra Decoction). A deep and short pulse with contracted scrotum indicates the accumulation of toxicity inside the abdomen. Hence it is necessary to induce diarrhea by prescribing *Cheng Qi Tang* (Order the Qi Decoction). If the administration of this formula is administered in haste,[45] only four out of five people will survive. If, after six to seven days of battling a Shang Han illness, simultaneous fever and chills occur with copious sweating, it signifies that the body is overcoming [a Jue Yin stage illness]. This can be compared to the *Yi Ching*-based concepts of "stagnation gives

---

45    "Haste" in this context refers to the administration of *Da Cheng Qi Tang* during the Jue Yin stage in situations when the scrotum has not contracted and the pulse isn't deep and short.

way to flow"[46] and encouraging "Water energy to flow upwards and Fire to flow downwards."[47]

諸手足逆冷은 皆屬厥陰하니 不可汗下나 然이나 有須汗須下者하니 謂手足이 雖逆冷하나 時有溫時하야 手足掌心이 必煖은 非正厥逆이니 當消息之니라.

[In the *Huoren Shu*, Zhu Gong also states that] since frigid hands and feet are a sign of Jue Yin stage illness, they should not be treated with diaphoretics or laxatives. Yet if the extremities occasionally feel warmer, while the palms and soles always feel warm, it may not necessarily indicate a genuine case of the above stage. In such cases, the aforementioned treatment methods may be necessary. Since this difference is easy to overlook, extreme caution should be taken.

李고이 曰舌卷厥逆에 冷過肘膝하며 小腹絞痛이면 三味蔘萸湯 四順湯을 主之하고 囊縮하며 手足이 乍冷乍溫하며 煩滿者는 大承氣湯을 主之니라.

Li Gao once stated that *San Wei Shen Yu Tang* (Three Flavors Ginseng and Evodia Fruit Decoction), *Si Shun Tang* (Four Ingredients Decoction to Smooth the Qi),[48] and other similar formulae are prescribed for symptoms such as a dry tongue with coldness of the extremities that radiates beyond the knees with a plugged-up, painful feeling in the lower abdomen. If the scrotum is contracted, the extremities alternate between feeling warm and cold, with an unsettled, full feeling in the chest, then *Da Cheng Qi Tang* (Major Order the Qi Decoction) should be administered.

---

46  The phrase "stagnation gives rise to flow" described the relationship between the 11th hexagram (entitled "Flowing") and the 12th hexagram (entitled "Stagnation") of the *Yi Ching* (周易, also known as the "I Ching" or "Zhou Yi"). They illustrate how, at its zenith, Yin will transform into Yang, and Yang will transform into Yin. Therefore, not only does stagnation give rise to flow, but flow will also eventually lead to stagnation. This is the ebb and flow of the ever-transforming universe.

47  The 11th hexagram, which represents flow, is depicted by the trigram for heaven, situated below the trigram for earth. This hexagram represents the descent of Yang (heaven) and the ascent of Yin (earth). Flow is achieved only by the interaction of Yin and Yang. Yang naturally flows upwards, while Yin flows downwards. If Yang, originally located above Yin, doesn't descend, there will be no interaction, and hence no flow. According to the *Yi Ching*, heaven's material manifestation is Fire, while earth's material manifestation is Water. Therefore, the phrase "Water energy flows upwards and Fire energy flows downwards" signifies the interaction and flow of Yin and Yang within the body.

48  Unlike the other formulae in this book, Lee Je-ma doesn't provide further information about *Si Shun Tang* (Four Ingredients Decoction to Smooth the Qi), and so its ingredients are provided here: Chuan Bei Mu (*Bulbus Fritillariae Cirrhosae*) 30g, Zhi Jie Geng (*Radix Platycodi*) 30g, Chai Hu (*Radix Bupleuri*) 30g and Zhi Gan Cao (*Radix Glycyrrhizae*) 15g. This formula was originally introduced by Xue Ji (1528) in his text *Waike Fahui* (*The Development of External Medicine*).

論曰張仲景所論에 厥陰病은 初無腹痛下利等證而六七日에 猝然而
厥하야 手足이 逐冷則此는 非陰證之類也오 乃少陰人이 太陽傷風하야
惡寒, 發熱, 汗自出之證이 正邪相持日久하야 當解가 不解而變爲此證
也니 此證은 當謂之太陽病厥陰證也니라. 此證에 不必用當歸四逆湯 桂麻
各半湯하며 而當用蔘茰湯 人蔘吳茱茰湯 獨蔘八物湯이오 不當用大承氣
湯하며 而當用巴豆니라.

Zhang Zhongjing referred to the initial stage of Jue Yin as a Yin category illness, which after six to seven days of Shang Han illness transfers from abdominal pain and diarrhea to sudden coldness of the extremities. From my perspective, this is not a Yin category illness, but instead the Tai Yang Shang Feng syndrome of the So Eum Individual, also characterized by simultaneous chills and fever, and spontaneous sweating.[49] This syndrome occurs after the *Zheng Qi* battles the pathogenic influence for days without rest, and should accurately be referred to as the Tai Yang Jue Yin stage illness. It should be treated with *Sam Yu Tang* (Lee Je-ma's Ginseng and Evodia Fruit Decoction), *San Wei Shen Yu Tang* (Three Flavors Ginseng and Evodia Fruit Decoction), or *Doksam Palmul Tang* (Lee Je-ma's Added Ginseng Eight Ingredient Gentlemen Decoction) rather than *Dang Gui Si Ni Tang* (Tangkuei Decoction for Frigid Extremities) or *Gui Ma Ge Ban Tang* (Combined Cinnamon Twig and Ephedra Decoction) [as mentioned above]. Moreover, *Padu Dan* (Lee Je-ma's Croton Seed Pill) should be used in place of *Da Cheng Qi Tang* (Major Order the Qi Decoction) [in case of restricted bowel flow].

凡少陰人이 外感病 六七日에 不得汗解而死者는 皆死於厥陰也니 四五
日에 觀其病勢하야 用黃芪桂枝湯 八物君子湯 三四貼하야 豫防이 可
也니라.

In general, the Jue Yin stage is the likeliest cause of death of a So Eum Individual who has battled with an External pathogen for six to seven days without sweating. To avoid this situation, administer three to five packets of *Huanggi Gyeji Tang* (Lee Je-ma's Cinnamon Twig Astragalus and Aconite Decoction) or *Palmul Gunja Tang* (Lee Je-ma's Eight Ingredient Gentlemen Decoction) for four to five days directly after detecting these symptoms.

49   In this sentence, Lee Je-ma distinguishes between the Jue Yin syndrome of the Tai Yang stage illness and the Jue Yin stage illness. The former syndrome is associated with Tai Yang stage symptoms such as chills, fever, and sweating. The latter syndrome includes fever but not sweating. Both syndromes, though, are associated with frigid extremities.

朱肱이 曰厥陰病 消渴은 氣上衝心하야 心中이 疼熱하고 飢不欲食하며 食則吐蚘니라.

Zhu Gong once said that Jue Yin syndrome is caused by the rebellious upward movement of *Xiao Ke*,[50] which slams against the chest causing chest pain and heat. A voracious appetite with the inability to eat is also a symptom of Jue Yin. In this case, parasite-infested vomit will occur after attempting to eat.

龔信이 曰傷寒에 有吐蚘者는 雖有大熱이나 忌下니 涼藥이 犯之면 必死라. 蓋胃中에 有寒則蚘가 不安所而上膈하나니 大凶之兆也니 急用理中湯이니라.

Gong Xin once stated that even if there is high fever accompanied by the vomiting of parasites, laxatives (Cold-natured herbs) should be avoided. If laxatives are used in this case, they will induce a fatal reaction with stomach coldness, causing internal parasites to escape upwards towards the chest. *Li Zhong Tang* (Regulate the Middle Decoction) should be prescribed immediately if so.

論曰此證에 當用理中湯하야 日三四服하고 又連日服하라. 或理中湯에 加陳皮 官桂 白何首烏니라. 重病과 危證에 藥不三四服則藥力이 不壯也오 又不連日服則病加於少愈也거나 或病愈而不快也니라. 連日服者는 或日再服하거나 或日一服 或日三服 或二三日連日服 或五六日連日服하고 或數十日連日服이니 觀其病勢하야 圖之니라.

From my perspective, three to four packs per day of *Li Zhong Tang* (Regulate the Middle Decoction) should be prescribed in this situation, with the addition of Chen Pi (*Pericarpium Citri Reticulatae*), Rou Gui (*Cortex Cinnamomi*), and Bai He Shou Wu (*Radix Polygoni Multiflori Alba*).[51] For serious and life-threatening situations, the effect will be limited if herbal tea is not continually ingested at least three to four times a day. At a lesser dosage, the symptoms will wax and wane. Whether administered throughout the day, once a day, two to three times a day, one to three days, five to six days, or even 20 or more days, this formula should be continued, no matter what, until the symptoms have clearly subsided.

---

50   *Xiao Ke* (消渴) translates literally as "wasting and thirsting" and closely resembles the symptoms of diabetes. There are three levels of *Xiao Ke*: *Shang Xiao Ke* (Upper *Jiao Xiao Ke*), *Zhong Xiao Ke* (Middle *Jiao Xiao Ke*), and *Xia Xiao Ke* (Lower *Jiao Xiao Ke*). *Shang Xiao Ke* involves the wasting away of lung Yin energy causing excessive thirst. *Zhong Xiao Ke* involves the wasting away of stomach Yin energy, causing excessive appetite with inability to eat. *Xia Xiao Ke* involves the wasting away of kidney Yin energy, leading to excessive urination.

51   When the above three ingredients are added to *Li Zhong Tang* (Regulate the Middle Decoction), Lee Je-ma also refers to it as *Baek Hasuoh Buja Yijung Tang* (Lee Je-ma's Fleeceflower and Aconite Regulate the Middle Decoction).

Table 6.5: Comparison between the three kidney Heat-induced Exterior syndromes of the So Eum Individual

| Syndrome | Tai Yang | Tai Yang Shang Feng (Tai Yang Jue Yin syndrome) | Yang Ming stage | | Jue Yin stage (transferred from Tai Yang—life threatening) |
|---|---|---|---|---|---|
| | | | Ul Kwang syndrome | Mang Yang syndrome | |
| Symptoms | Simultaneous chills and light fever, rhinitis | | No chills, or slight chills with increasing fever | | High fever |
| | No sweating | Spontaneous sweating | No sweating | Spontaneous sweating | No sweating |
| | No signs of internal issue such as constipation or difficult urination | Frigid extremities, contraction of scrotum | Stage 1: Emotional instability<br>Stage 2: *Wei Jia Shi* syndrome (constipation)<br>Stage 3: Tidal fever, incoherent speech, shortness of breath, and stupor | Stage 1: *Bi Yao* syndrome—light spontaneous sweating, little to no fever<br>Stage 2: Increasing fever and sweating<br>Stage 3: Copious sweating with high fever and difficult urination | Frigid extremities, contraction of scrotum<br>Critical stage: Vomiting of parasites, heat and pain in chest<br>(likeliest cause of death for the So Eum Individual) |
| Formula prescribed | *Gui Zhi Tang* (Cinnamon Twig Decoction)<br>*Gwakhyang Jeonggi San* (Lee Je-Ma's Agastache Powder to Rectify the Qi) | *Sam Yu Tang* (Lee Je-ma's Ginseng and Evodia Fruit Decoction)<br>*San Wei Shen Yu Tang* (Three Flavors Ginseng and Evodia Fruit Decoction), or *Doksam Palmul Tang* (Lee Je-Ma's Added Ginseng Eight Ingredient Gentlemen Decoction)<br>*Padu Dan* (if constipated) | *Palmul Gunja Tang* (Lee Je-ma's Eight Ingredient Gentlemen Decoction)<br>*Seungyang Ikgi Tang* (Lee Je-ma's Raise the Yang and Benefit the Qi Decoction)<br>*Padu Dan* (if constipated) | *Huanggi Gyeji Buja Tang* (Lee Je-ma's Cinnamon Twig Astralagus and Aconite Decoction)<br>*Insam Gyeji Buja Tang* (Lee Je-ma's Ginseng Cinnamon Twig and Aconite Decoction)<br>*Padu Dan* (if constipated) | *Baek Hasuob Buja Yijung Tang* (Lee Je-ma's Fleeceflower and Aconite Regulate the Middle Decoction) |
| Etiology (imbalanced *Song* emotion plus...) | External Cold invasion with *Zheng* (righteous) *Qi* still strong and intact | *Zheng Qi* battles the stagnant pathogenic influence for days without rest | Significant blockage of kidney Yang due to external Cold invasion with Yang still intact | External Cold invasion with prior spleen Yang deficiency | *Zheng Qi* battles the stagnant pathogenic influence for 6–7 days without sweating |

*Section 2*

# The Seo Eum Individual's Stomach Cold Causing Interior Cold Syndrome[1]

## 少陰人胃受寒裏寒病

張仲景이 曰太陰之證은 腹滿而吐하며 食不下하며 自利益甚하고 時腹自
痛이니라. 腹滿時痛하며 吐利不渴者는 爲太陰이니 宜四逆湯 理中湯이오
腹滿이 不減하며 減不足言하면 大承氣湯이니라. 傷寒에 自利不渴者는
屬太陰이니 以其臟有寒故也라 當溫之니 宜用四逆湯이니라 太陰證은 腹
痛, 自利, 不渴이니 宜理中湯 理中丸이오 四順理中湯丸도 亦主之니라.

According to Zhang Zhongjing, Tai Yin stage illness is marked by pain and fullness of the abdomen, postprandial vomiting, inability of food to descend through the digestive tract, and acute uncontrollable diarrhea. Zhang Zhongjing prescribed *Si Ni Tang* (Frigid Extremities Decoction) or *Li Zhong Tang* (Regulate the Middle Decoction) for the Tai Yin syndrome marked by abdominal distension with occasional pain, vomiting, and diarrhea without thirst. He prescribed *Da Cheng Qi Tang* (Major Order the Qi Decoction) when abdominal distension decreases only slightly or not at all. Uncontrollable diarrhea during Shang Han illness is due to the Internal Cold of the Tai Yin stage, for which warming methods should be introduced with *Si Ni Tang* (Frigid Extremities Decoction). The abdominal distension, uncontrollable diarrhea, and a lack of thirst of Tai Yin can be addressed with *Li Zhong Tang* (Regulate the Middle Decoction), *Li Zhong Wan* (Regulate the Middle Pill), or *Si Shun Li Zhong Tang* (Four Ingredients Decoction to Smooth and Regulate the Middle).

論曰右證에 當用理中湯 四順理中湯 四逆湯而古方이 草刱에 藥力이 不
具備일새니 此證에는 當用白何烏理中湯 白何烏附子理中湯이오 腹
滿不減하며 減不足言者는 有痼冷積滯也니 當用巴豆而不當用大承氣
湯이니라.

From my perspective, even though *Li Zhong Tang* (Regulate the Middle Decoction), *Si Shun Li Zhong Tang* (Four Ingredients Decoction to Smooth and Regulate the Middle), and *Si Ni Tang* (Frigid Extremities Decoction) are appropriate in cases of Tai Yin stage syndrome, they are based on outdated ancient herbal theories. For the aforementioned symptoms, I suggest the use of *Baek Hasuoh Yijung Tang* (Lee Je-ma's Fleeceflower Regulate the Middle Decoction) and *Baek Hasuoh Buja Yijung*

---

1    The So Eum Individual's Interior Cold syndrome is primarily due to the imbalance and sinking of joy, their *Jung* emotion, and the feeling of being neglected or unassisted. This affects the weakest area of their body, the Mid-Upper *Jiao*.

*Tang* (Lee Je-ma's Fleeceflower and Aconite Regulate the Middle Decoction). In cases of abdominal Cold stagnation[2] and distension, Ba Dou (*Semen Crotonis*), rather than *Da Cheng Qi Tang* (Major Order the Qi Decoction), is preferred.

張仲景이 曰病發於陰而反下之면 因作痞니라. 傷寒에 嘔而發熱者가 若心下滿이나 不痛하면 此爲痞니 半夏瀉心湯을 主之하고 胃虛氣逆者도 亦主之니라. 下後에 下利를 日數十行하고 穀不化하며 腹雷鳴하고 心下痞硬하며 乾嘔心煩은 此乃結熱이라. 乃胃中이 虛하야 客氣가 上逆故也니 甘草瀉心湯을 主之니라.

According to Zhang Zhongjing, *Bi* syndrome, characterized by a Shang Han illness accompanied by vomiting, fever, and epigastric fullness without pain, will occur if a Yin stage illness is treated with diuretic herbs, and should be addressed with *Ban Xia Xie Xin Tang* (Pinellia Decoction to Drain the Epigastrium). Stomach weakness and vexation are also symptoms of *Bi* syndrome and can be treated with this formula.

Continual diarrhea (over ten times) throughout a 24-hour period, indigestion, epigastric *Bi Ying* syndrome, incoherent speech, and fullness with vexation in the chest indicate the blockage of Internal Heat after the improper use of diuretic herbs. These symptoms may also be initiated by the attack of external "Guest Qi" which enters an already energetically compromised stomach, causing the reversal of "Host Qi." In this situation *Gan Cao Xie Xin Tang* (Licorice Decoction to Drain the Epigastrium) can be applied.

太陰證 下利淸穀을 若發汗則必脹滿이니 發汗後에 腹脹滿에는 宜用厚朴半夏湯이니라. 汗解後에 胃不和하야 心下痞硬하며 脇下에 有水氣하고 腹中雷鳴하며 下利者는 生薑瀉心湯을 主之니라. 傷寒에 下利하고 心下痞硬이어늘 服瀉心湯後에 以他藥으로 下之하니 利不止라 與理中湯하되 利益甚하면 赤石脂禹餘粮湯을 主之니라.

[According to Zhang Zhongjing,] Tai Yin stage syndrome is characterized by diarrhea with particles of undigested food. If diaphoretics are used here, the abdomen will be become distended and full. In this case, *Hou Po Ban Xia Tang* (Prepared Pinellia and Magnolia Bark Decoction) should be employed. If there is vexation with an unsettled stomach, epigastric *Bi Ying* syndrome, water retention below the ribcage, and borborygmus with diarrhea, then *Sheng Jiang Xie Xin Tang* (Ginger Decoction to Drain the Epigastrium) is chosen. Diarrhea with epigastric *Bi Ying* syndrome calls for *Xie Xin Tang* (Drain the Epigastrium Decoction).[3] In case of incessant

---

2   The Hot-natured Yang energy of the stomach is in charge of warming the entire body, yet the spleen and stomach-deficient So Eum Individual may experience Cold accumulation in the abdomen due to a lack of Yang energy.

3   Lee Je-ma doesn't give reference to *Xie Xin Tang* elsewhere in this text and so its ingredients are mentioned here: Da Huang (*Radix et Rhizoma Rhei*) 6g, Huang Qin (*Radix Scutellaria*) 3g, and Huang Lian (*Rhizoma Coptidis*) 3g. Source: Zhang Zhongjing's *Jin Gui* (*Golden Cabinet*).

diarrhea after taking diuretics, *Li Zhong Tang* (Regulate the Middle Decoction) is administered. If diarrhea still doesn't cease, then prescribe *Chi Shi Zhi Yu Yu Liang Tang* (Halloysite and Limonite Decoction).

論曰病發於陰而反下之云者는 病發於胃弱이니 當用藿香正氣散 而反用 大黃下之謂也라 麻黃 大黃은 自是太陰人藥이오 非少陰人藥則少陰人 病에 無論表裏하고 麻黃 大黃으로 汗下는 元非可論이라. 少陰人病에 下 利淸穀者는 積滯가 自解也니 太陰證下利淸穀者는 當用藿香正氣散 香砂 養胃湯 薑朮寬中湯하야 溫胃而降陰하고 少陰證下利淸穀者는 當用官桂 附子理中湯하야 健脾而降陰하니라. 藿香正氣散 香砂六君子湯 寬中湯 蘇 合元은 皆張仲景의 瀉心湯之變劑也니 此는 所謂靑於藍者 出於藍이라 噫라 靑雖自靑이나 若非其藍이면 靑何得靑이리오.

In my experience, if diuretic herbs, such as Da Huang (*Radix et Rhizoma Rhei*), are mistakenly applied during a Yin stage illness with weakened stomach energy, then *Gwakhyang Jeonggi San* (Lee Je-ma's Agastache Powder to Rectify the Qi) should be given as an antidote. Both Ma Huang (*Ephedra Sinica*) and Da Huang are herbs appropriate for the Tae Eum Individual. The So Eum Individual's illness is differentiated according to External and Internal influence, making it unnecessary to simply promote sweat or diarrhea with these herbs.[4] For the So Eum Individual, diarrhea with particles of indigested food is a sign that the body is recovering from accumulation and stagnation in the digestive tract. If there is diarrhea with undigested food particles during an illness of the Tai Yin stage, then *Gwakhyang Jeonggi San* (Lee Je-ma's Agastache Powder to Rectify the Qi), *Hyangsa Yangwi Tang* (Lee Je-ma's Cyperus and Hawthorn Enliven the stomach Decoction), or *Gangchul Gwanjung Tang* (Lee Je-ma's Ginger and Atractylodes Harmonize the Middle Decoction)[5] should be used to warm the stomach and descend the Yin energy. If there is diarrhea with undigested food particles during an illness of the Shao Yin stage, then *Gwangye Buja Yijung Tang* (Lee Je-ma's Cinnamon and Aconite Regulate the Middle Decoction) should be used to strengthen the spleen and descend the Yin energy. The four formulae *Huo Xiang Zheng Qi San* (Agastache Powder to Rectify the Qi), *Xiang Sha Liu Jun Zi Tang* (Six Gentlemen Decoction with Aucklandia and Amomum), *Kuan Zhong Tang* (Smooth the Middle Decoction), and *Su He Xiang Wan* (Liquid Styrax Pill) are variations of Zhang Zhongjing's *Xie Xin Tang* and can

---

4　Since the Tai Yin stage disorder of the So Eum Individual is considered an Internal illness, techniques that expel pathogenic influence from the Exterior, such as diaphoresis, or clear Heat from the Yang Ming stage through promoting bowel movement, are inappropriate.

5　Lee Je-ma doesn't give reference to *Gangchul Gwanjung Tang* elsewhere in this text and so its ingredients are mentioned here: Bai He Shou Wu (*Radix Polygoni Multiflori Alba*) 4g, Chi He Shou Wu (*Radix Polygoni Mult. Rubens*) 4g, Gao Liang Jiang (*Rhizoma Alpiniae Officinarum*) 4g, Gan Jiang (*Rhizoma Zingiberis*) 4g, Chen Pi (*Pericarpium Citri Reticulatae*) 4g, Qing Pi (*Pericarpium Citri Ret. Viridae*) 4g, Xiang Fu (*Rhizoma Cyperi*) 4g, Yi Zhi Ren (*Fructus Alpiniae Oxyphyllae*) 4g, Da Zao (*Fructus Zizyphi Jujubae*) 2 Pieces, and Bai Zhu (*Radix Atractylodis Macrocephalae*) 8–20g. Source: *Sasang Shinpyun (Revised Collection of Sasang Materia Medica)*.

be compared to the color of indigo, which although it is derived from the color blue, is even bluer.[6] Without indigo, how would we ever know the extent of blueness?[7]

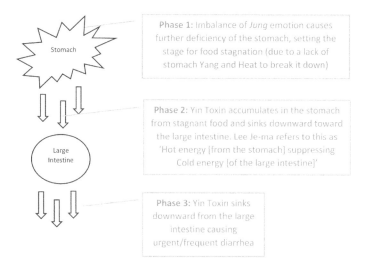

*Figure 6.5: The Tai Yin syndrome of the So Eum Individual*

張仲景이 日傷寒에 陰毒之病은 面靑하고 身痛如被杖하니 五日은 可治오 七日은 不治니라.

According to Zhang Zhongjing, cyanotic complexion and pain that feels like the entire body was beaten with a stick is caused by the Shang Han-induced *Yin Duo*[8] accumulation. This illness can be effectively treated even after five days of onset, but is incurable after seven days.

---

6    Lee Je-ma correlates these four modified formulae with the color indigo and Zhang Zhongjing's original formula, *Xie Xin Tang* (Drain the Epigrastrium Decoction), with the color blue. Although indigo may be considered blue, he refers to it as bluer than blue. Even though they appear similar, the former formulae are superior to that of *Xie Xin Tang*. Yet according to Lee Je-ma, even these formulae cannot compare to the effects of *Gwangye Buja Yijung Tang*.

7    Stagnation and accumulation that occur in the stomach will resolve if Yin energy flows downwards. One major difference between Tai Yin stage and Shao Yin stage formulae is the use of Fu Zi, which is needed to strengthen the spleen during the latter illness, and Sheng Jiang (*Rhizoma Zingiberis Recens*), Xiang Fu (*Rhizoma Cyperi*), and Huo Xiang (*Herba Pogostemonis*), which focus on warming the stomach during the former illness.

8    *Yin Duo* (陰毒), translated as "Yin toxin," is the accumulation of turbid energy and fluid within the body due to stagnation of food, phlegm, and/or Cold.

李┌이 曰三陰病이 深하면 必變爲陰毒이니 其證이 四肢厥冷하고 吐
利하나 不渴하며 靜踡而臥하며 甚則咽痛鄭聲하고 加以頭痛頭汗하며 眼
睛이 內痛하야 不欲見光하며 面脣指甲이 靑黑하고 身如被杖이니라. 又
此證은 面靑白黑하며 四肢厥冷하고 多睡니라.

According to Li Ting, if severe, the three Yin stage illnesses[9] eventually lead to
*Yin Duo* accumulation, which is marked by coldness of the extremities, vomiting,
diarrhea, and a lack of thirst. The body will curl up into a ball, and in severe cases,
throat pain with incoherent speech, headaches, sweating from the hair follicles
of the head, painful pupils with an aversion to light, dark blue lips, fingers, and
facial complexion, and body pain that feels like the entire body was beaten with a
stick. This syndrome may include a pale, bluish, or darker complexion with cold
extremities, and a constant desire to sleep.

論曰右證에 當用人蔘桂皮湯 人蔘附子理中湯이니라.

From my perspective, this syndrome can be treated with *Ren Shen Gui Zhi Tang*
(Cinnamon Twig Decoction with Ginseng) or *Li Zhong Tang* (Regulate the Middle
Decoction) with added Ren Shen (*Radix Ginseng*) and Fu Zi (*Radix Aconiti*).[10]

張仲景이 曰傷寒에 直中陰經은 初來에 無頭痛 無身熱 無渴하며 怕寒踡
臥하야 沈重欲眠하며 脣靑厥冷하며 脈微而欲絶하며 或脈伏이니 宜四逆
湯이니라. 四逆者는 四肢逆冷也니라.

According to Zhang Zhongjing, the first stage of Shang Han illness, which directly
enters the Yin channels, is marked by headache and fever without sweat, chills,
desire to lie down and curl up in a ball, stupor, fatigue, cyanotic lips, coldness
of the extremities, and a minute or hiding pulse (as if it is about to disappear).
He recommended the use of *Si Ni Tang* (Frigid Extremities Decoction) for this
syndrome to address extreme coldness of the extremities.

---

9    The three Yin stages refer to the Tai Yin, Shao Yin, and Jue Yin stages.

10   This formula is also referred in this text as *Doksam Buja Yijung Tang* (Lee Je-ma's Added Ginseng Regulate the
     Middle Decoction with Fu Zi).

論曰嘗治少陰人의 直中陰經하야 乾霍亂 關格之病할새 時屬中伏節
候라 少陰人 一人이 面部氣色이 或靑或白하야 如彈丸圈 四五點이 成
圈이로되 起居는 如常而坐於房室中倚壁하야 一身이 委靡無力而但欲
寐어늘 問其這間原委則曰數日前에 下利淸水一二行하고 仍爲便閉하야
至今爲兩晝夜로되 別無他故云어늘 問所飮食則曰食麥飯云하더라. 急用
巴豆如意丹하니 一半時刻에 其汗이 自人中穴出而達于面上하고 下利一
二度어늘 時當日暮에 觀其下利則淸水中에 雜穢物而出하더니 終夜에 下
利十餘行하고 翌日平明至日暮에 又十餘行下利하니 而淸穀麥粒이 皆如
黃豆大러라.

I once treated a So Eum Individual who, during the hottest period of the summer season, experienced a Shang Han illness that directly entered the Yin channels, leading to the onset of *Gan Huo Luan*[11] and *Guan Ge*[12] syndrome. He had a cyanotic complexion and what appeared to be four to five white spots randomly dispersed throughout his body that were shaped like small bullets. Although he was able to carry out day-to-day living, upon returning home, he always leaned against the wall, looking tired, and desired to sleep. Asked about the onset of his symptoms, he stated that the only event he could remember was having two bouts of watery diarrhea, afterwards becoming constant. This was followed by a two-week bout of constipation. He barely ate at all before this episode occurred. I immediately prescribed *Padu Yeowi Dan* (Lee Je-ma's Croton Seed Invigorate the Willpower Pill)[13] and within 30 minutes he started to sweat beneath his nose, at the *renzhong* (GV 26) acupuncture point location, which then spread throughout his face, and then experienced one or two bouts of diarrhea. I inspected his bowels after another bout of diarrhea later in the day and noticed that it was a greenish/blue color mixed with food byproduct. Throughout the evening, he had another ten bouts of diarrhea filled with undigested barley grains the size of a bean, making it apparent that this illness was due to food stagnation.

---

11  *Gan Huo Luan* (乾霍亂), translated literally as "dry heaves," is marked by sudden twisting pain in the stomach, with the urge to vomit and defecate to no avail.

12  *Guan Ge* (關格), translated literally as "trapped and blocked," is marked by sudden acute food stagnation causing blockage of blood and *Qi* in the chest leading to loss of consciousness.

13  This formula was originally introduced in the *Dongeui Bogam* (*Mirror of Eastern Medicine*), a Korean medical text published in 1610 and authored by Heo Jun.

其病이 爲食滯인 故로 連三日을 絶不穀食하고 日所食은 但進好熟冷一
二碗이러니 至第三日平明하야 病人이 面色則無不顯明而一身이 皆冷
하고 頭頸이 墜下하야 去地二三寸而不能仰擧하니 病證이 更重이라. 計
出無聊하야 仔細點檢病人一身則手足膀胱腰腹이 皆如氷冷하고 臍下
全腹이 堅硬如石而胸腹上中脘에 熱氣熏騰하야 炙手可熱하니 最爲可
觀이라.

For three days following this episode of food stagnation, he had absolutely no
appetite and ingested only water mixed with scorched rice.[14] On the third
day, his facial complexion improved but his whole body started to feel cold and
his neck drooped forward as if he could not lift his head.[15] It bewildered me that
his condition would suddenly take a turn for the worse. Careful examination
of his entire body showed that his hands, feet, bladder area, hips, and stomach
were as cold as ice and his lower abdomen was as hard as a rock. However,
there was a lot of Heat emanating from the *zhongwan* (CV 12) acupuncture point
location, which felt extremely Hot compared to his freezing cold hands.

至第五日平朝하야 一發吐淸沫而淸沫中에 雜米穀을 一朶而出하더니 自
此로 病勢가 大減하야 因進米飮聯服數碗하고 其翌日에 因爲粥食이러라
此病이 在窮村인 故로 未暇溫胃和解之藥이니라

To my surprise, on the fifth day he woke up in the middle of the night vomiting clear,
frothy fluid mixed with a single grain of rice. From that point onwards his condition
improved so much that he was able to eat several bowls of rice porridge over the next
few days. Since he was living in the middle of nowhere, it was impossible for me to
get hold of herbs that could warm his stomach.

其後에 又有少陰人 一人이 日下利數次而仍下淸水하고 全腹이 浮
腫이어늘 初用桂附藿陳理中湯에 倍加人蔘 官桂 各二錢, 附子二錢 或一
錢하야 日四服하고 數日後則日三服하야 至十餘日하니 遂下利淸穀이 連
三日에 三四十行而浮腫이 大減하니라.

Following this episode, another So Eum Individual had continuous bouts of
clear watery diarrhea with abdominal edema. At first I prescribed *Gyebu Gwakjin
Yijung Tang* (Lee Je-ma's Cinnamon Bark, Aconite, Agastache, and Tangerine Peel
Decoction to Regulate the Middle)[16] four times a day while doubling the dose of

---

14    Glutinous rice prepared by this method is called Nu Rung Ji (누룽지) in Korean. Rice is usually cooked with
      a stone pot until it hardens and then is scraped off and mixed with water while still hot.

15    Drooping forward of the neck is a hallmark sign of extreme Yang deficiency and is most commonly associated
      with advanced illness of the So Eum Individual.

16    Lee Je-ma doesn't give reference to *Gyebu Gwakjin Yijung Tang* elsewhere in this text and so its ingredients
      are mentioned here: Ren Shen (*Radix Ginseng*) 12g, Bai Zhu (*Radix Atractylodis Macrocephalae*) 8g, Pao Gan
      Jiang (*Rhizoma Zingiberis Preparata*) 8g, Rou Gui (*Cortex Cinnamomi*) 8g, Bai Shao Yao (*Radix Paeoniae
      Lactiflorae*) 4g, Chen Pi (*Pericarpium Citri Reticulatae*) 4g, Zhi Gan Cao (*Radix Gylcyrrhizae*) 4g, Huo Xiang
      (*Herba Pogostemonis*) 4g, Sha Ren (*Fructus Amomi*) 4g, and Pao Fu Zi (*Radix Aconiti Lateralis Praeparata*)
      4–8g. Source: *Sasang Jinryo Euijon* (*The Collection of Medical Prescription in Sasang Medicine*).

Ren Shen (*Radix Ginseng*) and Rou Gui (*Cortex Cinnamomi*) to 7.5g, with 3.75–7.5g of Fu Zi (*Radix Aconiti*). After several days, I reduced the dose to three times a day for ten days. On the tenth day, after about 30 to 40 bouts of diarrhea, his abdominal edema improved tremendously.

又少陰人 小兒 一人이 下利淸水하고 面色이 靑黯하며 氣陷如睡커늘 用 獨蔘湯에 加生薑 二錢 陳皮 砂仁 各一錢하야 日三四服하니 數日後에 下 利十餘行하고 大汗而解하니라.

There was another So Eum infantile patient who was in a constant stupor and suffered from bluish-green watery diarrhea with a dark complexion and fatigue. After taking *Doksam Tang* (Lee Je-ma's Ginseng Decoction)[17] with 7.5g of Sheng Jiang (*Rhizoma Zingiberis Recens*) and 3.75g of Chen Pi (*Pericarpium Citri Reticulatae*) and Sha Ren (*Fructus Amomi*) for a few days (three to four doses a day), he experienced ten frequent bouts of diarrhea and intense sweating, shortly after which he completely recovered.

蓋少陰人 霍亂關格病에 得人中汗者는 始免危也오 食滯大下者는 次免 危也오 自然能吐者는 快免危也니 禁進粥食하고 但進好熟冷하며 或米飮 者는 扶正抑邪之良方也니라. 宿滯之彌留者는 得好熟冷하야 乘熱溫進則 消火가 無異於飮食이리니 雖絶食二三四日이라도 不必爲慮니라.

Sweating at the *renzhong* (GV 26) acupuncture point location after the life-threatening symptoms of *Huo Luan* and/or *Guan Ge* syndrome is a sign of recovery. The occurrence of diarrhea or vomit after acute food stagnation is another sign of recovery. It is also advisable in such situations to refrain from eating except for the intake of rice gruel or scorched rice soup to strengthen the organs and ward off invasion from external pathogen. One should not have to worry even if there is no additional food intake for two, three, or even four days if warm soup made from scorched rice is ingested, because it can temporarily supply basic nutritional requirement during initial recovery.

張仲景이 曰少陰病은 脈微細하며 但欲寐ㅣ니라. 傷寒에 欲吐하나 不 吐하며 心煩하며 但欲寐라가 五六日에 自利而渴者는 屬少陰하니 小 便이 色白이면 宜四逆湯이니라. 少陰病에 身體痛하며 手足寒하며 骨 節痛하며 脈沈者는 附子湯을 主之니라. 下利하고 腹脹滿하며 身體疼 痛하면 先溫其裏하고 乃攻其表니 溫裏에는 宜四逆湯이오 攻表에는 宜 桂枝湯이니라.

Zhang Zhongjing stated that Shao Yin stage illness is marked by a minute pulse and constant desire to sleep. It also may manifest as a futile desire to vomit, fullness in the chest, five to six days of constant diarrhea, and thirst. If white-colored urine

---

17  *Doksam Tang* (Lee Je-ma's Ginseng Decoction) consists of 40–60g of Ren Shen (*Radix Ginseng*). Source: *Dongeui Bogam* (*Mirror of Eastern Medicine*).

accompanies the above symptoms, *Si Ni Tang* (Frigid Extremities Decoction) should be administered. *Fu Zi Tang* (Prepared Aconite Decoction) should be prescribed when the Shao Yin stage illness is accompanied by general body pain, cold hands and feet, painful joints, and a deep pulse. If diarrhea occurs with abdominal fullness and general body pain, it is first necessary to focus internally and warm the body with *Si Ni Tang* before moving onwards to treat the external aspect of Shao Yin illness, which is usually treated with *Gui Zhi Tang* (Cinnamon Twig Decoction).

論曰右證에 當用官桂附子理中湯이니라.

From my perspective, *Gwangye Buja Yijung Tang* (Lee Je-ma's Cinnamon and Aconite Regulate the Middle Decoction) should be prescribed for all of the above-described syndromes.

張仲景이 曰少陰病始得之에 反發熱하며 脈沈者는 麻黃附子細辛湯을 主之니라. 少陰病 一二日에 口中和하고 背惡寒이면 宜附子湯이니라. 少陰病 二三日에는 用麻黃附子甘草湯하야 微發之니 以二三日無證인 故로 微發汗也니 無證은 謂無吐利厥證也니라.

According to Zhang Zhongjing, if a Shao Yin stage illness is accompanied by the early onset of fever with a deep pulse, then *Ma Huang Fu Zi Xi Xin Tang* (Ephedra, Asarum, and Prepared Aconite Decoction) should be used. If there are chills but thirst after one to two days of Shao Yin illness, then *Fu Zi Tang* (Prepared Aconite Decoction) is preferred. If no vomiting, cold extremities, or diarrhea occur after two to three days of Shao Yin stage illness, then the mild diaphoretic action of *Ma Huang Fu Zi Gan Cao Tang* (Ephedra, Prepared Aconite, and Licorice Decoction) is to be employed.

下利하고 脈沈而遲하며 其人이 面小赤하며 身有微汗하며 下利淸穀이면 必鬱冒汗出而解니라 病人이 必微厥하리니 所以然者는 其面이 戴陽下虛인 故也니라. 少陰病에 脈細沈數은 病爲在裏니 不可發汗이오 少陰病에 但厥無汗而强發之면 必動其血하야 或從口鼻하며 或從目出하나니 是爲下厥上渴이니 難治니라.

[Zhang Zhongjing also stated that] if the patient experiences diarrhea with undigested food, a slightly reddish complexion, light sweating, and a deep/slow pulse, recovery is just around the corner. However, in the process, they will inevitably experience vertigo and further sweating. The patient will also have cold hands and feet with a slightly reddish complexion from weakness of the Lower *Jiao*. During a Shao Yin stage illness, a narrow, deep, and rapid pulse indicates that the illness is located internally. The absence of sweating further indicates an internal illness. If sweating is promoted in this situation, then the blood will be stirred up and exuded from the mouth, nose, or eyes, a syndrome referred to as "Lower Cold and Upper Exhaustion" that is difficult to treat.

**Table 6.6: Tai Yin syndrome**

| Syndrome | Due to | Common symptoms | Accompanying symptoms | Treated with | Approach |
|---|---|---|---|---|---|
| Tai Yin stage (Scenario A) | Constant overthinking and worry with stomach weakness and food stagnation causing Yin toxin accumulation, which sinks down to the intestines | | Stomach discomfort, vomiting after food intake, inability of food to descend through the digestive tract, abdominal distension, fatigue | **Non-acute:**<br><br>*Baek Hasuoh Yijung Tang* (Lee Je-ma's Fleeceflower Regulate the Middle Decoction)<br><br>**Acute:**<br><br>*Baek Hasuoh Buja Yijung Tang* (Lee Je-ma's Fleeceflower and Aconite Regulate the Middle Decoction)<br><br>Ba Dou (*Semen Crotonis*) | Strengthen and warm the stomach and encourage descent of Yin |
| Tai Yin stage (Scenario B) | Mistaken employment of Da Huang (laxatives/diuretics) or Ma Huang (diaphoretics) during a Yin stage illness and weakened stomach energy | Food stagnation, urgent diarrhea, full sensation of abdomen, no thirst | This formula is prescribed for the onset of Tai Yin stage symptoms due to excessive use of laxatives, diuretics, and/or diaphoretics | *Gwakhyang Jeonggi San* (Lee Je-ma's Agastache Powder to Rectify the Qi) | |
| Tai Yin stage (Scenario C) | Stomach weakness causing indigestion | | Diarrhea mixed with undigested food particles (The presence of food particles in diarrhea indicates improving condition) | *Gwakhyang Jeonggi San* (Lee Je-ma's Agastache Powder to Rectify the Qi)<br><br>*Hyangsa Yangwi Tang* (Lee Je-ma's Cyperus and Hawthorn Enliven the stomach Decoction)<br><br>*Gangchul Gwanjung Tang* (Lee Je-ma's Ginger and Atractylodes Harmonize the Middle Decoction) | |

143

| Syndrome | Due to | Common symptoms | Accompanying symptoms | Treated with | Approach |
|---|---|---|---|---|---|
| Tai Yin stage (Scenario D) | (A) Epidemic onset of Tai Yin stage disorder caused by direct transfer of pathogen<br><br>or<br><br>(B) Transfer of pathogen to Tai Yin stage after seven to eight days battling Shang Han | | Jaundice, difficult urination, abdominal *Bi* syndrome, edema | *Yin Chen Ju Pi Tang* (Artemisia Yinchenhao and Tangerine Peel Decoction)<br><br>*Yin Chen Fu Zi Tang* (Artemisia Yinchenhao and Poria Decoction)<br><br>*Yin Chen Si Ni Tang* (Artemisia Yinchenhao Decoction for Frigid Extremities) | Strengthen and warm the stomach and encourage descent of Yin |
| | | Food stagnation, urgent diarrhea, full sensation of abdomen, no thirst | | **Epidemic and acute disorders:**<br><br>*Zhang Dan Wan* (Epidemic Jaundice Pill)<br><br>Ba Dou (*Semen Crotonis*)<br><br>**Promote urination:**<br><br>Gan Jiang (*Rhizoma Zingiberis Officinalis*), Liang Jiang (*Rhizoma Alpiniae Officinarum*), Qing Pi (*Pericarpium Citri Ret. Viridae*), Chen Pi (*Pericarpium Citri Reticulatae*), Xiang Fu Zi (*Rhizoma Cyperi*), and Yi Zhi Ren (*Fructus Alpiniae Oxyphyllae*) | |

| Stage (Scenario) | Description | Symptoms | Formula |
|---|---|---|---|
| Tai Yin stage (Scenario E) | Acute onset of Tai Yin stage illness with significant stomach weakness and Cold accumulation leading to *Bi Ying* syndrome | Vexation with an unsettled stomach, (subjective) fullness of the epigastric area, a feeling of water retention below the ribs | *Gyeji Banha Senggang Tang* (Lee Je-ma's Cinnamon Pinellia and Ginger Decoction)<br>*Jok Hasuoh Guanjung Tang* (Lee Je-ma's Fleeceflower Smooth the Middle Decoction)<br>*San Wu Bai San* (Three Ingredients White Powder)<br>*Padu Dan* (Lee Je-ma's Croton Seed Pill) |
| Tai Yin stage (Scenario F) | Sudden acute onset of Tai Yin stage illness due to significant stomach deficiency (life threatening) | Continuous bouts of clear watery diarrhea with abdominal edema | *Gyebu Gwakjin Yijung Tang* (Lee Je-ma's Cinnamon Bark, Aconite, Agastache, and Tangerine Peel Decoction to Regulate the Middle) |
| Tai Yin stage (Scenario G)<br>This syndrome may also occur during Shao Yin stage illness (with thirst and fatigue) | Severe deficiency of stomach, food stagnation, and Cold toxin accumulation (life threatening) | Constant stupor, bluish-green watery diarrhea, dark complexion | *Doksam Tang* (Lee Je-ma's Ginseng Decoction) with 7.5g of Sheng Jiang (*Rhizoma Zingiberis Recens*) and 3.75 of Chen Pi (*Pericarpium Citri Reticulatae*) and Sha Ren (*Fructus Amomi*) |

論曰張仲景所論에 太陰病과 少陰病은 俱是少陰人의 胃氣虛弱 泄瀉之
證而太陰病泄瀉는 重證中 平證也오 少陰病泄瀉는 危證中 險證也니라.
人이 但見泄瀉하고 是一證而易於尋常做圖하나 少陰病泄瀉를 尋常做圖
則必不免死하리니 盖太陰病泄瀉는 大腸之泄瀉也오 少陰病泄瀉는 胃中
之泄瀉也니 太陰病泄瀉는 溫氣逐冷氣之泄瀉也오 少陰病泄瀉는 冷氣逼
溫氣之泄瀉也니라.

From my perspective, the Tai Yin and Shao Yin stage syndromes described by Zhang Zhongjing can be classified as the stomach deficiency with diarrhea syndrome of the So Eum Individual. Diarrhea during a Tai Yin stage illness can be seen as the least threatening stage of a serious illness, while diarrhea during a Shao Yin stage can be seen as an acute phase of a fatal illness.[18] Most of us would be inclined to think of diarrhea as a minor form of illness. However, overlooking the occurrence of diarrhea during a Shao Yin illness will definitely lead to fatality. For the most part, Tai Yin stage diarrhea correlates with the large intestine, while Shao Yin diarrhea correlates with the stomach.[19] The occurrence of diarrhea during the Tai Yin stage is the result of Warm energy chasing away Cold energy, while occurrence of diarrhea during the Shao Yin stage is the result of Cold energy suppressing Hot energy.[20]

少陰病이 欲自愈則面小赤하며 身有微汗하고 必鬱冒汗出而解인 故로 古
人이 有見於此하야 少陰病에 但厥無汗者를 亦以麻黃으로 强發汗하야
欲其自愈而反動其血하야 從口鼻出인 故로 於是乎 始爲戒懼하야 凡少陰
病에 不敢輕易用麻黃而少陰病始得之 一二日 二三日 初證에 以麻黃附子
甘草湯으로 微發之也니라 然이나 麻黃은 爲少陰病害藥則雖二三日 初
證이라도 必不可用麻黃發之也니라. 此證에 當用官桂附子理中湯이오 或
以桂枝로 易官桂니라.

[From my perspective] a slightly reddish complexion with minor sweating followed by vertigo and more intense sweating[21] indicates recovery from Shao Yin stage

---

18  Lee Je-ma classified illness into the following stages: moderate (輕, *kyung*), serious/significant (重, *jung*), and acute (急, *gup*). Each of these categories is further subdivided into non-life threatening (平, *pyung*), fatal/life threatening (危, *wi*), or critical (險, *hom*). He occasionally combines "life threatening" and "critical" into one category (危險, *wi hom*) to emphasize the extent and severity of the disease.

19  The large intestine is the Yang correlate of the kidney, the So Eum Individual's strongest organ, while the stomach is the Yang correlate of the spleen, the So Eum Individual's weakest organ. Hence disease of the large intestine is less severe than disease of the stomach.

20  The excessively Cold energy of the So Eum Individual is the culprit behind both Tai Yin and Shao Yin illness. In a Shao Yin stage illness, the Cold energy is so excessive that it presses down against Hot energy, causing it to eventually explode/rebel upwards, leading to thirst and fever. During a Tai Yin stage illness, the Cold energy accumulates but is pushed away by the remaining Warm energy within the body.

21  In this case, Lee Je-ma refers to sweating at the *renzhong* (DU 26) acupuncture point location and/or dripping sweat from the hairline. Clammy sweating throughout the body, on the other hand, is associated with loss of Yang during the occurrence of *Mang Yang* (Yang Collapse) syndrome.

illness. In ancient times, a lack of sweating with cold hands and feet was treated with diaphoretics. This approach caused bleeding from the mouth and nose from excessive stirring up of the blood. Without addressing the precise reasons why, they stopped using Ma Huang (*Ephedra Sinica*) during Shao Yin disease. Only afterwards did they reintroduce its use in *Ma Huang Fu Zi Gan Cao Tang* (Ephedra, Prepared Aconite, and Licorice Decoction) to promote slight sweating after two to three days from initial onset of Shao Yin stage illness [to release the exterior portion of the Shang Han illness]. Even if applied in this way, the use of Ma Huang to release the exterior is harmful and inappropriate during a Shao Yin stage illness. The use of *Gwangye Buja Yijung Tang* (Lee Je-ma's Cinnamon and Aconite Regulate the Middle Decoction), however, is appropriate for the above condition. When applying this formula, depending on the situation, Gui Zhi (*Ramulus Cinnamomi Cassiae*) can be used instead of Rou Gui (*Cortex Cinnamomi*) [to place further emphasis on eliminating the external component of Shao Yin illness].

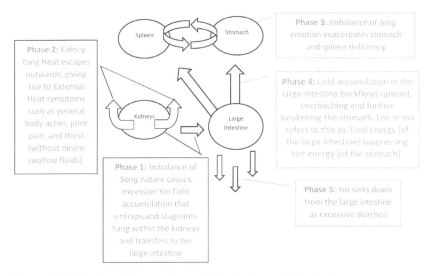

*Figure 6.6: The Shao Yin syndrome of the So Eum Individual*

少陰病은 初證에 因爲險證하야 繼而危證하니 此病은 初證에 早不辨證
而措置則危境이니라. 凡腹痛自利하며 無口渴하고 口中和者는 爲太陰
病이오 腹痛自利而有口渴하며 口中不和者는 爲少陰病이니 少陰病은 有
身體痛 骨節痛 表證하니 此則表裏俱病而大腸寒氣가 必勝胃中溫氣而上
升也라 太陰病은 無身體痛 骨節痛 表證하니 此는 則裏病이오 表不病而
胃中溫氣가 猶勝大腸寒氣而下降이니라.

From its onset, Shao Yin stage illness, which is marked by stomach pain, uncontrollable diarrhea, thirst, and an uncomfortable feeling inside the mouth, is classified as a life-threatening illness, and if not treated in a timely manner, will lead to fatality. Although some may consider the presence of general body aches and joint pain to be signs of an external illness,[22] Shao Yin stage illness is actually a combination of external and internal illness, as a result of large intestinal Cold that extinguishes the warmth of the stomach as it rises upwards. The internal nature of Tai Yin stage illness is marked by a lack of exterior symptoms such as general body and joint pain, and is due to stomach Heat that descends and eliminates the Cold of the intestines.[23]

張仲景이 曰少陰病에 自利純靑水하며 心下痛하며 口燥乾者는 宜大承氣
湯이니라.

Zhang Zhongjing recommends *Da Cheng Qi Tang* (Major Order the Qi Decoction) during Shao Yin stage illness when there is pure blue diarrhea, pain in the epigastric area, and dry mouth-related symptoms.

朱肱이 曰少陰病에 口燥 咽乾而渴은 宜急下之니 非若陽明이면 宜下而
可緩也니라.

According to Zhu Gong, if a Shao Yin stage illness is accompanied by thirst and a dry throat, then laxatives should be immediately prescribed. He asserts that the laxative approach during a Shao Yin stage illness, however, should be more subtle than during a Yang Ming stage illness.

---

22   Body aches and joint pain are primarily associated with Tai Yang and Yang Ming stage illnesses, but here they are accompanied by the classic signs of Shao Yin stage illness: fatigue, thirst with the inability to drink fluids, and diarrhea.

23   The So Eum Individual's strongest Yang organ, the large intestine, is the source of Cold energy, while the stomach, their weakest Yang organ, is the source of Hot energy. Shao Yin stage illness is marked by excessive coldness, which chases the Heat of the stomach away, while Tai Yin illness is caused by the stagnation of food in the stomach, leading to the accumulation of Heat due to friction. This Heat eventually travels down to the intestines and chases away its Cold energy. The former is more acute than the latter situation, since the So Eum Individual's Cold energy of the Intestine is much stronger and capable of causing greater damage to the system. In this case, intestinal Cold energy accumulates, causing Yang energy to stagnate and inhibiting its ascent. Instead, accumulation will cause Yin energy to rise up to the stomach.

李杲 東垣書에 曰少陰證은 口中辨이니 口中이 和者는 當溫이오 口中이 乾燥者는 當下니라. 少陰證은 下利辨이니 色不靑者는 當溫이오 色靑 者는 當下니라.

Li Gao states in his *Dong Yuan Shu* (*The Writings of Li Dongyuan*)[24] that the treatment approach for Shao Yin stage illness can be determined by mouth sensation. If there is no discomfort inside the mouth, then warming methods should be employed, but if the mouth feels dry and uncomfortable, then bowel movement should be promoted. He maintains that the treatment approach for Shao Yin stage illness can also be determined by the appearance of diarrhea. If its color is not bluish-green, then warming methods should be employed, but if the color of diarrhea is bluish-green, bowel movement should be promoted.

李ㄱ이 曰舌乾口燥하며 或下利靑水하다가 譫語便閉어든 宜小承氣湯이오 脣靑하고 四肢厥冷하며 指甲이 靑黑이어든 宜薑附湯이니라.

Li Ting once stated that *Xiao Cheng Qi Tang* (Minor Guide the Qi Decoction) should be used for mouth and tongue dryness, occasional clear watery diarrhea with constipation, and incoherent speech. *Jiang Fu Tang* (Ginger Aconite Decoction) should be used for cyanotic lips, Cold extremities, and bluish-black fingertips.

論曰下利靑水者를 欲下之則當用巴豆하고 溫之則當用官桂附子理 中湯하며 下利靑水라가 仍爲便閉者는 先用巴豆하고 後用薑朮寬中 湯이니라.

From my perspective, [when treating a Yin stage illness] Ba Dou (*Semen Crotonis*) together with *Gwangye Buja Yijung Tang* (Lee Je-ma's Cinnamon and Aconite Regulate the Middle Decoction) should be employed to promote warmth in cases of bluish-green diarrhea. If constipation follows bouts of bluish-green diarrhea then Ba Dou (*Semen Crotonis*) should be prescribed immediately to promote bowel flow, followed by *Gangchul Gwanjung Tang* (Lee Je-ma's Ginger and Atractylodes Harmonize the Middle Decoction).

**Table 6.7: General treatment strategy for bluish-green diarrhea**

| Bluish-green diarrhea followed by constipation | Bluish-green diarrhea without constipation |
| --- | --- |
| Ba Dou (*Semen Crotonis*) | |
| Ba Dou should be prescribed beforehand to promote bowel flow, followed by *Gangchul Gwanjung Tang* (Lee Je-ma's Ginger and Atractylodes Harmonize the Middle Decoction) | Ba Dou together with *Gwangye Buja Yijung Tang* (Cinnamon and Aconite Regulate the Middle Decoction) |

---

24 The *Dong Yuan Shu* (*The Writings of Li Dongyuan*), published in 1529, is a collection of twelve essays by various influential physicians including Li Gao, also known as Li Dongyuan (1180–1252).

**Table 6.8: Shao Yin syndrome**

| Syndrome | Due to | Common symptoms | Accompanying symptoms | Treated with | Approach |
|---|---|---|---|---|---|
| Tai Yang/Shao Yin stage (Scenario A) | Pathogenic influence directly entering the Shao Yin stage | | General body pain, cold hands and feet, painful joints, possible white-colored urine, and fever without sweating | *Gwangye Buja Yijung Tang* (Cinnamon and Aconite Regulate the Middle Decoction) | |
| Shao Yin stage (Scenario B) | Transfer of pathogenic influence from Tai Yin to Shao Yin stage | | Diarrhea with undigested food particles | *Gwangye Buja Yijung Tang* (Cinnamon and Aconite Regulate the Middle Decoction) | Strengthen spleen and stomach, raise Yang energy, and descend Yin energy |
| Shao Yin stage (Scenario C) This syndrome may also occur during critical Tai Yin stage illness (without thirst or fever) | Sudden acute onset of Shao Yin stage illness due to significant stomach and spleen deficiency (life threatening) | Minute pulse and constant desire to sleep, desire to vomit but to no avail, chest fullness, stomach pain, five to six days or more of constant uncontrollable diarrhea, fever, thirst, and an uncomfortable feeling in the mouth | Continuous bouts of clear watery diarrhea with abdominal edema | *Gyebu Gwakjin Yijung Tang* (Lee Je-ma's Cinnamon Bark, Aconite, Agastache, and Tangerine Peel Decoction to Regulate the Middle)<br><br>*Doksam Buja Yijung Tang* (Lee Je-Ma's Added Ginseng Regulate the Middle Decoction with Fu Zi) | |
| Shao Yin stage (Scenario D) This syndrome may also occur during Tai Yin stage illness (without thirst or fever) | Severe deficiency of stomach and spleen, food stagnation, and Cold toxin accumulation (life threatening) | | Constant stupor, bluish-green watery diarrhea, dark complexion, fatigue | *Doksam Tang* (Lee Je-ma's Ginseng Decoction) with 7.5g of Sheng Jiang (*Rhizoma Zingiberis Recens*) and 3.75g of Chen Pi (*Pericarpium Citri Reticulatae*) and Sha Ren (*Fructus Amomi*) | |

嘗見少陰人 十歲兒가 思慮耗氣하야 每有憂愁하고 二日則必腹痛泄
瀉하거늘 一二日에 用白何烏理中湯 二三四貼하며 或甚則附子理中湯 一
二貼則泄瀉가 必愈矣니라. 忽一日에 此兒가 心有憂愁하야 氣度가 不平
數日인 故로 預治次로 用白何烏理中湯 二貼則泄瀉가 因作하야 下利靑
水어늘 連用六貼이로되 靑水不止하야 急用附子理中湯六貼하니 靑水變
爲黑水하고 又二貼하니 黑水泄瀉가 亦愈키로 又二三貼하야 調理하니라.
以此로 觀之則下利靑水者는 病人이 有霍亂 關格而後에 成此病也ㅣ니
此證에 當用巴豆하야 破積滯痼冷은 自是無疑니라. 此兒는 十歲冬十二
月에 有下利靑水病이러니 十一歲春二月에 又得亡陽病하니라.

I once treated a ten-year-old So Eum Individual who exhausted his vital energy by constantly overthinking and worrying. After two to three days of worrying, he would always experience a stomach ache and diarrhea. I prescribed two to three days (four packs) of *Baek Hasuoh Yijung Tang* (Lee Je-ma's Fleeceflower Regulate the Middle Decoction) when his symptoms were less acute. If his symptoms became worse, I prescribed *Baek Hasuoh Buja Yijung Tang* (Lee Je-ma's Fleeceflower and Aconite Regulate the Middle Decoction). After only two packs, his diarrhea always improved. One day, he reported to me that he felt uncomfortable after a few days of worrying. In order to prevent the situation from getting worse, I prescribed two packs *Baek Hasuoh Yijung Tang* (Lee Je-ma's Fleeceflower Regulate the Middle Decoction). Shortly afterwards, he started to experience bluish-green watery diarrhea, which didn't cease even after six packs of the above formula. For this, I immediately prescribed six packs of *Baek Hasuoh Buja Yijung Tang* (Lee Je-ma's Fleeceflower and Aconite Regulate the Middle Decoction), which caused his watery diarrhea to turn black. After another two packs of this formula, he stopped experiencing black-watery diarrhea. Finally, after an additional two packs, he recovered completely. As this case illustrates, bluish-green watery diarrhea results from *Huo Luan* and *Guan Ge* syndromes. There is no doubt that Ba Dou (*Semen Crotonis*) can remove Cold stagnation and food accumulation in such situations. In December of the same year, the above-mentioned child experienced another bout of bluish-green watery diarrhea, and then in February of the following year, he experienced *Mang Yang* syndrome.

朱肱이 曰躁無暫定而厥者는 爲藏厥이니라.

Zhu Gong held that a constant feeling of vexation, anxiousness, and fidgetiness with cold extremities is referred to as *Zhang Jue*[25] syndrome.

---

25   *Zhang Jue* (exhaustion of the *Zhang* organs) is a syndrome marked by extremely cold extremities due to Yang exhaustion of the *Zhang* organs. It is one of several *Han Jue* (Cold-induced *Jue*) syndromes.

李┌이 曰藏厥者는 發躁하야 無休息時이니 發熱七八日에 脈微하며 膚冷
而躁하며 或吐 或瀉하야 無時暫安者는 乃厥陰眞藏氣가 絶인 故로 曰藏
厥이니라 仲景이 無治法而四逆湯을 冷飮하야 救之며 又少陰病에 厥而
吐利 發躁者는 亦不治而三味蔘萸湯으로 救之니라.

Li Ting stated that *Zhang Jue* syndrome is marked by a constant inability to feel
calm with cold extremities, seven to eight days of fever, a minute pulse, Cold skin
(to the touch), and a feeling of fullness and vexation in the chest. If these symptoms
are accompanied by diarrhea and constant anxiety, then it is a sign of Jue Yin stage
illness, in which the *Zhen Zhang Qi*[26] has already been severed. This syndrome
can also be referred to as *Zhang Jue*. Zhang Zhongjing mentioned that there is
no treatment for such a severe illness. Li Ting has successfully prescribed *Si Ni
Tang* (Frigid Extremities Decoction) for this. Zhang Zhongjing also maintained
that there was no cure for Shao Yin illness accompanied by vomit, diarrhea, and
vexation. Li Ting has successfully prescribed *San Wei Shen Yu Tang* (Three Flavors
Ginseng and Evodia Fruit Decoction) in this situation.

論曰少陰人이 喜好不定而計窮力屈則心煩躁也니 少陰病傷寒에 欲吐不
吐하며 心煩하며 但欲寐者는 此非計窮力屈者之病乎아 蓋喜好者는 所慾
也니 何故로 至於計窮力屈而得此少陰病乎아 何不早用君子寬平心乎아
然이나 初證傷寒에 欲吐不吐하며 心煩하며 但欲寐者를 早用藥則猶可
免死也니라. 其病이 至於躁無暫定而厥則勢在極危也니 其不可憐乎아 此
證에 當用蔘萸湯 四逆湯 官桂附子理中湯 吳茱萸附子理中湯이니라.

In my experience, the So Eum Individual's uneasiness and fullness in the chest is
a result of the inability to control their sense of happiness and joy.[27] This feeling
eventually leads to the inability to face failure and plan a way out of their situation.
Wouldn't it be natural that Shao Yin stage symptoms such as an urge to vomit to no
avail, fullness in the chest, and/or constant fatigue would be a result of this inability?[28]

---

26  *Zhen Zhang Qi* (眞藏氣) is translated as the "true," "foundational," or "upright" energy of the *Zhang* organs.

27  The inability to control one's desire for joy is referred to as *Gyegung Yukgul* (計窮力屈). It literally translates
    as "a loss of energy after exhausting all of one's strategy." As mentioned in Chapter 1, *Bang Ryak* (strategic
    planning) resides in the buttocks. This area correlates with the Lower *Jiao* and the kidneys, the So Eum
    Individual's strongest organ. Hence the So Eum Individual's stronger kidneys give them a profound ability to
    strategize and think carefully before taking action. If the So Eum Individual's strategy doesn't come to fruition,
    it is difficult for them to feel calm. If the So Eum Individual doesn't control their emotions and balance their
    predominant temperament of calmness, then they will experience an explosion of unbalanced joy. Unbalanced
    joy will manifest as (a) losing touch with reality, and/or (b) an extreme desire to remain joyful that inevitably
    leads to vexation.

28  Generally speaking, the Internal illness of the So Eum Individual is marked by the stagnation of Mid-Upper
    *Jiao* Yin and inability of Yin to descend from the spleen, which, due to the occasional sinking of Yin, may
    lead to diarrhea. The External syndrome of the So Eum Individual is marked by the stagnation and inability
    of Yang to ascend from the kidneys, which may lead to clammy sweating from the upwards and outwards
    escape of Yang. If either of these situations becomes acute, they can exhibit both Internal and External
    symptoms. Hence even though the Shao Yin stage is marked by Internal illness, in acute cases it may also
    exhibit symptoms of Yang escaping upwards, such as dry heaves, vexation, and fullness in the chest.

Although we know that the So Eum Individual's selfishness results in constant desire for joy, how is it that they let this situation get so out of control that it becomes a Shao Yin stage illness? Why can't the So Eum Individual attempt to express the open-mindedness and harmonious thoughts of a Gentleman [rather than getting themselves into such a life-threatening situation]? What a pity it is, having to administer medicine in order to avoid fatality when a patient experiences dry heaves, fullness in the chest, and a constant desire to sleep [knowing that such an extreme situation could have been avoided had they controlled their desire for joy]. The situation will worsen quickly if medicine is not given immediately, and hands and feet become frigid. In this case *Sam Yu Tang* (Lee Je-ma's Ginseng and Evodia Fruit Decoction), *Si Ni Tang* (Frigid Extremities Decoction), *Gwangye Buja Yijung Tang* (Lee Je-ma's Cinnamon and Aconite Regulate the Middle Decoction), or *Ohsuyu Buja Yijung Tang* (Lee Je-ma's Evodia Fruit and Aconite Regulate the Middle Decoction) can be prescribed.

朱肱이 日病人이 身冷하며 脈沈細而疾하고 煩躁而不飲水者는 陰盛隔陽也라 若飲水者는 非此證也니 厥陰病에 渴欲飲水者는 小小與之면 愈니라.

Zhu Gong once stated that the Yin Excess Overwhelming Yang[29] syndrome, as seen in Jue Yin Stage illness, is marked by chills, a minute, narrow, and rapid pulse, fullness in the chest, vexation, and a lack of thirst. Initial recovery from Jue Yin stage illness is shown by a desire to drink small amounts of fluid.

成無己가 日煩은 謂心中鬱煩也오 躁는 謂氣外熱躁也니 但煩不躁 及先煩後躁者는 皆可治오 但躁不煩及先躁後煩者는 皆不可治니라. 先躁後煩은 謂┌┌然하야 更作躁悶이니 此는 陰盛隔陽也라 雖大躁하야 欲於泥水中臥라도 但水不得入口가 是也니 此는 氣欲絶而爭이니 譬如燈將滅而暴明이니라.

Cheng Wuji[30] once stated that the two Chinese characters that form the phrase *Bon Jo* (煩躁) have distinct meanings. The first character, *Bon* (煩), signifies fullness and congestion in the chest. The second character, *Jo* (躁), signifies excessive Heat in the

---

29  The Yin Excess Overwhelming Yang syndrome (陰盛隔陽) is due to the extreme accumulation of Yin and Cold within the body leading to extreme deficiency of Yang, which gets pushed outwards to the extremities, resulting in Heat-related symptoms such as thirst, skin that is Warm/Hot (to the touch), restless extremities, and a full pulse. Yet these are also accompanied by Cold-related symptoms such as the desire to wear thick clothing, stay under a thick blanket, and an inability to drink fluids with a desire to simply gargle with warm water. Although the extremities may feel warm to the touch, they will often feel extremely cold from the inside.

30  Chen Wuji was a medical doctor and scholar of the latter Jin Dynasty who devoted himself to the study of the *Shang Han Lun*. His focus was on clearly deciphering between Shang Han diseases related to exterior, interior, excess, and deficiency. Chen Wuji wrote three texts entitled *Zhu Jie Shang Han Lun* (*The Annotated Shang Han Lun*)—ten volumes, *Shang Han Ming Li Lun* (*A Logical Interpretation of the Shang Han Lun*)—three volumes, and the *Shang Han Lun Fang* (*Formulae of the Shang Han Lun*)—one volume.

hands and feet [, which is pushed out to the extremities from Cold stirring in the Interior]. [Since both of these symptoms often occur together, they are collectively referred to as *Bon Jo*.] The occurrence of *Bon* symptoms before *Jo* results in a favorable prognosis. If there are only *Jo* symptoms, or if they precede *Bon* symptoms, then the prognosis is unfavorable. Yin Excess Overwhelming Yang occurs when *Jo* precedes *Bon*, and is marked by a reddish and lustrous complexion with fullness in the chest and vexation. *Jo* is also characterized by extreme thirst without the desire to drink fluids.[31] These symptoms signify the body's desperate attempt to survive despite its waning energy and can be compared to the bright flicker of a candle light right before it burns out.

李ㄷ이 曰傷寒에 陰盛隔陽은 其證이 身冷하나 反躁하야 欲投井中하며 脣靑面黑하며 渴欲飮水하나 復吐하며 大便이 自利黑水하며 六脈이 沈細而疾커나 或無脈이면 陰盛隔陽 大虛證也라 宜霹靂散이오 又曰厥逆 煩躁者는 不治니라.

Li Chan once stated that despite the fact that the body feels frozen during Yin Excess Overwhelming Yang syndrome, there will be so much thirst due to *Jo* that jumping into a well may seem appealing. Extreme deficiency caused by Yin Excess Overwhelming Yang includes the above symptoms, accompanied by cyanotic lips, dark complexion, dry throat and thirst with an inability to keep fluids down, dark watery diarrhea, and a deep (or minute to the point of absence) and rapid pulse. In this case, *Pi Li San* (Thunderbolt Powder) should be prescribed. Yet he believed that there is no cure for *Bon Jo* occurrence with cold extremities.

論曰此證에 當用官桂附子理中湯 吳茱萸附子理中湯 或用 霹靂散이니라. 藏厥與陰盛隔陽은 病情이 大同小異로되 俱在極危하니 如存一髮이면 措手難及이니라. 若論此病之可治하면 上策이 莫如此證未成之前에 早用官桂附子理中湯 吳茱萸附子理中湯이니라.

From my perspective, the above syndrome should be treated with *Gwangye Buja Yijung Tang* (Lee Je-ma's Cinnamon and Aconite Regulate the Middle Decoction) and *Ohsuyu Buja Yijung Tang* (Lee Je-ma's Evodia Fruit and Aconite Regulate the Middle Decoction). *Pi Li San* (Thunderbolt Powder) can also be prescribed.

*Zhang Jue* and Yin Excess Overwhelming Yang are similar syndromes with equally fatal effects. It is very challenging to treat these syndromes after even the slightest delay. *Gwangye Buja Yijung Tang* (Lee Je-ma's Cinnamon and Aconite Regulate the Middle Decoction) or *Ohsuyu Buja Yijung Tang* (Lee Je-ma's Evodia Fruit and

---

31    Thirst without the ability to drink fluids is characterized by a desire to moisten the mouth with warm fluid without actually ingesting it. This is a reflection of Yin Overwhelming Yang syndrome, in which Yang-related symptoms are due to deficient Yang escaping Yin, rather than excess itself. Hence these symptoms are often referred to as "False" or "Fake" Heat in Oriental medicine.

Aconite Regulate the Middle Decoction) should be administered immediately, even at the slightest hint of onset.

**Table 6.9: Jue Yin syndrome**

| Syndrome | Due to | Symptoms | Treated with | Approach |
|---|---|---|---|---|
| Jue Yin stage (Scenario A) | Delayed treatment during Shao Yin stage, lack of controlling one's desire for joy (also referred to as Yin Excess Overwhelming yang) | Dry heaves, fullness in the chest, a constant desire to sleep, frigid hands and feet | *Sam Yu Tang* (Lee Je-ma's Ginseng and Evodia Fruit Decoction) *Si Ni Tang* (Frigid Extremities Decoction) *Gwangye Buja Yijung Tang* (Lee Je-ma's Cinnamon and Aconite Regulate the Middle Decoction) *Ohsuyu Buja Yijung Tang* (Lee Je-ma's Evodia Fruit and Aconite Regulate the Middle Decoction) | Strengthen the spleen and stomach, rescue Yang energy, and descend Yin energy |
| Jue Yin stage (Scenario B) | Critical stage leading to the occurrence of *Bon* and *Jo* syndromes (also referred to as *Zhang Jue*) | Whole body feels frozen to touch but patient is so thirsty that they may desire to jump into a well, cyanotic lips, dark complexion, dry throat and thirst with an inability to keep fluids down, dark watery diarrhea, a deep (or minute to the point of absence) and rapid pulse | *Gwangye Buja Yijung Tang* (Lee Je-ma's Cinnamon and Aconite Regulate the Middle Decoction) *Ohsuyu Buja Yijung Tang* (Lee Je-ma's Evodia Fruit and Aconite Regulate the Middle Decoction) *Pi Li San* (Thunderbolt Powder) | |

凡觀少陰人病에 泄瀉初證者는 當觀於心煩與不煩也니 心煩則口渴而口中이 不和也오 心不煩則口不渴而口中이 和也니라. 觀少陰人病에 危證者는 當觀於躁之有定無定也니 欲觀躁之有定無定則必占心之範圍의 有定無定也니 心之範圍가 綽綽者는 心之有定而躁之有定也오 心之範圍 耿耿者는 心之無定而躁之無定也라 心雖耿耿忽忽이라도 猶有一半時刻을 綽綽卓卓則其病은 可治니 可治者는 用薑 附而可效也니라.

During the initial stages of Shao Yin stage illness, it should be determined whether or not there are *Bon*-related symptoms, such as fullness of the chest. Fullness in the chest will inevitably be accompanied by thirst and an uncomfortable feeling in the mouth. If there is no fullness in the chest, then accompanying symptoms such as thirst and an uneasy feeling in the mouth will also be absent. During the acute stages of Shao Yin stage illness, one must determine whether or not there are *Jo*-related symptoms, such as extreme thirst. In order to assess the extent of damage caused by *Jo*, it is necessary to observe the condition of the mind. Calmness of the mind indicates a lack of *Jo*-related symptoms, while an unsettled mind is a sign of an exacerbation of *Jo*-related symptoms. If medicine is administered within 30 minutes of the symptomatic onset, there is a chance of recovery. Fu Zi (*Radix Aconiti*) and Gan Jiang (*Rhizoma Zingiberis Officinalis*) are effective in such cases.

凡少陰人의 泄瀉가 日三度는 重於一二度也오 四五度는 重於二三度也 而日四度泄瀉則太重也며 泄瀉一日은 輕於二日也오 二日은 輕於三日也 而連三日泄瀉則太重也니라. 少陰人 平人이 一月間에 或泄瀉二三次則不 可謂輕病人也며 一日間에 乾便三四度 則不可謂輕病人也니라 下利淸穀 者는 雖日數十行이라도 口中이 必不燥乾而冷氣外解也오 下利淸水者는 腹中에 必有靑水也오 若下利黃水則非淸水而又必雜穢物也니라.

Diarrhea that occurs three times a day during a Shao Yin stage illness indicates a worse condition than only two times a day. If it occurs four times a day, it indicates an extremely serious condition—even more serious than three times a day. Diarrhea occurring for a single day indicates a lighter situation than over a two-day period. A two-day occurrence of diarrhea is still better than three days, evidence of an extremely serious condition. If an otherwise healthy So Eum Individual experiences two to three bouts of diarrhea a month, it would be considered a mild issue. But if they experience three to four bouts of dry stools in a given day, it would not be considered just a mild issue. Continuous clear-watery diarrhea throughout the day without thirst indicates the release of excessive Cold accumulation through the stools. This condition is always accompanied by the accumulation of bluish-green fluids[32] in the abdomen. Yellowish diarrhea contrasts significantly with clear diarrhea, since it will always be mixed with dregs.

張仲景이 日傷寒七八日에 身黃如梔子色하며 小便不利하며 腹微滿은 屬太陰이니 宜茵蔯蒿湯이오 傷寒에 但頭汗出하고 餘無汗하며 劑頸而 還하고 小便이 不利하면 身必發黃이니라.

Zhang Zhongjing stated that *Yin Chen Hao Tang* (Artemisia Yinchenhao Decoction) should be prescribed when, after seven to eight days of Shang Han illness, the body turns as yellow as Zhi Zi (*Fructus Gardeniae Jasminoidis*) with the inability to urinate

---

32  Bluish-green fluid accumulation in the abdomen indicates stagnation of food and Cold toxin. Yellow or red fluid accumulation would be a sign of Heat toxin.

and slight swelling of the abdomen. Jaundice will definitely occur if, during Shang Han illness, there is dysuria and sweating only from the neck upwards.

李ㄱ이 曰天行疫癘에 亦能發黃하나니 謂之瘟黃이라 殺人最急하니 宜瘴疽丸이니라.

Li Chan stated that jaundice resulting from an epidemic disease is referred to as *Wen Huang* (溫黃, Epidemic Jaundice); this is a life-threatening situation that must be treated immediately with *Zhang Dan Wan* (Epidemic Jaundice Pill).

論曰右證에 當用茵蔯橘皮湯 茵蔯附子湯 茵蔯四逆湯 瘴疽丸이오 或用巴豆丹이니라.

From my perspective, the above condition should be treated with *Yin Chen Ju Pi Tang* (Artemisia Yinchenhao and Tangerine Peel Decoction), *Yin Chen Fu Zi Tang* (Artemisia Yinchenhao and Poria Decoction), *Yin Chen Si Ni Tang* (Artemisia Yinchenhao Decoction for Frigid Extremities), or *Zhang Dan Wan* (Epidemic Jaundice Pill). Ba Dou (*Semen Crotonis*) can also be prescribed [to promote bowel movement].

醫學綱目에 曰但結胸하고 無大熱者는 此爲水結이오 但頭汗出을 名曰水結胸이니 小半夏湯을 主之니라.

The *Yixue Gangmu* (*Compendium of Medicine*) states that the occurrence of *Jie Xiong*[33] syndrome without high fever indicates Water stagnation and accumulation. If this is accompanied by sweating only from the neck upwards it is referred to as *Shui Jie Xiong*[34] syndrome, a condition that is treated with *Xiao Ban Xia Tang* (Minor Pinellia Decoction).[35]

龔信이 曰寒實結胸하고 無熱證者는 宜三物白散이니라.

Gong Xin once stated that *San Wu Bai San* (Three Ingredients White Powder) should be prescribed for *Jie Xiong* syndrome due to excessive Cold without fever.

---

33   *Jie Xiong* (結胸) translates literally as "blockage in the chest" and is marked by a hardening of the epigastric area as a result of an Exterior pathogenic influence, which directly becomes a Yin stage illness of the So Eum Individual. According to Lee Je-ma, this is a syndrome typical of the So Yang Individual, and not the So Eum Individual. If, in rare cases, the So Eum does experience *Jie Xiong*, it is then referred to as *Zhang Jie*, a life-threatening situation.

34   *Shui Jie Xiong* (水結胸) translates as "water blockage and accumulation in the chest." It is the acute stage of *Jie Xiong* in which the pathogenic influence and the upper body's natural defense system, *Zhen* (righteous) *Qi*, battle for an extended period of time, resulting in the accumulation of fluids in the chest cavity.

35   Lee Je-ma doesn't mention the ingredients of *Xiao Ban Xia Tang* elsewhere in this text, so they are listed here: Zhi Ban Xia (*Rhizoma Pinelliae Preparatum*) 9–24g, and Sheng Jiang (*Rhizoma Zingiberis Recens*) 9–24g. Source: *Jing Gui Yao Lue* (*Essential Prescriptions from the Golden Cabinet*), written by Zhang Zhongjing.

論曰右證에 當用桂枝半夏生薑湯 赤白何烏寬中湯 三物白散이오 或用巴
豆丹이니라. 少陽人病에 心下結硬者를 名曰結胸病이니 其病은 可治也오
少陰人病에 心下結硬者를 名曰藏結病이니 其病은 不治也ㅣ니라. 醫學綱
目과 醫鑑所論에 水結胸과 寒實結胸證藥은 俱是少陰人 太陰病而與張仲
景 茵蔯蒿湯證으로 相類則此病은 想必非眞結硬於心下而卽痞滿於心下
者也니라. 張仲景의 瀉心湯證에 傷寒下利하고 心下痞硬하며 汗解後에
心下痞硬云者는 亦皆痞滿於心下거나 或臍上近處에 結硬也而非眞結硬
於心下者也니라. 若少陰人病而心下右邊에 結硬則不治니라.

From my perspective, *Gyeji Banha Senggang Tang* (Lee Je-ma's Cinnamon Pinellia and Ginger Decoction), *Jok Hasuoh Gwanjung Tang* (Lee Je-ma's Fleeceflower Smooth the Middle Decoction), *San Wu Bai San* (Three Ingredients White Powder), or *Padu Dan* (Lee Je-ma's Croton Seed Pill) can be used for the above condition.

The *Jie Xiong* syndrome, which is marked by hardening of the epigastric area, is curable only for the So Yang Individual. In the So Eum Individual's case, hardening of the epigastric area is referred to as *Zhang Jie*[36] syndrome and is incurable. The formulae for *Shui Jie Xiong* and *Jie Xiong* syndromes due to Cold excess mentioned in the *Yixue Gangmu* (*Compendium of Medicine*) and the *Gujin Yijian* (*Newly Amended Mirror of Ancient and Modern Medicine*) can be classified as treatments for the Tai Yin syndrome of the So Eum Individual. These formulae also resemble Zhang Zhongjing's *Yin Chen Hao Tang* (Artemisia Yinchenhao Decoction). With further inquiry, these formulae are not actually used for hardness of the epigastric area,[37] which is characteristic of *Jie Xiong*, but for a full and stifling sensation in the chest. Zhang Zhongjing's *Yin Chen Hao Tang* syndrome is marked by a Shang Han[38] influence causing diarrhea and epigastric *Bi* syndrome[39] [without hardening of the epigastrium]. If there is hardness around the umbilicus after sweating is promoted [by improper treatment] along with the above symptoms, it is still not considered *Jie Xiong* syndrome. If, indeed, a So Eum Individual experiences *Jie Xiong* syndrome with hardening and tightening of the right-side epigastrium, it is a grave situation.

---

36  *Zhang Jie* (臟結) literally translates as "hardening of the organs" and is a life-threatening syndrome marked by a hardening of the epigastric area during a Yin stage illness of the So Eum Individual. It occurs as a result of waning Yang energy and a severe blockage of Cold toxin within the stomach and epigastrium.

37  Although Lee Je-ma refers to this situation as "epigastric *Bi Ying*," the epigastrium isn't hard to the touch, as seen in true epigastric *Bi Ying* and *Jie Xiong* syndromes.

38  In this sentence, Lee Je-ma is referring to a Tai Yang stage illness, which may cause subjective fullness in the chest but not objective hardness of the right-side epigastric area (as in *Jie Xiong* syndrome), detected with only a light touch.

39  Epigastric *Bi* syndrome is marked by a stifling and full sensation in the epigastric area. This syndrome differs from true epigastric *Bi Ying* syndrome, since there is no objective feeling of hardness in the epigastric area.

張仲景이 曰病有結胸하며 有藏結하니 其狀이 如何오 曰按之痛하며
寸脈이 浮하며 關脈이 沈을 名曰結胸也ㅣ라. 何謂藏結인고 曰如結胸
狀하고 飮食이 如故하며 時時下利하며 寸脈이 浮하고 關脈이 細小沈
緊을 名曰藏結이니 舌上에 白胎滑者는 難治니라. 病人의 胸中에 素有
痞하야 連在臍傍이라가 引入小腹하야 入陰筋者를 此名藏結이니 死니라.

When asked what the difference between *Jie Xiong* and *Zhang Jie* was, Zhang Zhongjing replied that *Jie Xiong* is marked by epigastric pain when pressure is applied, superficial pulses in the bilateral *cun* (inch) positions, and deep/sinking pulses in the bilateral *guan* (bar) positions. He also stated that *Zhang Jie* shares the same symptoms as *Jie Xiong* except for the occasional occurrence of diarrhea while consuming the same amount of food prior to onset, and small, thin, deep, rapid, tight, and bound pulses in the bilateral *guan* positions. There is no cure for *Zhang Jie* if these symptoms are accompanied by a greasy and thick white tongue coating. *Zhang Jie* may also be characterized by the sudden hardening (to the touch) around the umbilicus and genitals after the occurrence of chest *Bi* syndrome, in which case there is no chance of recovery.

朱肱이 曰藏結은 狀如結胸하고 飮食이 如故하며 時時下利而舌上白
胎니라.
歌曰飮食이 如常하나 時下利하고 更加舌上白胎時라 連臍腹痛引陰筋
者니 此疾이 元來死不醫니라.

Zhu Gong once stated that *Zhang Jie* syndrome is similar to *Jie Xiong* except for occasional diarrhea with a consistent appetite, and a thick white tongue coating. There is a tenet stating that when the appetite continues but there is occasional diarrhea and the tongue has a thick white coating, be aware of whether or not there is an accompanying pulling sensation and pain around the umbilicus that spreads to the genitals, because recovery from this condition is impossible.

論曰嘗見少陰人 一人이 心下右邊에 結硬하야 百藥이 無效어늘 與巴
豆如意丹호니 反劇하야 搖頭하며 動風하다가 有頃而止러니 數月後에
死하고 其後에 又有少陰人 一人이 有此證者를 用巴豆丹호니 面上과 身
上에 有汗而獨上脣人中穴左右邊에 無汗하더니 此人이 一週年後에 亦
死니라. 凡少陰人이 心下結硬하며 有此證者를 目睹四五人하니 或은 半
年 或은 一年에 針灸醫藥이 無不周至而個個無回生之望하니 此는 卽藏
結病而少陰人病이니라.

I once attempted to assist a So Eum Individual with hardening of the right-side epigastrium, but no matter how much I tried, it was without success. At one point I prescribed *Padu Yeowi Dan* (Lee Je-ma's Croton Seed Invigorate the Willpower Pill), but his symptoms became worse and his head shook uncontrollably from Wind stirring internally. Unfortunately, he passed away a few months later. Afterwards, I attempted to help another So Eum Individual with the same symptoms. He began to sweat profusely from his face (especially at the *renzhong* (GV 26) acupuncture point location)[40] and body after taking *Padu Dan* (Lee Je-ma's Croton Seed Pill). However, he died after a year went by. Even after six months to one year of extensive herbal and acupuncture treatment, I was not able to save the lives of up to five So Eum Individuals who experienced hardening of the epigastric area. The above cases surely illustrate the challenges of addressing *Zhang Jie* syndrome of the So Eum Individual.

**Table 6.10: Combined three stage syndromes**

| Syndrome | Due to | Symptoms | Treated with | Approach |
|---|---|---|---|---|
| Combined Tai Yin, Shao Yin, and Jue Yin syndromes | Yin/Cold toxin accumulation from spleen and stomach deficiency and food stagnation | Coldness of the extremities, vomiting, diarrhea, a lack of thirst. If severe there will also be throat pain with incoherent speech, headaches, sweating from the hair follicles of the head, painful pupils with an aversion to light, dark blue lips, fingers, and facial complexion, body pain which feels like the entire body was beaten with a stick, pale, bluish, or darker complexion with cold extremities, and a constant desire to sleep | *Ren Shen Gui Zhi Tang* (Cinnamon Twig Decoction with Ginseng) *Doksam Buja Yijung Tang* (Lee Je-Ma's Added Ginseng Regulate the Middle Decoction with Fu Zi) | Warm the stomach, clear Cold toxin |
| Combined Tai Yin, Shao Yin, and Jue Yin syndromes (acute onset) | Direct transfer to Three Yin stage illness from a Tai Yang stage illness, acute Yin toxic accumulation | Sudden acute food stagnation causing twisting pain in the stomach with the urge to vomit and defecate to no avail, cyanotic complexion, constant desire to sleep, acute loss of appetite, and watery diarrhea followed by constipation | *Padu Yeowi Dan* (Lee Je-ma's Croton Seed Invigorate the Willpower Pill) | Warm the stomach, purge Yin toxin |

---

40  As mentioned earlier in this chapter, if the So Eum Individual sweats at the *renzhong* acupuncture point location, situated at the centerline of the body halfway between the nose and the upper lip, after battling with illness, it is a sign of recovery.

張仲景이 曰黃疸之病은 當以十八日로 爲期하니 十日以上에 宜差로대
反劇은 爲難治니라. 發於陰部면 其人이 必嘔오 發於陽部면 其人이 振寒
而發熱이니라. 諸疸에 小便이 黃赤色者는 爲濕熱이니 當作濕熱治오 小
便이 色白하야 不可除熱者는 無熱也니 若有虛寒證이면 當作虛勞治니라.
腹脹滿하며 面萎黃하면 躁不得睡니라.

According to Zhang Zhongjing, the symptoms of jaundice often improve within
18 days, and recovery almost always begins after ten days. If symptoms get worse
after ten days, jaundice will be difficult to treat. Yin jaundice is associated with
vomiting, whereas Yang jaundice occurs with spontaneous chills and fever. Damp
Heat jaundice is characterized by yellowish-brown urine. In this case, treatment
should be focused on eliminating Dampness and clearing Heat. If the urine is
whitish in color, then Heat is unlikely to be an issue. If jaundice is accompanied
by deficient Cold-related symptoms, then tonification should be the focus. [If
treatment is not administered in time,] fullness and distension of the stomach and a
yellowish complexion will eventually lead to fullness in the chest and vexation with
dry heaves.[41]

黃家는 日晡時에 當發熱이어늘 反惡寒은 此爲女勞得之니 膀胱이
急하며 小腹이 滿하며 一身이 盡黃하되 額上이 黑하며 足下에 熱하면
因作黑疸이라. 腹脹이 如水狀하며 大便이 黑하며 或時溏이면 此는 女勞
之病이오 非水也ㅣ니 腹滿者는 難治니라.

[According to Zhang Zhongjing,] fever in the evening occurs as a matter of course
after the onset of jaundice. Yet, if chills occur instead of fever, it is a sure sign of
*Nu Lao*[42] syndrome. *He Dan*[43] occurs if *Nu Lao*-related symptoms are accompanied
by extreme fullness of the bladder, as if it were to explode, swelling of the lower
abdomen—which may appear as if filled with water—yellowish skin with a
darkened forehead complexion, and a sensation of heat radiating from the feet.
There may also be black-colored stool and occasional diarrhea with fullness and pain
in the abdomen. These symptoms, associated with *Nu Lao*, are due to the effects of
jaundice, rather than water retention. If this syndrome is accompanied by a severely
distended abdomen, treatment will be difficult.

---

41  In this sentence, Lee Je-ma is describing the progression of a Shao Yin stage illness from non-life threatening
(平, *pyung*) or fatal/life threatening (險, *hom*).

42  *Nu Lao* (女勞), literally translated as "woman fatigue" syndrome, is the result of excessive sexual activity,
which causes exhaustion due to the waning of vital Yang energy.

43  *He Dan* (黑疸), literally translated as "black jaundice," occurs after a long-term episode of jaundice, leading
to a dark facial complexion, and occurs when diarrhea is mistakenly induced to treat *Nu Lao* syndrome. *He
Dan* is considered a symptom of advanced-stage *Nu Lao* syndrome.

朱肱이 曰陰黃은 煩躁하며 喘嘔不渴이니 宜用茵蔯橘皮湯이니라 一人이
傷寒에 發黃하고 脈微弱하며 身冷이어늘 次第用藥하야 至茵蔯四逆
湯하니 大效하고 一人이 傷寒에 發黃하야 脈沈細遲無力이어늘 次第用
藥하야 至茵蔯附子湯하니 大效니라.

Zhu Gong once asserted that *Yin Huang*[44] is marked by fullness in the chest, vexation, shortness of breath, and vomiting without thirst and suggested *Yin Chen Ju Pi Tang* (Artemisia Yinchenhao and Tangerine Peel Decoction) for this situation. Zhu Gong once used *Yin Chen Si Ni Tang* (Artemisia Yinchenhao Decoction for Frigid Extremities) to successfully treat an individual whose skin was yellow, whose pulse was minute and weak, and who was extremely cold due to a Shang Han influence. He assisted another individual with *Yin Chen Fu Zi Tang* (Artemisia Yinchenhao and Poria Decoction) who suffered from a Shang Han influence that led to jaundice, fatigue, and a deep, narrow, and slow pulse.

醫學綱目에 曰濕家之黃은 色暗不明하며 一身이 不痛하고 熱家之黃은
如橘子하며 一身이 盡痛이니라.

In the *Yixue Gangmu* (*Compendium of Medicine*) jaundice caused by Dampness results in a darker skin complexion without general body pain. Jaundice caused by Heat results in tangerine-colored skin with pain.

王好古가 曰凡病에 當汗而不汗커나 當利小便而不利하면 亦生黃이니라.

Wang Hao Gu said that all sickness can be cured by the promotion of sweat or urination. He is referring to the fact that jaundice results from an inability to sweat or urinate efficiently.

朱震亨이 曰黃疸에 因食積者는 下其食積하고 其餘는 但利小便이니 小
便이 利白이면 其黃이 自退니라.

Zhu Zhenheng once stated that jaundice is caused by food stagnation and is cured by promoting digestion and urination. Smoother and clearer urination is a sign of recovery.

李梴이 曰黃疸十日以上에 入腹하야 喘滿 煩渴하며 面黑者는 死니라.

Li Chan maintained that after ten days of jaundice, if a patient has a blackish complexion with shortness of breath, fullness in the chest, vexation, and thirst, he or she will not survive.

---

44  *Yin Huang* (陰黃), literally translated as "Yin yellow," is a term used to describe jaundice caused by excessive Yin and Cold accumulation within the body.

王叔和 脈經에 曰黃家에 寸口脈이 近掌無脈하며 口鼻冷하며 黑色이면 竝不可治니라.

Wang Shu He states in his *Mai Jing* (*The Pulse Classic*)[45] that if the radial pulse is not detected, the mouth and nose are cold to touch, and the complexion is black, then a cure is impossible.

論曰陰黃은 卽少陰人病也니 當用朱氏茵蔯橘皮湯 茵蔯四逆湯이오 女勞 之黃과 熱家之黃과 利小便之黃은 想或 非少陰人病而余所經驗이 未嘗 一遇黃疸而治之인 故로 未得仔細裏許나 然이나 痞滿과 黃疸과 浮腫이 同出一證而有輕重하니 若欲利小便則乾薑 良薑 陳皮 靑皮 香附子 益智 仁이 能利少陰人小便이오 荊芥 防風 羌活 獨活 茯苓 澤瀉가 能利少陽人 小便이니라.

From my perspective, Yin jaundice is an illness that is exclusively associated with the So Eum Individual, which can be treated with Zhu Zhenheng's *Yin Chen Ju Pi Tang* (Artemisia Yinchenhao and Tangerine Peel Decoction) or *Yin Chen Si Ni Tang* (Artemisia Yinchenhao Decoction for Frigid Extremities). I would also speculate that jaundice caused by *Nu Lao* or Heat is also exclusively an issue of the So Eum Individual. To be honest, I have not even once treated an individual with jaundice and therefore am not directly familiar with a precise treatment approach. Abdominal *Bi* syndrome, jaundice, and edema can all be classified in the same category of illness, but into different levels of severity. Herbs such as Gan Jiang (*Rhizoma Zingiberis Officinalis*), Liang Jiang (*Rhizoma Alpiniae Officinarum*), Qing Pi (*Pericarpium Citri Ret. Viridae*), Chen Pi (*Pericarpium Citri Reticulatae*), Xiang Fu Zi (*Rhizoma Cyperi*), and Yi Zhi Ren (*Fructus Alpiniae Oxyphyllae*) can be prescribed to promote urination as a treatment for the So Eum Individual's jaundice. Jing Jie (*Herba Schizonepetae*), Fang Feng (*Radix Saposhnikoviae*), Qiang Huo (*Rhizoma et Radix Notoperygii*), Du Huo (*Radix Angelicae Pubescentis*), Fu Ling (*Poria Alba*), and/or Ze Xie (*Rhizoma Alismatis*) can be prescribed to promote urination of the So Yang Individual.

---

45  The *Mai Jing* (脈經, *The Pulse Classic*), written by Wang Shu He (265–316 AD) of the Western Jin Dynasty, consists of ten volumes that describe a total of 24 different pulses in great detail.

# A Synopsis of So Eum Illness
## 泛論

論曰發熱惡寒者는 爲太陽病이오 發熱不惡寒者는 爲陽明病이니 太陽 陽明之發熱形證은 一也而惡寒不惡寒之間에 相去가 遠甚而陽氣之進退强弱도 泰山之比岡陵也라 自利而不渴者는 爲太陰病이오 自利而渴者는 爲少陰病이니 太陰과 少陰之自利形證은 一也而渴不渴之間에 相去가 遠甚而冷氣之聚散輕重도 雲夢之比瀦澤也니라.

Spontaneous chills and fever are a result of Tai Yang stage illness, whereas a lack of chills results from Yang Ming stage illness. Even though both of these syndromes are marked by the occurrence of fever, they are clearly differentiated by whether or not chills are present. This difference can help decipher whether Yang *Qi* is retreating or advancing, strong or weak, and can be likened to that of a high mountain compared to a small hill. Moreover, diarrhea that occurs without thirst is a result of Tai Yin illness, while diarrhea with thirst is a hallmark sign of Shao Yin illness. Even though both of these syndromes are marked by diarrhea, it is the presence or absence of thirst that differentiates them. The presence or lack of thirst indicates whether or not the illness is retreating or advancing, severe, or less severe—like the difference between a huge lake and a tiny marsh.

是故로 藿香正氣散 香砂養胃湯之證勢는 平地駿馬之病勢也오 獨蔘八物湯 桂附理中湯之證勢는 太行短⌐之病勢也니라. 若使一天下 少陰人 稟賦者로 自知其病之陽明少陰證이 如太行之險路하야 得之可畏오 救之不易하야 攝身療病하면 戒懼謹愼之道가 有若大路然而不迷則其庶幾乎인저.

Therefore, the ease of addressing syndromes involving the use of *Gwakhyang Jeonggi San* (Lee Je-ma's Agastache Powder to Rectify the Qi) and *Hyangsa Yangwi Tang* (Lee Je-ma's Cyperus and Hawthorn Enliven the stomach Decoction)[46] can be compared to a swift horse galloping on flat land. Yet the difficulty of addressing syndromes involving the use of *Doksam Palmul Tang* (Lee Je-ma's Added Ginseng Eight Ingredient Gentlemen Decoction) and *Gwangye Buja Yijung Tang* (Lee Je-ma's Cinnamon and Aconite Regulate the Middle Decoction)[47] can be compared to hiking a dangerously steep mountain with a walking stick that is too short. As for the So Eum Individual, one must clearly distinguish between Yang Ming and

---

46  Both of these formulae are used to treat Tai Yang/Yang Ming stage syndromes, indicating that the pathogen is still in the Exterior and the body's *Zheng Qi* is still intact.

47  Both of these formulae are used to treat acute Yin stage syndromes, indicating that the pathogen has already entered the Interior, and the body's spleen and stomach *Qi* and Yang have already significantly weakened.

Shao Yin stage illnesses. Only then could he or she climb a dangerous mountain without mishap. Taking precaution and preserving one's energy before the onset of even a minor illness results in the ability to stay on course and be clear of the illness's further progression.

太陽病汗出은 熱氣卻寒氣之汗出也오 陽明病汗出은 寒氣犯熱氣之汗出也며 太陰病下利는 溫氣逐冷氣之下利也오 少陰病下利는 冷氣逼溫氣之下利也니라. 少陰人病이 有二吉證하니 人中汗이 一吉證也오 能飮水가 一吉證也ㅣ니라. 少陰人病에 有二急證하니 發熱汗多가 一急證也오 下利淸水가 一急證也니라.

Sweat during a Tai Yang stage illness is a sign of Hot energy pushing Cold energy[48] away from the body. Sweating during a Yang Ming stage illness is a sign of Cold energy pushing Hot energy away from the body.[49] Diarrhea during a Tai Yin stage illness is a sign of Warm energy chasing away Cool energy within the body.[50] Diarrhea during a Shao Yin stage illness is a sign of Cool energy suppressing Warm energy.[51] There are two signs of recovery from a Shao Yin stage illness. The first sign is sweating from the *renzhong* (GV 26) acupuncture point location, and the second is the ability to drink water. There are two signs that Shao Yin stage illness is getting worse. The first sign is excessive sweating with fever, and the second is diarrhea of clear fluids.

少陰人病에 有六大證하니 一曰少陰病이오 二曰陽明病이오 三曰太陰病陰毒證也오 四曰太陽病 厥陰證也오 五曰太陰病 黃疸證也오 六曰太陽病胃家實證也니라.

There are six major syndromes associated with the So Eum Individual. The first is Shao Yin syndrome, the second is Yang Ming syndrome, the third is an accumulation of *Yin Duo* [from food stagnation of the] Tai Yin syndrome, the fourth is the *Jue Yin*

---

48    "Hot energy" refers to the integrity of the So Eum Individual's *Zheng Qi*, while "Cold energy" refers to the strength of pathogenic influence. The spleen and stomach are the source of Heat within the body. In the Tai Yang stage, there is enough Heat, or spleen and stomach energy, to fight off and "push away" the Cold-natured pathogen.

49    In this case, the pathogenic Cold of the Yang Ming stage is quickly and efficiently fighting off, or pushing away, the So Eum Individual's *Zheng Qi*—a result of spleen and stomach weakness, which produce and store Hot energy. If not addressed immediately, the sudden accumulation of Cold energy can quickly destroy the So Eum's remaining Yang energy and eventually lead to death.

50    In this case, the So Eum Individual may not be able to build up enough Hot energy, as in Tai Yang stage illness, because of blockage of the stomach and spleen, but they can accumulate Warm energy (from lungs and esophagus) to chase away the Cold pathogen.

51    Unlike the abrupt nature of the Yang Ming stage's Cold pathogen, the Cold pathogenic influence of the Shao Yin stage slowly suppresses the remaining Heat, or Warm nature, of the lungs and esophagus. The accumulation of Cold energy can destroy the So Eum's remaining Yang energy and eventually lead to death if not addressed appropriately.

syndrome of the Tai Yang stage,[52] the fifth is jaundice of the Tai Yin stage, and the sixth is the *Wei Jia Shi* syndrome of the Tai Yang stage.[53]

發熱汗出則病必解也而發熱汗出而病益甚者는 陽明病也오 通滯下利則病
必解也而通滯下利而病益甚者는 少陰病也니
陽明과 少陰은 以邪犯正之病이니 不可不急用藥也니라. 惡寒汗出則病必
盡解也而惡寒汗出而其病이 半解不解者는 厥陰之漸也오
腹痛下利則病必盡解也而腹痛下利而其病이 半解不解者는 陰毒之漸也니
厥陰과 陰毒은 正邪相傾之病이니 不可不預用藥也니라

Sweating that occurs during an episode of fever will, in most cases, lead to recovery. Fever that gets worse even after sweating is a sign of Yang Ming stage syndrome. Diarrhea following food stagnation will, in most cases, lead to recovery. Illness that gets worse even after diarrhea points to the onset of a Shao Yin stage syndrome. Immediate herbal treatment should be administered if Yang Ming or Shao Yin stage illness of the So Eum Individual occurs, indicating that *Zheng Qi*[54] has been invaded by pathogenic *Qi*. Sweating during an episode of chills will, in most cases, lead to recovery. If only half of an illness is cured while the other half stubbornly remains even after sweating, it signifies Jue Yin stage illness. Stomach pain, in most cases, is cured by the promotion of diarrhea [with herbs such as Ba Dou (*Semen Crotonis*)]. If a stomach ache is only half resolved after promoting diarrhea, it is a sign of *Yin Duo*[55] accumulation. The syndromes of Jue Yin and *Yin Duo* involve a battle between the *Zhang* organs and a pathogenic influence. In order to avoid injury to the organs, it is crucial that medicine be administered as soon as possible.

發熱 一汗而病卽解者는 太陽之輕病也오 食滯一下而病卽解者는 太陰之
輕病也니太陽과 太陰之輕病은 不用藥而亦自愈也니라.

If fever goes down after a bout of sweating, it is considered a minor Tai Yang stage illness. If bowel movement occurs after a bout of food stagnation, then it is considered a minor Tai Yin stage illness. These syndromes are self-resolving and do not need intervention.

---

52  It is necessary to differentiate between the Jue Yin stage and Jue Yin syndrome of the Tai Yang stage. The Tai Yang stage Jue Yin syndrome is marked by extremely cold hands and feet with simultaneous chills and fever. The Jue Yin stage is also marked by extremely cold hands and feet with pronounced fever, but no chills. The absence of chills and presence of fever indicates an Internal, rather than External, pathogenic influence. The So Eum Individual's spleen Yang energy is still intact during the Tai Yang stage but is severely deficient in the event of a Jue Yin stage illness.

53  As mentioned earlier in this chapter, *Wei Jia Shi* may also occur during the Yang Ming and Tai Yin stages. Actually, *Wei Jia Shi* is the hallmark syndrome of the Yang Ming stage, despite the fact that lesser acute *Wei Jia Shi* signs, such as moderate constipation, can be detected during the Tai Yang stage.

54  *Zheng Qi* (正氣) is translated as righteous *Qi*.

55  *Yin Duo* (陰毒) translates as "Yin toxin."

發熱三日에 不得汗解者는 太陽之尤病也오食滯三日에 不能化下者는 太
陰之尤病也니 太陽과 太陰之尤病은 已不可謂輕證而用藥二三貼으로 亦
自愈也오 發熱六日에 不得汗解하며 食滯六日에도 不能化下者는 太陽과
太陰之胃家實과 黃疸病也니 太陽과 太陰之胃家實 黃疸은 正邪壅錮之
病이니 不可不大用藥也니라.

If fever without sweating is present after three days of Tai Yang stage onset, it means that the illness has taken a turn for the worse. If after three days of food stagnation there is no bowel movement, it is a sign that the Tai Yin stage illness is taking a turn for the worse. Even though these cases are not minor, they will still resolve after administering two to three packs of herbs. *Wei Jia Shi* [from Yang Ming syndrome] occurs after battling a Tai Yang stage illness without sweating for six days. Jaundice occurs after six days of battling a Tai Yin stage illness without sufficient bowel movement. These illnesses occur due to a fight between *Zheng Qi* and pathogenic *Qi*, and should be treated with a significant amount of medicine.

太陽과 太陰之病은 六七日에 或成危證하며 或成重證而十日內에 必有
險證이오 陽明과 少陰之病은 自始發로 已爲重證而二三日內에 亦致險
證하나니 是故로 陽明과 少陰之病은 不可不察於始發也오 太陽과 太陰
之病은 不可不察於四五日間也니라.

Six to seven days of lingering Tai Yang or Tai Yin stage illness indicate that it has become life threatening,[56] and after ten days it would be considered critical.[57] Even from their onset, Yang Ming and Shao Yin stage illnesses are considered severe.[58] After only two to three days of onset they can become critical.[59] These syndromes should therefore be treated immediately and with great care as soon as they are detected. The same level of precaution should be taken after four to five days of lingering Tai Yang or Tai Yin stage illness.

太陽과 太陰之病은 病勢緩而能曠日持久인 故로 變證이 多也오 陽明과
少陰之病은 病勢急而不能曠日持久인 故로 變證이 少也ㅣ니라. 蓋陽明과
少陰病은 過一日而至二日則不可不用藥也오 太陽과 太陰病은 過四日而
至五日則不可不用藥也오 太陽과 太陰之厥陰과 陰毒은 皆六七日之死境
也니 尤不可不謹也니라.

Chronic Tai Yang and Tai Yin stage syndromes tend to transform into more acute phases after several days without recovery. Yet due to their intrinsic severity, both Yang Ming and Shao Yin stage illnesses do not transfer into other phases after several days from onset. In order to increase the odds of recovery, medicine should be

---

56    Lee Je-ma classifies this stage as the *wi* (危, life threatening) level of a *jung* (重, serious) illness.

57    Lee Je-ma classifies this stage as the *hom* (險, critical) level of a *jung* (重, serious) illness.

58    The word "severe" in this sentence is a translation of *jung* (重).

59    The term "critical" in this sentence is a translation of *hom* (險).

administered after one to two days of onset for Yang Ming and Shao Yin stage illness, and four to five days from onset for the Tai Yang and Tai Yin stages. If Tai Yang or Tai Yin stage illness leads to Jue Yin or *Yin Duo* syndromes and lingers for six to seven days, there is no chance of survival. Hence it crucial that precautionary steps be taken.

陽明과 太陽之危者는 獨蔘八物湯 補中益氣湯이 可以解之而病勢危時에 若非日三四服而又連日服則難解也오 少陰과 太陰之危者는 獨蔘附子理中湯 桂附藿陳理中湯으로 可以解之而病勢危時에 若非日三四服而又連日服則難解也니라

*Doksam Palmul Tang* (Lee Je-ma's Added Ginseng Eight Ingredient Gentlemen Decoction) and *Bochung Ikgi Tang* (Lee Je-ma's Tonify the Middle and Augment the Qi Decoction) can be used to address life-threatening cases of Yang Ming and Tai Yang stage illness, and once detected, medicine should be administered three to four times a day in order to attempt recovery. It only takes a few days of such illnesses to claim the life of an individual.

   *Doksam Buja Yijung Tang* (Lee Je-ma's Added Ginseng Regulate the Middle Decoction with Fu Zi)[60] and *Gyebu Gwakjin Yijung Tang* (Lee Je-ma's Cinnamon Bark, Aconite, Agastache, and Tangerine Peel Decoction to Regulate the Middle) can help alleviate the effects of a life-threatening Shao Yin or Tai Yin stage syndrome. But even in such cases, medicine should be administered three to four times a day to avoid loss of life.

病勢極危時는 日四服하며 病勢半危時는 日三服하며 病勢不減則日二服하고 病勢少減則二日三服거나 而一日則一服 一日則二服하며 病勢大減則日一服하며 病勢又大減則間二三四五日 一服이니라.

For a life-threatening illness, medicine should be administered four times a day. If the illness is 50 percent less urgent, then dosage can be reduced to three times a day. If the illness lingers on, reducing dosage to two times a day will avoid overuse. If there is a slight indication of recovery, then intake can be reduced to three doses over a two-day period, or one to two doses over the course of a day. A single dose would suffice once recovery is significant, and once recovery is complete, a dose every two to five days should be administered.[61]

---

60   Lee Je-ma doesn't mention the ingredients of *Doksam Buja Yijung Tang* elsewhere in this text, so they are listed here: Ren Shen (*Radix Ginseng*) 20g, Bai Zhu (*Radix Atractylodis Macrocephalae*) 8g, Gan Jiang (*Rhizoma Zingiberis Officinalis*) 8g, Bai Shao Yao (*Radix Paeoniae Lactiflorae*) 8g, Chen Pi (*Pericarpium Citri Reticulatae*) 4g, Zhi Gan Cao (*Radix Glycyrrhizae*) 4g, Da Zao (*Fructus Zizyphi Jujubae*) 2 Pieces, and Fu Zi (*Radix Aconiti*) 1–4g.

61   In case of life-threatening illness, the administration of herbal medicine isn't to be discontinued despite the cessation of symptoms. After symptoms have ceased, intake frequency is consistently reduced but continued until full recovery is established.

蓋有病者가 可以服藥이오 無病者는 不可以服藥하며 重病에 可以重藥이오 輕病에 不可以重藥이니 若輕病에 好用重藥커나 無病者가 好服藥하면 臟氣脆弱하야 益招病矣니라. 膏粱이 雖則助味나 常食則損味하고 羊裘가 雖則禦寒하나 常着則攝寒하나니 膏粱과 羊裘도 猶不可以常食常着어든 況藥乎아 若論常服藥之有害則反爲百倍於全不服藥之無利也니라. 蓋有病者는 明知其證則必不可不服藥이로되 無病者는 雖明知其證이라도 必不可服藥이니라. 歷觀於世之服 鴉片烟 水銀 山蔘 鹿茸者컨대 屢服則無不促壽者하니 以此占之則可知矣니라.

In general, medicine is only to be administered in the presence of illness [and not for the sake of simply supporting health]. For serious[62] illness, stronger medicines should be administered, which should not be applied to moderate[63] illness. Organ energy runs the risk of depletion if a doctor prefers using stronger medications for minor illnesses or for the sake of simply supporting his/her patient's health. Even though rich-tasting foods are pleasant to the taste, over-indulgence will eventually ruin our ability to appreciate other types of foods. Even though wool can protect us from the cold, wearing it constantly can trap in the cold[64] [and cause illness]. Just as there are appropriate times to eat richer foods [to nourish the body] and wear wool [to protect from the cold], how could the administration of herbs be any different? Generally speaking, an injury sustained from the continuous use of incompatible herbs is 100 times worse than abstaining from them entirely. If an illness occurs, only after thorough examination should it be attended to with herbs. Even if close examination of symptoms yields no significant illness, the use of herbs should be abstained from. I have witnessed many individuals who have shortened their lifespan through the frequent use of opium, mercury-containing herbs, wild ginseng, and deer antlers. From this you can well imagine that [herbs are not to be administered without due consideration].

少陰人 吐血에 當用獨蔘八物湯이오 咽喉痛에 當用獨蔘官桂理中湯이니라.

*Doksam Palmul Tang* (Lee Je-ma's Added Ginseng Eight Ingredient Gentlemen Decoction) is appropriate when the So Eum Individual vomits blood. *Doksam Gwangye Yijung Tang* (Lee Je-ma's Cinnamon Regulate the Middle Decoction with Added Ginseng)[65] can be prescribed for a painful and swollen throat.

---

62    The word "serious" in this sentence is a translation of *jung* (重).

63    The word "moderate" in this sentence is a translation of *kyung* (經).

64    "Cold" in this sentence refers to the So Eum Individual's stronger kidney Yin energy, which produces ample Cold energy. Constant use of excessively warm clothing can trap the Cold energy of the kidneys within the body.

65    Lee Je-ma doesn't mention the ingredients of *Doksam Gwangye Yijung Tang* elsewhere in this text, so they are listed here: Ren Shen (*Radix Ginseng*) 20g, Huang Qi (*Radix Astragali Membranacei*) 12g, Bai Zhu (*Radix Atractylodis Macrocephalae*) 4g, Bai Shao Yao (*Radix Paeoniae Lactiflorae*) 4g, Dang Gui (*Radix Angelicae Sinensis*) 4g, Chuan Xiong (*Radix Ligustici Chuanxiong*) 4g, Guan Gui (*Cortex Cinnamomi Cassiae*) 4g, and Zhi Gan Cao (*Radix Glycyrrhizae*) 4g. Source: *Sasang Shinpyun* (*Revised Collection of Sasang Materia Medica*).

嘗見少陰人이 飲食倍常하고 口味甚甘하더니 不過一月에 其人이 浮腫而 死하니 少陰人食消는 卽浮腫之屬而危證也라 不可不急治니 當用芎歸蔥 蘇理中湯이니라.

I once witnessed a So Eum Individual with a voracious appetite who started craving sweet foods while eating twice his normal amount. He died after one month with severe edema. The So Eum Individual's voracious and unsatiated appetite[66] is a sure sign of edema and indicates a life-threatening situation that needs to be treated right away with *Gunggui Chongso Yijung Tang* (Lee Je-ma's Regulate the Middle Decoction with Lovage, Angelica, Scallion, and Perilla Leaf).[67]

嘗見少陰人의 浮腫에 獐肝一部를 切片作膾하야 一服盡하기를 連用 五部하니 其病이 卽效하고 又有少陰人이 服獐肝一部하니 眼力이 倍 常하고 眞氣가 湧出하더라. 少陽人이 虛勞病에 服獐肝一部하니 其人이 吐血而死하니라.

Another So Eum Individual overcame a case of edema by consuming five slices of raw deer liver. I also witnessed a So Eum Individual whose eyesight and *Zheng Qi* dramatically improved after consuming one slice of raw deer liver, while a So Yang Individual ingested one slice of raw deer liver after suffering from fatigue. Soon after ingestion, he vomited blood and passed away.[68]

嘗見少陰人의 浮腫에 有醫가 敎以服海鹽自然汁 日半匙라하야 四五日 服하니 浮腫이 大減하고 一月服하니 永爲完健하야 病不再發하니라.

A So Eum Individual once overcame edema after being prescribed a half spoonful of salt water per day for four to five days. After one month of continuing this regime, his health greatly improved, with no return of edema.

---

66  The So Eum Individual's voracious and unsatiated appetite is referred to in this text as *Shi Xiao* (食消), or "food-related wasting and thirsting disorder." It is a result of long-term deficient Heat stagnation and accumulation in the stomach causing *Qi* and *Jin Ye* fluid deficiency due to the So Eum Individual's *Wei Jia Shi* syndrome. *Shi Xiao* syndrome is another term used for *Zhong Xiao*, or "Middle *Jiao* wasting and thirsting disorder," also interpreted as "Middle *Jiao* diabetes."

67  Lee Je-ma doesn't mention the ingredients of to *Gunggui Chongso Yijung Tang* elsewhere in this text, so they are listed here: Ren Shen (*Radix Ginseng*) 20g, Bai Zhu (*Radix Atractylodis Macrocephalae*) 4g, Pao Gan Jiang (*Rhizoma Zingiberis Preparata*) 4g, Guan Gui (*Cortex Cinnamomi Cassiae*) 4g, Bai Shao Yao (*Radix Paeoniae Lactiflorae*) 4g, Chen Pi (*Pericarpium Citri Reticulatae*) 4g, Zhi Gan Cao (*Radix Glycyrrhizae*) 4g, Fu Zi (*Radix Aconiti*) 4–6g, Chuan Xiong (*Radix Ligustici Chuanxiong*) 3g, Dang Gui (*Radix Angelicae Sinensis*) 3g, Zi Su Ye (*Folium Perillae*) 3g, and Cong Bai (*Radix Allii*) 3g. Source: *Sasang Shinpyun* (*Revised Collection of Sasang Materia Medica*).

68  In this sentence, Lee Je-ma illustrates how all medicines have constitutionally specific properties, and could result in significant health issues if given to the wrong constitution type.

嘗見少陰人의 咽喉痛이 經年不愈어늘 有醫가 教以服金蛇酒 卽效라하니 金蛇酒는 卽金色黃章蛇로 釀酒者也라.

A So Eum Individual who suffered over a month of throat pain improved after being given golden-snake wine.[69] This remedy is prepared by steeping a snake with yellowish-golden spots in rice wine.

嘗見少陰人의 痢疾에 有醫가 教以服項赤蛇煎湯 卽效라하니 項赤蛇를 去頭斷尾하야 納二疊細囊中하고 藥缸內에 別設橫木하야 懸空掛之하고 用水五碗하야 煎取一碗하야 服하라. 二疊細囊에 懸空掛煎者는 恐犯蛇骨 故也니 蛇骨이 有毒이니라.

There was once a So Eum Individual cured of dysentery by a boiled concoction from red-naped snake.[70] The red-naped snake is prepared by cutting off the head and tail and inserting it into a double-folded, silk-lined pouch that is placed into a jar with two Wooden skewers pierced into it, in a criss-cross configuration. The pouch is then boiled with five bowls of water and simmered for a long period until only one bowl is left. The pouch is necessary because this snake has poisonous bones.

嘗見少陰人의 痢疾에 有醫가 教以大蒜三顆와 淸蜜半匙를 同煎하야 三日服하니 卽效하니라.

I have once witnessed a So Eum Individual cured of dysentery by three cloves of garlic and one half spoonful of honey taken for three days.

嘗見少陰人의 乳房近脇에 有漏瘡하야 歷七八月한데 瘡口不合하며 惡汁이 常流어늘 有醫가 教以山蔘 熊膽末 各一分을 傅之 卽效라하고 又少陰人 一人이 滿身有瘡에 以人蔘末로 塗傅하니 卽效니라.

I once witnessed a So Eum Individual with a mammary cyst located on the lateral side of the breast causing a seeping gash in her skin, which continued to suppurate even after seven to eight months from onset. One doctor successfully treated this condition with .375g of Wild Ginseng (*Radix Ginseng*) and Xiong Dan Powder (*Vesica Fellea Ursi*). Another So Eum Individual given powdered ginseng to place on boils that spread throughout his body was soon cured.

---

69    The golden-snake remedy is not currently utilized in Sasang medicine.

70    Red-naped snake is no longer used for this condition due to its extremely high level of toxicity. Instead, Lee Je-ma often prescribes Ba Dou (*Semen Crotonis*) in acute situations to regulate bowel movement for the So Eum Individual.

嘗見少陰人의 乳傍近脇에 發內癰이어늘 有醫가 教以火針取膿하니라. 醫
曰內癰은 外證이 惡寒發熱하야 似傷寒而有痛處也니 察其痛處하야 明知
有膿則不可不用火針이니라.

There was once a So Eum Individual who was cured of her non-elevated mammary abscess by the use of the Fire Acupuncture technique[71] in order to exude the pus. According to the treating physician, this is the only way to treat internal abscesses accompanied by Shang Han-induced chills, fever, and pain at the abscess location. Fire Acupuncture is inserted at the site of pain.

嘗見少陰人의 背癰에 有醫가 教以火刀裂瘡하니라. 醫曰火刀裂瘡은 宜早
也니 若疑訝而緩不及事則全背堅硬하나니 悔之無及이니라.

A So Eum Individual's spinal cyst was successfully excised by the Fire Knife technique.[72] According to the treating physician, this technique is to be performed in the early stages, and if this technique is carried out too late, the cyst will harden and get worse. How pitiful it is to regret the delay of treatment as a physician hopes that the cyst will resolve on its own accord!

嘗見少陰人의 半身不遂病에 有醫가 教以服鐵液水 得效하니라.

There was once a So Eum Individual who suffered from hemiplegia and was successfully treated with the Iron Water Acupuncture technique.[73]

嘗見少陰人 小兒의 腹瘧病에 有醫가 教以瘧病將發之早朝에 用火煅金頂
砒하되 極細末六厘를 生甘草湯에 調下하니 卽效하니라. 醫曰砒藥은 必
金頂砒然後에 可用而又火煅然後에 可用也오 必不可過六厘而又不可不
及六厘也니 過六厘則藥毒이 太過也오 不及六厘則瘧不愈也니 此藥은 屢
試屢驗而有一服에 愈이어늘 後에 瘧又再發者는 又用之則其病이 益甚而
危하니 蓋此藥은 可以一服이오 不可再服云하니라.

---

71　The Fire Acupuncture technique involves placing needles directly into a flame until red-hot before insertion. This technique was historically practiced for sanitary reasons as well as to remove (bacterial) toxins from the local area. The So Eum Individual responds well to Heat-related therapies due to the systemic accumulation of Yin Cold within the body.

72　The Fire Knife technique is similar to the Fire Acupuncture technique, but was utilized for larger cysts and abscesses that were more difficult to access and/or remove. It involves placing a knife directly into a flame until red-hot before insertion.

73　The Iron Water Acupuncture technique involves dipping needles into water that has been boiled in a cast iron kettle before insertion.

There was once a So Eum Individual who suffered from Abdominal Malaria syndrome.[74] He was successfully treated with .225g of finely grated Fire-heated arsenic[75] and fresh Gan Cao (*Radix Glycyrrhizae*). This combination was boiled in water early in the morning before the symptoms of malaria fully manifested. According to the treating physician, life-threatening situations always call for the use of arsenic, which must be fire-heated beforehand and prescribed at exactly .225g in a single dose. Lower dosages have no effect on malaria while higher dosages can lead to medically induced toxicity. He tested the use of arsenic several times and discovered that there was only one case of disease recurrence, which quickly became worse after a second dose. He concluded that arsenic can only be prescribed once, and if ineffective, it cannot be given a second time.

聽醫言而究其理則一服愈而瘧不再發者는 皆少陰人小兒也오 一服愈而 瘧又再發者는 皆非少陰人小兒也니 惟少陰人兒의 腹瘧病 難治者에 用此 藥이오 尋常瘧은 不必用此不祥之藥이니라. 少陰人의 尋常間日瘧은 惡寒 時에 用川芎桂枝湯 二三貼則亦無不愈오 又腹中에 實滿而大便硬하며 瘧 發者는 亦可用巴豆니라.

From my experience with the use of fire-heated arsenic, when it is prescribed only once for the So Eum child, there is no recurrence of malaria. Recurrence occurs only in adults. Yet such a strong medicine should only be applied in acute Abdominal Malaria syndrome, and should never be used for any other type of malaria. *Cheongung Gyeji Tang* (Lee Je-ma's Lovage Root and Cinnamon Twig Decoction) should be used for less acute cases of malaria, accompanied by continuous chills during the first few days of onset. Recovery is certain after only a few days of using this formula. Ba Dou (*Semen Crotonis*) can also be used with malaria involving constipation and fullness of the upper abdomen.

百藥이 莫非善藥而惟少陰人의 信砒藥과 太陰人의 瓜蒂藥이 最爲惡藥 也ㅣ라 何哉오 少陰人의 信砒藥을 百病에 用之면 皆殆而祇有治瘧之一 能者나 亦有名無實하야 不無危慮니 萬不如桂枝 人蔘 白芍藥 三四服 之하야 治瘧則此非天下萬害無用之藥乎아 太陰人의 瓜蒂藥을 百病에 用 之면 皆殆而祇有治痰涎壅塞之一能者나 亦有名無實하야 不無危慮니 萬 不如桔梗 麥門冬 五味子 三四服之하야 治痰涎壅塞則 此非天下萬害無用 之藥乎아 此二藥은 外治에 可用而內服은 不可用이니라.

---

74 "Abdominal Malaria syndrome," or *Fu Nue Bing* (腹瘧病), is marked by malaria-induced swelling of the spleen, forming a turtle-shaped protrusion above the abdominal area, accompanied by extreme alternating chills and fever. Most, if not all, other forms of malaria tend to affect the So Yang rather than So Eum Individual.

75 Arsenic is no longer used for this condition due to its extremely high level of toxicity.

Even though herbs can be life saving, they can also be life threatening. Arsenic for the So Eum Individual and Gua Di (*Pedicellus Cucumeris Melonis*) for the Tae Eum Individual are the most dangerous of all medicines, no matter what illness they are used for. Hence there is no need to worry about using such approaches because they are limited to the treatment of only one condition. Even if arsenic is somewhat effective in the treatment of Abdominal Malaria of the So Eum Individual, it cannot compare to the effects of taking three to four doses of Gui Zhi (*Ramulus Cinnamomi Cassiae*), Ren Shen (*Radix Ginseng*), and Bai Shao Yao (*Radix Paeoniae Lactiflorae*). If the latter approach is available, why would anyone want to risk the life of their patient by prescribing a dangerous herb that may not yield the desired effects? Since Gua Di (*Pedicellus Cucumeris Melonis*) is a dangerous herb that is used solely for the Tae Eum Individual's phlegm obstruction, why would anyone in their right mind want to use it? The Tae Eum Individual's phlegm obstruction can be effectively and safely treated with three to four doses of Jie Geng (*Radix Platycodi*), Mai Men Dong (*Tuber Ophiopogonis*), and Wu Wei Zi (*Fructus Shizandrae*). This formula is ten thousand times safer than Gua Di (*Pedicellus Cucumeris Melonis*), making the latter useless in comparison. To avoid danger, arsenic and Gua Di (*Pedicellus Cucumeris Melonis*) should be applied for topical use only.

嘗見少陰人의 中氣病에 舌卷不語이어늘 有醫가 針合谷穴而其效如 神하고 其他諸病之藥이 不能速效者를 針能速效者가 有之니 蓋針穴도 亦有太少陰陽四象人 應用之穴而必有升降緩速之妙하나니 繫是不可不 察하야 敬俟後之謹厚而好活人者하노라.

There was a So Eum Individual who suffered from *Zhong Qi* syndrome[76] that was treated with the *hegu* (LI 4) acupuncture point, yielding surprisingly positive results. From my experience, acupuncture is always useful if herbal medicines have not yielded quick and effective results. There are likely specific acupuncture protocols, which have yet to be discovered, that promote the raising/lowering and quickening/slowing of energy according to each constitution. The discovery of such methods by a prudent and benevolent doctor who devotes himself to helping others is yet to come. I graciously await this opportunity.

---

76  *Zhong Qi* (中氣) syndrome, especially affecting the So Eum Individual, is a result of spleen and stomach deficiency. It manifests as food stagnation, distension, and flatulence from the inability to process food efficiently.

# The So Eum Individual's 23 Formulae from Zhang Zhongjing's *Shang Han Lun*

### Gui Zhi Tang
*Cinnamon Twig Decoction*

| Gui Zhi | *Ramulus Cinnamomi Cassiae* | 11.25g |
| Bai Shao Yao | *Radix Paeoniae Lactiflorae* | 7.5g |
| Gan Cao | *Radix Glycyrrhizae* | 3.75g |
| Sheng Jiang | *Rhizoma Zingiberis Recens* | 3 Slices |
| Da Zao | *Fructus Jujubae* | 2 Pieces |

### Li Zhong Wan
*Regulate the Middle Pill*

| Ren Shen | *Radix Ginseng* | 7.5g | |
| Bai Zhu | *Radix Atractylodis Macrocephalae* | 7.5g | |
| Gan Jiang | *Rhizoma Zingiberis Officinalis* | 7.5g | (Sun-dried) |
| Zhi Gan Cao | *Radix Glycrrhizae* | 3.75g | (Dry-fried with honey) |

### Jiang Fu Tang
*Ginger Aconite Decoction*

| Pao Gan Jiang | *Rhizoma Zingiberis* | 37.5g | (Dry-fried until blackened) |
| Pao Fu Zi | *Radix Aconiti Lateralis Praeparata* | 18.75g | (Dry-fried until blackened) |

Thinly slice the Pao Fu Zi before dry-frying. Prepare both ingredients as a decoction. When fresh Fu Zi is used, the formula is referred to as *Bai Tong Tang* (White Penetrating Decoction).

### Si Shun Li Zhong Tang
*Four Ingredients Decoction to Smooth and Regulate the Middle*

| Ren Shen | *Radix Ginseng* | 7.5g | |
| Bai Zhu | *Radix Atractylodis Macrocephalae* | 7.5g | |
| Gan Jiang | *Rhizoma Zingiberis Officinalis* | 7.5g | |
| Zhi Gan Cao | *Radix Glycrrhizae* | 7.5g | (Dry-fried with honey) |

### Gui Zhi Ren Shen Tang
*Cinnamon Twig Ginseng Decoction*

| | | | |
|---|---|---|---|
| Zhi Gan Cao | *Radix Glycrrhizae* | 6.75g | (Dry-fried with honey) |
| Gui Zhi | *Ramulus Cinnamomi Cassiae* | 6.75g | |
| Bai Zhu Radix | *Atractylodis Macrocephalae* | 5.625g | |
| Ren Shen | *Radix Ginseng* | 5.625g | |
| Gan Jiang | *Rhizoma Zingiberis Officinalis* | 5.625g | (Sun-dried) |

### Si Ni San
*Frigid Extremities Powder*

| | | | |
|---|---|---|---|
| Zhi Gan Cao | *Radix Glycrrhizae* | 22.5g | (Dry-fried with honey) |
| Pao Gan Jiang | *Rhizoma Zingiberis* | 18.75g | (Dry-fried until blackened) |
| Sheng Fu Zi | *Radix Aconiti* | 1 Slice | |

The above formula is divided into two packs before decocting.

### Hou Po Ban Xia Tang
*Prepared Pinellia and Magnolia Bark Decoction*

| | | |
|---|---|---|
| Hou Po | *Cortex Magnoliae Officinalis* | 11.25g |
| Ren Shen | *Radix Ginseng* | 5.625g |
| Ban Xia | *Rhizoma Pinelliae* | 5.625g |
| Gan Cao | *Radix Glycyrrhizae* | 2.625g |
| Sheng Jiang | *Rhizoma Zingiberis* | 7 Slices |

### Ban Xia Tang
*Prepared Pinellia Decoction*

| | | | |
|---|---|---|---|
| Zhi Ban Xia | *Rhizoma Pinelliae* | 7.5g | (Prepared with ginger to reduce toxicity) |
| Zhi Gan Cao | *Radix Glycrrhizae* | 7.5g | (Dry-fried with honey) |
| Gui Zhi | *Ramulus Cinnamomi Cassiae* | 7.5g | |

### Chi Shi Zhi Yu Yu Liang Tang
*Halloysite and Limonite Decoction*

| | | |
|---|---|---|
| Chi Shi Zhi | *Halloysitum Rubrum* | 9.375g |
| Yu Yu Liang | *Limonitum Cum Terra* | 9.375g |

### Fu Zi Tang
*Prepared Aconite Decoction*

| Bai Zhu | *Radix Atractylodis Macrocephalae* | 15g | |
| Bai Shao Yao | *Radix Paeoniae Lactiflorae* | 11.25g | |
| Bai Fu Ling | *Poria Alba* | 11.25g | |
| Pao Fu Zi | *Radix Aconiti Lateralis Praeparata* | 7.5g | (Dry-fried until blackened) |
| Ren Shen | *Radix Ginseng* | 7.5g | |

### Ma Huang Fu Zi Xi Xin Tang
*Ephedra, Asarum, and Prepared Aconite Decoction*

| Ma Huang | *Herba Ephedrae* | 7.5g | |
| Xi Xin | *Herba Asari* | 7.5g | |
| Pao Fu Zi | *Radix Aconiti Lateralis Praeparata* | 3.75g | (Dry-fried until blackened) |

### Ma Huang Fu Zi Gan Cao Tang
*Ephedra, Prepared Aconite, and Licorice Decoction*

| Ma Huang | *Herba Ephedrae* | 11.25g | |
| Gan Cao | *Radix Glycyrrhizae* | 11.25g | |
| Pao Fu Zi | *Radix Aconiti Lateralis Praeparata* | 3.75g | (Dry-fried until blackened) |

### Dang Gui Si Ni Tang
*Tangkuei Decoction for Frigid Extremities*

| Bai Shao Yao | *Radix Paeoniae Lactiflorae* | 7.5g |
| Dang Gui | *Radix Angelica Sinensis* | 7.5g |
| Gui Zhi | *Ramulus Cinnamomi Cassiae* | 5.625g |
| Xi Xin | *Herba Asari* | 3.75g |
| Tong Cao | *Medulla Tetrapanacis* | 3.75g |
| Gan Cao | *Radix Glycyrrhizae* | 3.75g |

### Ban Xia Xie Xin Tang
*Pinellia Decoction to Drain the Epigastrium*

| Zhi Ban Xia | *Rhizoma Pinelliae* | 7.5g | (Prepared with ginger to reduce toxicity) |

| Ren Shen | *Radix Ginseng* | 5.625g | |
| Gan Cao | *Radix Glycyrrhizae* | 5.625g | |
| Huang Qin | *Radix Scutellariae* | 5.625g | |
| Gan Jiang | *Rhizoma Zingiberis Officinalis* | 3.75g | (Sun-dried) |
| Huang Lian | *Rhizoma Coptidis* | 1.875g | |
| Sheng Jiang | *Rhizoma Zingiberis* | 3 Slices | |
| Da Zao | *Fructus Jujubae* | 2 Pieces | |

### Sheng Jiang Xie Xin Tang
*Ginger Decoction to Drain the Epigastrium*

| Sheng Jiang | *Rhizoma Zingiberis* | 7.5g | |
| Ban Xia | *Rhizoma Pinelliae* | 7.5g | |
| Ren Shen | *Radix Ginseng* | 5.625g | |
| Gan Jiang | *Rhizoma Zingiberis Officinalis* | 5.625g | (Sun-dried) |
| Huang Lian | *Rhizoma Coptidis* | 3.75g | |
| Gan Cao | *Radix Glycyrrhizae* | 3.75g | |
| Huang Qin | *Radix Scutellariae* | 1.875g | |
| Da Zao | *Fructus Jujubae* | 3 Pieces | |

### Gan Cao Xie Xin Tang
*Licorice Decoction to Drain the Epigastrium*

| Gan Cao | *Radix Glycyrrhizae* | 7.5g | |
| Gan Jiang | *Rhizoma Zingiberis Officinalis* | 5.625g | (Sun-dried) |
| Huang Qin | *Radix Scutellariae* | 5.625g | |
| Zhi Ban Xia | *Rhizoma Pinelliae* | 3.75g | (Prepared with ginger to reduce toxicity) |
| Ren Shen | *Radix Ginseng* | 3.75g | |
| Da Zao | *Fructus Jujubae* | 3 Pieces | |

### Yin Chen Hao Tang
*Artemisia Yinchenhao Decoction*

| Yin Chen Hao | *Herba Artemisiae Scopariae* | 37.5g |
| Da Huang | *Radix et Rhizoma Rhei* | 18.75g |
| Zhi Zi | *Fructus Gardeniae* | 7.5g |

Decoct Yin Chen Hao until half of the water remains and then add the next two ingredients until half of this water is left. Ingest twice a day. This formula will help reduce abdominal distension, eradicate hematuria, and eliminate jaundice by promoting urination.

### Di Dang Tang
*Rhubarb and Leech Decoction*

| Shui Zhi | *Hirudo* | 10 Pieces | |
| Meng Chong | *Tabanus* | 10 Pieces | (Legs and wings removed) |
| Tao Ren | *Semen Persicae* | 10 Pieces | |
| Da Huang | *Radix et Rhizoma Rhei* | 11.25g | |

### Tao Ren Cheng Qi Tang
*Guide the Qi Formula with Persica*

| Da Huang | *Radix et Rhizoma Rhei* | 11.25g |
| Gui Shim | *Ramulus Cinnamomi* | 7.5g |
| Mang Xiao | *Natrii Sulfas* | 7.5g |
| Gan Cao | *Radix Glycyrrhizae* | 3.75g |
| Tao Ren | *Semen Persicae* | 10 Pieces |

### Ma Ren Tang
*Persica Formula*

| Da Huang | *Radix et Rhizoma Rhei* | 150g |
| Zhi Shi | *Fructus Aurantii Immaturus* | 75g |
| Hou Po | *Cortex Magnoliae Officinalis* | 75g |
| Chi Shao Yao | *Radix Paeoniae Rubra* | 75g |
| Ma Zhi Ren | *Fructus Cannabis* | 56.25g |
| Xing Ren | *Semen Armeniacae Amarum* | 46.875g |

Grind the above herbs into powder and combine with honey to make empress tree seed-sized[77] pills. Ingest 50 pills in one serving on an empty stomach with warm water.

### Mi Dao Fa
*Honey-based Purgative Method*

This method should be administered when the patient is constipated but unable to ingest medicine because of a frail constitution or advanced age. Mi Dao Fa consists of boiled honey

---

77   Empress tree seeds are approximately ¼ inch in diameter.

mixed with small amounts of Zao Jiao (*Gleditsia Sinensis*) and then made into small pills, the size of an empress tree seed. Stools will certainly pass if the pills are inserted directly into the anus.

### Da Cheng Qi Tang
*Major Order the Qi Decoction*

| Da Huang | *Radix et Rhizoma Rhei* | 15g |
| Hou Po | *Cortex Magnoliae Officinalis* | 7.5g |
| Zhi Shi | *Fructus Aurantii Immaturus* | 7.5g |
| Mang Xiao | *Natrii Sulfas* | 7.5g |

At first, boil Zhi Shi and Hou Po with two cups of water and let simmer until only one cup remains. Then add Da Huang and bring to a boil. Remove the dregs after simmering for seven minutes. Then add Mang Xiao, bring to a boil, and drink while still warm.

### Xiao Cheng Qi Tang
*Minor Order the Qi Decoction*

| Da Huang | *Radix et Rhizoma Rhei* | 15g |
| Hou Po | *Cortex Magnoliae Officinalis* | 5.625g |
| Zhi Shi | *Fructus Aurantii Immaturus* | 5.625g |

Make sure herbs are thinly sliced and prepare as a single pack to be ingested as a decoction.

## The So Eum Individual's 13 Formulae Presented by Doctors of the Song, Yuan, and Ming Dynasties— with Six Containing Ba Dou (*Semen Crotonis*)
### Shi Quan Da Bu Tang
*All-Inclusive Great Tonifying Decoction*

| Ren Shen | *Radix Ginseng* | 3.75g | |
| Bai Zhu | *Radix Atractylodis Macrocephalae* | 3.75g | |
| Bai Shao Yao | *Radix Paeoniae Lactiflorae* | 3.75g | |
| Zhi Gan Cao | *Radix Glycrrhizae* | 3.75g | (Dry-fried with honey) |
| Huang Qi | *Radix Astragali Membranacei* | 3.75g | |
| Gui Shim | *Cortex Cinnamomi* | 3.75g | |
| Dang Gui | *Radix Angelicae Sinensis* | 3.75g | |
| Chuan Xiong | *Radix Ligustici Chuanxiong* | 3.75g | |
| Fu Ling | *Poria Alba* | 3.75g | |
| Shu Di Huang | *Radix Rehmanniae Preparata* | 3.75g | |

| Shen Xiang | *Rhizoma Zingiberis Recens* | 3 Slices |
| Da Zao | *Fructus Jujubae* | 2 Pieces |

This formula, mentioned in Wang Hao Gu's text entitled *Hai Zang Shu*, is indicated for deficiency and fatigue.

My own accumulated clinical experience has shown me [that] Fu Ling (*Poria Alba*) and Shu Di Huang (*Radix Rehmanniae Preparata*) [are for the So Yang Individual] and should therefore be replaced with Sha Ren (*Fructus Amomi*) and Chen Pi (*Pericarpium Citri Reticulatae*).

### Bu Zhong Yi Qi Tang
*Tonify the Middle and Augment the Qi Decoction*

| Huang Qi | *Radix Astragali* | 5.625g | |
| Zhi Gan Cao | *Radix Glycrrhizae* | 3.75g | (Dry-fried with honey) |
| Ren Shen | *Radix Ginseng* | 3.75g | |
| Bai Zhu | *Radix Atractylodis Macrocephalae* | 3.75g | |
| Dang Gui | *Radix Angelicae Sinensis* | 2.625g | |
| Chen Pi | *Pericarpium Citri Reticulatae* | 2.625g | |
| Sheng Ma | *Rhizoma Cimicifugae* | 1.125g | |
| Chai Hu | *Radix Bupleuri* | 1.125g | |
| Sheng Jiang | *Rhizoma Zingiberis Recens* | 3 Slices | |
| Da Zao | *Fructus Jujubae* | 2 Pieces | |

This formula, mentioned in Li Gao's text *Dong Yuan Shu*, is indicated for overwork and exhaustion leading to *Lao Juan*,[78] and overall fatigue.

My own accumulated clinical experience tells me that the dosage of Huang Qi (*Radix Astragali Membranacei*) should be increased to 11.25g, and since Chai Hu (*Radix Bupleuri*) and Sheng Ma (*Rhizoma Cimicifugae*) [are for the So Yang and Tae Eum Individuals respectively], they should be replaced by Huo Xiang (*Herba Pogostemonis*) and Zi Su Ye (*Folium Perillae*).

### Xiang Sha Liu Jun Zi Tang
*Six Gentlemen Decoction with Aucklandia and Amomum*

| Xiang Fu Zi | *Rhizoma Cyperi* | 3.75g |
| Bai Zhu | *Radix Atractylodis Macrocephalae* | 3.75g |
| Bai Fu Ling | *Poria Alba* | 3.75g |

---

78  The two Chinese characters of *Lao* (勞) and *Juan* (倦) literally translate as "overwork" and "laziness." Together, these characters represent the desire to disconnect with one's environment as a result of excessive worry and anxiety. As mentioned in the second chapter, the stronger kidneys of the So Eum Individual correlate with *rak* (樂), or calmness, and they also correlate with the buttocks, which are associated with planned action. Hence, if events do not go as planned and the So Eum Individual cannot achieve satisfaction and calmness, then he or she may disengage and retreat into their own fantasy world.

| Ban Xia | *Rhizoma Pinelliae* | 3.75g | |
| Chen Pi | *Pericarpium Citri Reticulatae* | 3.75g | |
| Hou Po | *Cortex Magnoliae Officinalis* | 3.75g | |
| Bai Dou Kou | *Fructus Amomi Rotundus* | 3.75g | |
| Ren Shen | *Radix Ginseng* | 1.875g | |
| Gan Cao | *Radix Glycyrrhizae* | 1.875g | |
| Mu Xiang | *Radix Aucklandiae* | 1.875g | |
| Sha Ren | *Fructus Amomi* | 1.875g | |
| Yi Zhi Ren | *Semen Alpiniae Oxyphyllae* | 1.875g | |
| Sheng Jiang | *Rhizoma Zingiberis Recens* | 3 Slices | |
| Da Zao | *Fructus Jujubae* | 2 Pieces | |

This formula, mentioned in Gong Xin's text entitled *Yijianshu* (*Mirror of Eastern Medicine*), is indicated for lack of appetite, indigestion, bloating, and belching after eating.

In my own accumulated clinical experience over the years, Fu Ling (*Poria Alba*) [is prescribed for the So Yang Individual] and should therefore be replaced with He Shou Wu (*Polygoni Multiflori Alba*).

## Mu Xiang Shun Qi San
*Smooth the Qi Decoction with Aucklandia*

| Wu Yao | *Radix Linderae* | 3.75g | |
| Xiang Fu Zi | *Rhizoma Cyperi* | 3.75g | |
| Chong Pi | *Pericarpium Citri Ret. Viridae* | 3.75g | |
| Chen Pi | *Pericarpium Citri Reticulatae* | 3.75g | |
| Hou Po | *Cortex Magnoliae Officinalis* | 3.75g | |
| Zhi Ke | *Fructus Aurantii* | 3.75g | |
| Ban Xia | *Rhizoma Pinelliae* | 3.75g | |
| Mu Xiang | *Radix Aucklandiae* | 1.875g | |
| Sha Ren | *Fructus Amomi* | 1.875g | |
| Gui Pi | *Cortex Cinnamomi* | 1.125g | |
| Gan Jiang | *Rhizoma Zingiberis* | 1.125g | (Sun-dried) |
| Zhi Gan Cao | *Radix Glycrrhizae* | 1.125g | (Dry-fried with honey) |
| Sheng Jiang | *Rhizoma Zingiberis* | 3 Slices | (Sun-dried) |
| Da Zao | *Fructus Jujubae* | 2 Pieces | |

This formula, mentioned in Gong Xin's text entitled *Wan Bing Hui Chun* (*Restoring Health from Tens of Thousands of Diseases*), is indicated for *Zhong Qi* (Central *Qi*) syndrome, in which dizziness and fainting occur after extreme anger or shock. Sheng Jiang (*Rhizoma Zingiberis*) tea should be administered beforehand to calm the patient before administering the above formula.

### *Su He Xiang Wan*
*Liquid Styrax Pill*

| Bai Zhu | *Radix Atractylodis Macrocephalae* | 3.75g |
|---|---|---|
| Mu Xiang | *Radix Aucklandiae* | 1.875g |
| Chen Xiang | *Lignum Aquilariae Resinatum* | 75g |
| She Xiang | *Moschus* | 75g |
| Ding Xiang | *Flos Caryophylli* | 75g |
| An Xi Xiang | *Benzoinum* | 75g |
| Tan Xiang | *Lignum Santali Albi* | 75g |
| He Zi | *Fructus Chebulae* | 75g |
| Xiang Fu Zi | *Rhizoma Cyperi* | 3.75g |
| Bi Bo | *Fructus Piperis Longi* | 75g |
| Xi Jiao | *Cornu Rhinoceri* | 75g |
| Zhu Sha | *Cinnabaris* | 75g |
| Ru Xiang | *Resina Olibani* | 37.5g |
| Bing Pian | *Borneolum* | 37.5g |

Grind the above into thin powder and mix with the above dosage of An Xi Xiang (*Benzoinum*) fried with honey (until honey is evaporated and sticks to An Xi Xiang), and make into a total of 40, 37.5g pills. Ingest two to three pills per dose with well water collected before dawn or simply with warm water.

This formula, presented in the *Ju Fang* (*Formularies of the Bureau of People's Welfare Pharmacies*), is indicated for numerous *Qi*-related disorders such as boils, tumors, abscesses, reversal of *Qi*, dizziness, *Qi Yu* syndrome,[79] and blockage of *Qi* causing pain.

Xu Shu-wei states in his text, *Benshifang* (*Prescriptions of Universal Benefit from My Own Practice*), that excessive joy causes depletion of Yang *Qi*, and excessive anger causes depletion of the Yin *Qi*. Long-term overwork and anxiety will generally lead to *Jue Ni* syndrome,[80] which calls for medicine. If this situation is hastily treated as a *Zhong Feng*[81] illness, then it will endanger the patient's life.

In Wei Yi-lin's text entitled *Dexiaofang* (*Collection of Effective Prescriptions*), he states that when *Zhong Feng* occurs, the pulse will be superficial, the body will feel warm (vs. cold as in *Jue Ni* syndrome), with copious phlegm [accumulation in the mouth]. Yet, if *Zhong Qi* occurs, there will be a sinking pulse, the body will feel cold, with no sign of copious phlegm accumulation in the mouth.

---

79　*Qi Yu* (氣鬱) syndrome is the result of *Qi* stagnation in the upper body due to excessive worry, sadness, and/ or loneliness. Symptoms include a full and uncomfortable sensation in the chest, tenderness in the flank area, and a lack of appetite. For the So Eum Individual, the above emotions lead to a lack of Yin descent from the spleen to kidneys, causing stagnation in the upper body.

80　*Jue Ni* (厥逆) syndrome is due to the reversal of *Qi* movement, leading to a minute (or absent) pulse, freezing cold hands and feet, and loss of consciousness. This life-threatening syndrome may occur during a pathogenic influence of the Tai Yang, Yang Ming, Tai Yin, or Jue Yin stages, but is most commonly seen during the latter stage of illness. In the So Eum Individual, *Jue Ni* occurs when extreme suppression of Yang *Qi* within the spleen and kidney leads to rebellion (aka explosion) of Yang *Qi* upwards and outwards.

81　*Zhong Feng* (中風) is also referred to as *Tai Yang Zhong Feng* syndrome, and occurs during the first stage of a Shang Han (Cold-induced) illness.

In my own clinical experience, She Xiang (*Moschus*), Xi Jiao (*Cornu Rhinoceri*), and Bing Pian (*Borneolum*) [which are prescribed for the Tae Eum Individual], and Zhu Sha (*Cinnabaris*) and Ru Xiang (*Resina Olibani*) [which are prescribed for the So Yang Individual], should be omitted and Huo Xiang (*Herba Pogostemonis*), Xiao Hui Xiang (*Fructus Foeniculi*), Gui Pi (*Cortex Cinnamomi*), Wu Ling Zhi (*Faeces Trogopterorum*), and Yan Hu Suo (*Rhizoma Corydalis*) should be added.

### Huo Xiang Zheng Qi San
*Agastache Powder to Rectify the Qi*

| | | |
|---|---|---|
| Huo Xiang | *Herba Pogostemonis* | 5.625g |
| Zi Su Ye | *Folium Perillae* | 3.75g |
| Hou Po | *Cortex Magnoliae Officinalis* | 1.875g |
| Da Fu Pi | *Pericarpium Arecae* | 1.875g |
| Bai Zhu | *Radix Atractylodis Macrocephalae* | 1.875g |
| Chen Pi | *Pericarpium Citri Reticulatae* | 1.875g |
| Ban Xia | *Rhizoma Pinelliae* | 1.875g |
| Gan Cao | *Radix Glycyrrhizae* | 1.875g |
| Jie Geng | *Radix Platycodi* | 1.875g |
| Bai Zhi | *Radix Angelicae Dahuricae* | 1.875g |
| Bai Fu Ling | *Poria Alba* | 1.875g |
| Sheng Jiang | *Rhizoma Zingiberis Recens* | 3 Slices |
| Da Zao | *Fructus Jujubae* | 2 Pieces |

This formula, in Gong Xin's work entitled *Yijianshu* (*Mirror of Eastern Medicine*), is prescribed as a remedy for Shang Han illness.

As I found in the course of my own clinical experience, Jie Geng (*Radix Platycodi*) and Bai Zhi (*Radix Angelicae Dahuricae*) [which are prescribed for the Tae Eum Individual], and Bai Fu Ling (*Poria Alba*) [, which is prescribed for the So Yang Individual], should be omitted and replaced with Gui Pi (*Cortex Cinnamomi*), Gan Jiang (*Rhizoma Zingiberis Officinalis*), and Yi Zhi Ren (*Fructus Alpiniae Oxyphyllae*).

### Xiang Su San
*Cyperus and Perilla Leaf Powder*

| | | |
|---|---|---|
| Xiang Fu Zi | *Rhizoma Cyperi* | 11.25g |
| Zi Su Ye | *Folium Perillae* | 9.375g |
| Chen Pi | *Pericarpium Citri Reticulatae* | 5.625g |
| Cang Zhu | *Rhizoma Atractylodis* | 3.75g |
| Gan Cao | *Radix Glycyrrhizae* | 3.75g |
| Sheng Jiang | *Rhizoma Zingiberis Recens* | 3 Slices |
| Cong Bai | *Radix Allii* | 2 Stems |

This formula, mentioned in Wei Yi-lin's *Dexiaofang* (*Collection of Effective Prescriptions*), is prescribed for epidemic diseases that occur during any of the four seasons. The *Ju Fang* (*Formularies of the Bureau of People's Welfare Pharmacies*) tells of an elderly man who prescribed this formula for all members of a village that was stricken by an epidemic disease, with everyone recovering shortly afterwards.

### Gui Zhi Fu Zi Tang
*Cinnamon Twig and Poria Pill*

| | | | |
|---|---|---|---|
| Pao Fu Zi | *Radix Aconiti Lateralis Praeparata* | 11.25g | (Dry-fried until blackened) |
| Gui Zhi | *Ramulus Cinnamomi Cassiae* | 11.25g | |
| Bai Shao Yao | *Radix Paeoniae Lactiflorae* | 7.5g | |
| Zhi Gan Cao | *Radix Glycrrhizae* | 3.75g | (Dry-fried with honey) |
| Sheng Jiang | *Rhizoma Zingiberis Recens* | 3 Slices | |
| Da Zao | *Fructus Jujubae* | 2 Pieces | |

This formula, appearing in Li Chan's text *Yixuefang* (*Introduction to Medicine*), is prescribed for a lack of sweating and stiffness of the extremities, with difficulty flexing and extending the arms and feet.

### Yin Chen Si Ni Tang
*Artemisia Yinchenhao Decoction for Frigid Extremities*

| | | | |
|---|---|---|---|
| Yin Chen Hao | *Herba Artemisiae Scopariae* | 37.5g | |
| Pao Fu Zi | *Radix Aconiti Lateralis Praeparata* | 3.75g | (Dry-fried until blackened) |
| Pao Gan Jiang | *Rhizoma Zingiberis* | 3.75g | (Dry-fried until blackened) |
| Zhi Gan Cao | *Radix Glycrrhizae* | 3.75g | (Dry-fried with honey) |

This formula, within Zhu Gong's text *Hourenshu* (*Revive the People*), is prescribed for Yin jaundice with continuous flow of sweat due to [Yang] deficiency.

### Yin Chen Fu Zi Tang
*Artemisia Yinchenhao and Poria Decoction*

| | | | |
|---|---|---|---|
| Yin Chen Hao | *Herba Artemisiae Scopariae* | 37.5g | |
| Pao Fu Zi | *Radix Aconiti Lateralis Praeparata* | 3.75g | (Dry-fried until blackened) |
| Zhi Gan Cao | *Radix Glycrrhizae* | 3.75g | (Dry-fried with honey) |

This formula, within Zhu Gong's text *Hourenshu* (*Revive the People*), is prescribed for Yin jaundice accompanied by cold sweating.

### Yin Chen Ju Pi Tang
*Artemisia Yinchenhao and Tangerine Peel Decoction*

| Yin Chen Hao | *Herba Artemisiae Scopariae* | 37.5g |
|---|---|---|
| Chen Pi | *Pericarpium Citri Reticulatae* | 3.75g |
| Bai Zhu | *Radix Atractylodis Macrocephalae* | 3.75g |
| Ban Xia | *Rhizoma Pinelliae* | 3.75g |
| Sheng Jiang | *Rhizoma Zingiberis Recens* | 3.75g |

This formula, presented in Zhu Gong's *Hourenshu* (*Revive the People*), is prescribed for Yin jaundice with shortness of breath and dry heaves without thirst.

### San Wei Shen Yu Tang
*Three Flavors Ginseng and Evodia Fruit Decoction*

| Wu Zhu Yu | *Fructus Evodiae* | 11.25g |
|---|---|---|
| Ren Shen | *Radix Ginseng* | 7.5g |
| Sheng Jiang | *Rhizoma Zingiberis Recens* | 4 Slices |
| Da Zao | *Fructus Jujubae* | 2 Pieces |

This formula, given in Li Chan's text *Yuxuerumen* (*Introduction to Medicine*), is prescribed for Jue Yin syndrome characterized by an unsettled stomach with vomiting of frothy sputum. It can also be used with great results for Shao Yin Stage ice-cold extremities, shortness of breath, and vexation, or post-prandial vomiting due to Yang Ming Stage syndrome.

### Pi Li San
*Thunderbolt Powder*

| Pao Fu Zi | *Radix Aconiti Lateralis Praeparata* | 1 Piece | (Dry-fried until blackened) |
|---|---|---|---|

Dry-fry Fu Zi (*Radix Aconiti*) until it turns black, then immerse in cold ashes for 30 minutes. Cut into thin slices and boil with 3.75g of green tea (made with young tea leaves) and one cup of water for six minutes. Strain the herbs and tea and then mix in half a tablespoon of honey. Drink while warm. Recovery from tightness of the chest and vexation will follow shortly after ingesting this tea. Full recovery from illness will occur the next morning after night sweating.

This formula, from Li Chan's *Yuxuerumen* (*Introduction to Medicine*), is prescribed when abundant Internal Yin chases the weakened Yang outwards to the Exterior.

## Wen Bai Yuan
### Warm the White Pill

| | | | |
|---|---|---|---|
| Pao Chuan Wu | *Radix Aconiti Carmichaeli* | 93.75g | (Dry-fried until blackened) |
| Wu Zhu Yu | *Fructus Evodiae* | 18.75g | |
| Jie Geng | *Radix Platycodi* | 18.75g | |
| Chai Hu | *Radix Bupleuri* | 18.75g | |
| Shi Chang Pu | *Rhizoma Apori Graminei* | 18.75g | |
| Zi Wan | *Radix Asteris* | 18.75g | |
| Huang Lian | *Rhizoma Coptidis* | 18.75g | |
| Pao Gan Jiang | *Rhizoma Zingiberis* | 18.75g | (Dry-fried until blackened) |
| Rou Gui | *Cortex Cinnamomi* | 18.75g | |
| Chuan Jiao | *Pericarpium Zanthoxyli* | 18.75g | (Stir-fried with honey) |
| Chi Fu Ling | *Poria Rubra* | 18.75g | |
| Zao Jiao | *Spina Gleditsiae* | 18.75g | |
| Hou Po | *Cortex Magnoliae Officinalis* | 18.75g | |
| Ren Shen | *Radix Ginseng* | 18.75g | |
| Ba Dou | *Semen Crotonis Pulveratum* | 18.75g | |

Grind the above ingredients into a powder and combine with honey to make empress tree seed-sized pills. Ingest three to seven pills on an empty stomach with warm ginger tea.

This formula, in the *Ju Fang* (*Formularies of the Bureau of People's Welfare Pharmacies*), is indicated for hypochondriac and abdominal masses from long-term food stagnation, jaundice, abdominal distension, ten types of diseases due to water retention, nine types of cardiac-related issues, eight types of *Bi* syndrome, five types of gonorrhea, and chronic malaria.

Gong Xin states in the *Yijianshu* (*Mirror of Eastern Medicine*): "This formula will bring foreseeable relief for the female suffering from abdominal masses the size of a full-term pregnancy, lack of appetite, exhaustion and fatigue, or sudden singing and crying as if she has lost her mind. If this medicine is taken after a long-term illness, the patient will excrete parasites, turbid phlegm, and other pathogens."

### *Zhang Dan Wan*
*Epidemic Jaundice Pill*

| | | |
|---|---|---|
| Yin Chen Hao | *Herba Artemisiae Scopariae* | 37.5g |
| Zhi Zi | *Fructus Gardenia* | 37.5g |
| Da Huang | *Radix et Rhizoma Rhei* | 37.5g |
| Mang Xiao | *Natrii Sulfas* | 37.5g |
| Xing Ren | *Semen Armeniacae Amarum* | 22.5g |
| Chang Shan | *Radix Dichroae* | 15g |
| Bie Jia | *Carapax Trionycis* | 15g |
| Ba Dou | *Semen Crotonis Pulveratum* | 15g |
| Dan Dou Chi | *Semen Sojae Praeparatum* | 7.5g |

Grind the above into powder and combine with rice cake mix[82] to make empress tree seed-sized pills. Ingest three to seven pills on an empty stomach with warm water.

This formula, from Wei Yi-lin's text entitled *Dexiaofang* (*Collection of Effective Prescriptions*), is prescribed for epidemic disease, chronic malaria, jaundice, and Damp Heat disorders. It is also referred to as *Yin Chen Wan* (Artemisia Pill).

### *San Leng Xiao Ji Wan*
*Scirpus Eliminate the Accumulation Decoction*

| | | | |
|---|---|---|---|
| San Leng | *Rhizoma Sparganii* | 26.25g | |
| E Zhu | *Rhizoma Zedoariae* | 26.25g | |
| Shen Qu | *Massa Medicata Fermentata* | 26.25g | |
| Ba Dou | *Semen Crotonis Pulveratum* | 18.75g | (Stir-fry the Ba Dou peel with rice until blackened, then discard the rice) |
| Qing Pi | *Pericarpium Citri Ret. Viridae* | 18.75g | |
| Chen Pi | *Pericarpium Citri Reticulatae* | 18.75g | |
| Xiao Hui Xiang | *Fructus Foeniculi* | 18.75g | |
| Ding Xiang Pi | *Pericarpium Flos Caryophylii* | 11.25g | |
| Yi Zhi Ren | *Fructus Alpiniae Oxyphyllae* | 11.25g | |

Grind the above into powder and combine with vinegar to make a paste, then form into empress tree seed-sized pills. Ingest 30 to 40 pills on an empty stomach with warm water.

This formula, which Li Gao presents in his *Dong Yuan Shu*, is indicated for indigestion and fullness after the intake of raw and/or cold foods.

---

82   Rice cake mix, or *Jung Byoung* (蒸餅) in Korean, is a form of powdered rice used to make Korean rice cakes called *Duk*.

## Bi Fang Hwa Zhi Wan
*Secret Transform Stagnation Pill*

| | | | |
|---|---|---|---|
| Ba Dou | *Semen Crotonis Pulveratum* | 22.5g | (Place inside vinegar and let sit overnight, then boil down until dry) |
| San Leng | *Rhizoma Sparganii* | 18g | |
| E Zhu | *Rhizoma Zedoariae* | 18g | (Roasted in hot ashes) |
| Ban Xia Qu | *Rhizoma Pinelliae Fermentata* | 9.375g | |
| Mu Xiang | *Radix Aucklandiae* | 9.375g | |
| Ding Xiang | *Flos Caryophylli* | 9.375g | |
| Qing Pi | *Pericarpium Citri Ret. Viridae* | 9.375g | |
| Chen Pi | *Pericarpium Citri Reticulatae* | 9.375g | (Discard white inner peel) |
| Huang Lian | *Rhizoma Coptidis* | 9.375g | |

Grind the above into powder and combine with Wu Mei (*Fructus Mume*) powder and a small amount of wheat flour to make a paste, then form into oat-sized pills. Ingest five to ten pills on an empty stomach. Swallow with warm water to induce diarrhea. To reduce size of abdominal mass, take with Chen Pi (*Pericarpium Citri Reticulatae*) tea. Swallow with cool water to stop continuous diarrhea.

This formula, in Zhu Zhenheng's *Danxi Xinfa* (*The Teachings of Danxi*), is prescribed for all types of chronic and sudden *Qi* stagnation and mass accumulation. It has a profound ability to promote the flow of *Qi* and balance Yin and Yang by simultaneously sedating and tonifying as needed.

## San Wu Bai San
*Three Ingredients White Powder*

| | | | |
|---|---|---|---|
| Jie Geng | *Radix Platycodi* | 11.25g | |
| Bei Mu | *Fritillariae Cirrhosae Hulbus* | 11.25g | |
| Ba Dou | *Semen Crotonis Pulveratum* | 3.74g | (Discard shell and pound in mortar) |

Grind the above into fine powder to mix all ingredients thoroughly. Ingest 2g of this formula with warm water. Reduce dosage by one half in case of significant deficiency. This formula, mentioned in Li Chan's *Yuxuerumen* (*Introduction to Medicine*), may induce diarrhea and/or vomiting [to expel blockage]. If there is no sign of diarrhea, then one bowl of warm rice porridge should be provided, while one bowl of cool rice porridge will stop continuous diarrhea.

### Ru Yi Dan
*Invigorate the Willpower Pill*

| | | | |
|---|---|---|---|
| Pao Chuan Wu | *Radix Aconiti Carmichaeli* | 30g | (Dry-fried until blackened) |
| Bin Lang | *Semen Aracae* | 18.75g | |
| Ren Shen | *Radix Ginseng* | 18.75g | |
| Chai Hu | *Radix Bupleuri* | 18.75g | |
| Wu Zhu Yu | *Fructus Evodiae* | 18.75g | |
| Chuan Jiao | *Pericarpium Zanthoxyli* | 18.75g | |
| Bai Fu Ling | *Poria Alba* | 18.75g | |
| Sheng Jiang | *Rhizoma Zingiberis Recens* | 18.75g | |
| Huang Lian | *Rhizoma Coptidis* | 18.75g | |
| Zi Wan | *Radix Asteris* | 18.75g | |
| Hou Po | *Cortex Magnoliae Officinalis* | 18.75g | |
| Rou Gui | *Cortex Cinnamomi* | 18.75g | |
| Dang Gui | *Radix Angelicae Sinensis* | 18.75g | |
| Jie Geng | *Radix Platycodi* | 18.75g | |
| Zao Jiao | *Spina Gleditsiae* | 18.75g | |
| Shi Chang Pu | *Rhizoma Apori Graminei* | 18.75g | |
| Ba Dou | *Semen Crotonis Pulveratum* | 9.375g | (Defatted croton seed powder) |

Grind the above into powder and combine with boiled-down honey to make empress tree seed-sized pills and coat with Zhu Sha (*Cinnabaris*).[83] Ingest five to seven pills with warm ginger tea.

This formula, from Li Chan's text *Yuxuerumen* (*Introduction to Medicine*), is generally prescribed for febrile disease and sudden onset of psychosis.

From my perspective, the above six formulae containing Ba Dou (*Semen Crotonis Pulveratum*) are the result of the accumulated experience of ancient doctors. There is no doubt that all of these doctors agreed that Ba Dou is the most powerful ingredient in each formula. Since Ba Dou is such a powerful herb for the So Eum Individual, it should not be haphazardly prescribed for any of the other body types. However, there is no doubt regarding its effects. These six formulae are therefore handed down to us through extensive experience and are suitable for a skilled practitioner who does not use it in haste.

---

83    Zhu Sha (*Cinnabaris*) contains significant amounts of mercury and is therefore considered highly toxic. Hence it is no longer used for coating pills.

## 24 Newly Discovered Formulae for the So Eum Individual (Formulated by Lee Je-ma)

### *Huanggi Gyeji Buja Tang*

*Lee Je-ma's Astragalus Cinnamon Twig and Aconite Decoction (Modified Gui Zhi Fu Zi Tang)*

| | | | |
|---|---|---|---|
| Gui Zhi | *Ramulus Cinnamomi* | 11.25g | |
| Huang Qi | *Radix Astragali Membranacei* | 11.25g | |
| Bai Shao Yao | *Radix Paeoniae Lactiflorae* | 7.5g | |
| Dang Gui | *Radix Angelicae Sinensis* | 3.75g | |
| Zhi Gan Cao | *Radix Glycrrhizae* | 3.75g | (Dry-fried with honey) |
| Pao Fu Zi | *Radix Aconiti Lateralis Praeparata* | 3.75–7.5g | (Dry-fried until blackened) |
| Sheng Jiang | *Rhizoma Zingiberis Recens* | 3 Slices | |
| Da Zao | *Fructus Jujubae* | 2 Pieces | |

### *Insam Gyeji Buja Tang*

*Lee Je-ma's Ginseng Cinnamon Twig and Aconite Decoction (Modified Gui Zhi Fu Zi Tang)*

| | | | |
|---|---|---|---|
| Ren Shen | *Radix Ginseng* | 15g | |
| Gui Zhi | *Ramulus Cinnamomi* | 11.25g | |
| Bai Shao Yao | *Radix Paeoniae Lactiflorae* | 7.5g | |
| Huang Qi | *Radix Astragali Membranacei* | 7.5g | |
| Dang Gui | *Radix Angelicae Sinensis* | 3.75g | |
| Zhi Gan Cao | *Radix Glycrrhizae* | 3.75g | (Dry-fried with honey) |
| Pao Fu Zi | *Radix Aconiti Lateralis Praeparata* | 3.75–7.5g | (Dry-fried until blackened) |
| Sheng Jiang | *Rhizoma Zingiberis Recens* | 3 Slices | |
| Da Zao | *Fructus Jujubae* | 2 Pieces | |

### Seungyang Ikgi Buja Tang
*Lee Je-ma's Raise the Yang Support the Qi Aconite Decoction*

| Ren Shen | *Radix Ginseng* | 7.5g | |
|---|---|---|---|
| Gui Zhi | *Ramulus Cinnamomi* | 7.5g | |
| Bai Shao Yao | *Radix Paeoniae Lactiflorae* | 7.5g | |
| Huang Qi | *Radix Astragali Membranacei* | 7.5g | |
| Bai He Shou Wu | *Radix Polygoni Multiflori Alba* | 3.75g | |
| Gui Pi | *Cortex Cinnamomi* | 3.75g | |
| Dang Gui | *Radix Angelicae Sinensis* | 3.75g | |
| Zhi Gan Cao | *Radix Glycrrhizae* | 3.75g | (Dry-fried with honey) |
| Pao Fu Zi | *Radix Aconiti Lateralis Praeparata* | 3.75–7.5g | (Dry-fried until blackened) |
| Sheng Jiang | *Rhizoma Zingiberis Recens* | 3 Slices | |
| Da Zao | *Fructus Jujubae* | 2 Pieces | |

### Insam Gwangye Buja Tang
*Lee Je-ma's Ginseng Cinnamon Bark and Aconite Decoction*

| Ren Shen | *Radix Ginseng* | 18.75–37.5g | |
|---|---|---|---|
| Gui Pi | *Cortex Cinnamomi* | 11.25g | |
| Huang Qi | *Radix Astragali Membranacei* | 11.25g | |
| Bai Shao Yao | *Radix Paeoniae Lactiflorae* | 7.5g | |
| Pao Fu Zi | *Radix Aconiti Lateralis Praeparata* | 7.5–9.375g | (Dry-fried until blackened) |
| Dang Gui | *Radix Angelicae Sinensis* | 3.75g | |
| Zhi Gan Cao | *Radix Glycrrhizae* | 3.75g | (Dry-fried with honey) |
| Sheng Jiang | *Rhizoma Zingiberis Recens* | 3 Slices | |
| Da Zao | *Fructus Jujubae* | 2 Pieces | |

The four prescriptions mentioned above are prescribed when Yang *Qi* is severely deficient [as in *Mang Yang* syndrome]. If there is whitish cloudy frequent urine, the situation is considered somewhat critical and therefore 3.75g of Pao Fu Zi (*Radix Aconiti Lateralis Praeparata*) should be ingested two times a day. Reddish infrequent urine indicates a life-threatening situation and therefore 7.5g of Pao Fu Zi (*Radix Aconiti Lateralis Praeparata*) should be ingested two to three times a day. If there are signs that this illness is becoming critical, then 3.75g of Pao Fu Zi (*Radix Aconiti Lateralis Praeparata*) should be ingested two to three times a day. If the illness is no longer life threatening, then 3.75g of Pao Fu Zi (*Radix Aconiti Lateralis Praeparata*) should be ingested two to three times a day. After complete recovery from illness, 3.75g of Pao Fu Zi (*Radix Aconiti Lateralis Praeparata*) should be ingested two times a day to nurse the patient back to optimum health.

### Seungyang Ikgi Tang
*Lee Je-ma's Raise the Yang Support the Qi Decoction*
*(Modified Bu Zhong Yi Qi Tang)*

| Ren Shen | Radix Ginseng | 7.5g | |
|---|---|---|---|
| Gui Zhi | Ramulus Cinnamomi | 7.5g | |
| Huang Qi | Radix Astragali Membranacei | 7.5g | |
| Bai Shao Yao | Radix Paeoniae Lactiflorae | 7.5g | |
| Bai He Shou Wu | Radix Polygoni Multiflori Alba | 3.75g | |
| Gui Pi | Cortex Cinnamomi | 3.75g | |
| Dang Gui | Radix Angelicae Sinensis | 3.75g | |
| Zhi Gan Cao | Radix Glycrrhizae | 3.75g | (Dry-fried with honey) |
| Sheng Jiang | Rhizoma Zingiberis Recens | 3 Slices | |
| Da Zao | Fructus Jujubae | 2 Pieces | |

### Bochung Ikgi Tang
*Lee Je-ma's Tonify the Middle and Augment the Qi Decoction*
*(Modified Bu Zhong Yi Qi Tang)*

| Ren Shen | Radix Ginseng | 3.75g | |
|---|---|---|---|
| Huang Qi | Radix Astragali Membranacei | 3.75g | |
| Zhi Gan Cao | Radix Glycrrhizae | 3.75g | (Dry-fried with honey) |
| Bai Zhu | Radix Atractylodis Macrocephalae | 3.75g | |
| Dang Gui | Radix Angelicae Sinensis | 3.75g | |
| Chen Pi | Pericarpium Citri Reticulatae | 3.75g | |
| Huo Xiang | Herba Pogostemonis | 1.125–1.875g | |
| Zi Su Ye | Folium Perillae | 1.125–1.875g | |
| Sheng Jiang | Rhizoma Zingiberis Recens | 3 Slices | |
| Da Zao | Fructus Jujubae | 2 Pieces | |

### Huanggi Gyeji Tang

*Lee Je-ma's Astragalus and Cinnamon Twig Decoction (Modified Gui Zhi Tang)*

| Gui Zhi | *Ramulus Cinnamomi* | 11.25g | |
|---|---|---|---|
| Bai Shao Yao | *Radix Paeoniae Lactiflorae* | 7.5g | |
| Huang Qi | *Radix Astragali Membranacei* | 7.5g | |
| Bai He Shou Wu | *Radix Polygoni Multiflori Alba* | 3.75g | |
| Dang Gui | *Radix Angelicae Sinensis* | 3.75g | |
| Zhi Gan Cao | *Radix Glycrrhizae* | 3.75g | (Dry-fried with honey) |
| Sheng Jiang | *Rhizoma Zingiberis Recens* | 3 Slices | |
| Da Zao | *Fructus Jujubae* | 2 Pieces | |

### Cheongung Gyeji Tang

*Lee Je-ma's Lovage Root and Cinnamon Twig Decoction (Modified Gui Zhi Tang)*

| Gui Zhi | *Ramulus Cinnamomi Cassiae* | 11.25g | |
|---|---|---|---|
| Bai Shao Yao | *Radix Paeoniae Lactiflorae* | 7.5g | |
| Chuan Xiong | *Radix Ligustici Chuanxiong* | 3.75g | |
| Cang Zhu | *Rhizoma Atractylodis* | 3.75g | |
| Chen Pi | *Pericarpium Citri Reticulatae* | 3.75g | |
| Zhi Gan Cao | *Radix Glycrrhizae* | 3.75g | (Dry-fried with honey) |
| Sheng Jiang | *Rhizoma Zingiberis Recens* | 3 Slices | |
| Da Zao | *Fructus Jujubae* | 2 Pieces | |

### Gunggwi Hyangsu San

*Lee Je-ma's Cyperus and Perilla Leaf Powder with Lovage and Angelica Root (Modified Xiang Su San)*

| Xiang Fu Zi | *Rhizoma Cyperi* | 7.5g | |
|---|---|---|---|
| Zi Su Ye | *Folium Perillae* | 3.75g | |
| Chuan Xiong | *Radix Ligustici Chuanxiong* | 3.75g | |
| Dang Gui | *Radix Angelicae Sinensis* | 3.75g | |
| Cang Zhu | *Rhizoma Atractylodis* | 3.75g | |
| Chen Pi | *Pericarpium Citri Reticulatae* | 3.75g | |
| Zhi Gan Cao | *Radix Glycrrhizae* | 3.75g | (Dry-fried with honey) |
| Cong Bai | *Radix Allii* | 5 Stems | |
| Sheng Jiang | *Rhizoma Zingiberis Recens* | 3 Slices | |
| Da Zao | *Fructus Jujubae* | 2 Pieces | |

### Gwakhyang Jeonggi San
*Lee Je-ma's Agastache Powder to Rectify the Qi (Modified Huo Xiang Zheng Qi San)*

| | | | |
|---|---|---|---|
| Huo Xiang | *Herba Pogostemonis* | 5.625g | |
| Zi Su Ye | *Folium Perillae* | 3.75g | |
| Cang Zhu | *Rhizoma Atractylodis* | 1.875g | |
| Bai Zhu | *Radix Atractylodis Macrocephalae* | 1.875g | |
| Ban Xia | *Rhizoma Pinelliae* | 1.875g | |
| Chen Pi | *Pericarpium Citri Reticulatae* | 1.875g | |
| Qing Pi | *Pericarpium Citri Ret. Viridae* | 1.875g | |
| Da Fu Pi | *Pericarpium Arecae* | 1.875g | |
| Gui Pi | *Cortex Cinnamomi* | 1.875g | |
| Gan Jiang | *Rhizoma Zingiberis Officinalis* | 1.875g | (Sun-dried) |
| Yi Zhi Ren | *Fructus Alpiniae Oxyphyllae* | 1.875g | |
| Zhi Gan Cao | *Radix Glycrrhizae* | 1.875g | (Dry-fried with honey) |
| Sheng Jiang | *Rhizoma Zingiberis Recens* | 3 Slices | |
| Da Zao | *Fructus Jujubae* | 2 Pieces | |

### Palmul Gunja Tang
*Lee Je-ma's Eight Ingredient Gentlemen Decoction (Modified Si Jun Zi Tang)*

| | | | |
|---|---|---|---|
| Ren Shen | *Radix Ginseng* | 7.5g | |
| Huang Qi | *Radix Astragali Membranacei* | 7.5g | |
| Bai Zhu | *Radix Atractylodis Macrocephalae* | 3.75g | |
| Bai Shao Yao | *Radix Paeoniae Lactiflorae* | 3.75g | |
| Dang Gui | *Radix Angelicae Sinensis* | 3.75g | |
| Chuan Xiong | *Radix Ligustici Chuanxiong* | 3.75g | |
| Chen Pi | *Pericarpium Citri Reticulatae* | 3.75g | |
| Zhi Gan Cao | *Radix Glycrrhizae* | 3.75g | (Dry-fried with honey) |
| Sheng Jiang | *Rhizoma Zingiberis Recens* | 3 Slices | |
| Da Zao | *Fructus Jujubae* | 2 Pieces | |

If Ren Shen (*Radix Ginseng*) is replaced with Bai He Shou Wu (*Radix Polygoni Multiflori Alba*), this formula is referred to as *Baek Hasuoh Gunja Tang* (Lee Je-ma's Fleeceflower Gentlemen Decoction). If 3.75g of Ren Shen (*Radix Ginseng*), Bai He Shou Wu (*Radix Polygoni Multiflori Alba*), and Rou Gui (*Cortex Cinnamomi*) are added, then it is referred to as *Shipjun Daebo Tang* (Lee Je-ma's All-Inclusive Great Tonifying Decoction). If 37.5g of Ren Shen (*Radix Ginseng*) and 3.75g of Huang Qi (*Radix Astragali Membranacei*) are used, this formula is called *Doksam Palmul Tang* (Lee Je-ma's Added Ginseng Eight Ingredient Gentlemen Decoction).

### Hyang Buja Palmul Tang

*Lee Je-ma's Eight Ingredient Decoction with Cyperus Tuber*

| Xiang Fu Zi | *Rhizoma Cyperi* | 7.5g | |
|---|---|---|---|
| Dang Gui | *Radix Angelicae Sinensis* | 7.5g | |
| Bai Shao Yao | *Radix Paeoniae Lactiflorae* | 7.5g | |
| Bai Zhu | *Radix Atractylodis Macrocephalae* | 3.75g | |
| Bai He Shou Wu | *Radix Polygoni Multiflori Alba* | 3.75g | |
| Chuan Xiong | *Radix Ligustici Chuanxiong* | 3.75g | |
| Chen Pi | *Pericarpium Citri Reticulatae* | 3.75g | |
| Zhi Gan Cao | *Radix Glycrrhizae* | 3.75g | (Dry-fried with honey) |
| Sheng Jiang | *Rhizoma Zingiberis Recens* | 3 Slices | |
| Da Zao | *Fructus Jujubae* | 2 Pieces | |

I once treated a So Eum Individual who suffered from spleen injury due to emotional stress leading to dryness of the throat and tongue and minor headaches. This formula provided amazing results.

### Gyeji Banha Senggang Tang

*Lee Je-ma's Cinnamon Pinellia and Ginger Decoction*
*(Modified Gui Zhi Ban Xia Sheng Jiang Tang)*

| Sheng Jiang | *Rhizoma Zingiberis Recens* | 11.25g | |
|---|---|---|---|
| Gui Zhi | *Ramulus Cinnamomi Cassiae* | 7.5g | |
| Ban Xia | *Rhizoma Pinelliae* | 7.5g | |
| Bai Shao Yao | *Radix Paeoniae Lactiflorae* | 3.75g | |
| Bai Zhu | *Radix Atractylodis Macrocephalae* | 3.75g | |
| Chen Pi | *Pericarpium Citri Reticulatae* | 3.75g | |
| Zhi Gan Cao | *Radix Glycrrhizae* | 3.75g | (Dry-fried with honey) |

This formula is prescribed for deficiency-related Cold-induced disorders, vomiting, and *Shui Jie Xiong* syndrome.

### Hyangsa Yangwi Tang
*Lee Je-ma's Cyperus and Hawthorn Enliven the Stomach Decoction*

| | | | |
|---|---|---|---|
| Ren Shen | *Radix Ginseng* | 3.75g | |
| Bai Zhu | *Radix Atractylodis Macrocephalae* | 3.75g | |
| Bai Shao Yao | *Radix Paeoniae Lactiflorae* | 3.75g | |
| Zhi Gan Cao | *Radix Glycrrhizae* | 3.75g | (Dry-fried with honey) |
| Ban Xia | *Rhizoma Pinelliae* | 3.75g | |
| Xiang Fu Zi | *Rhizoma Cyperi* | 3.75g | |
| Chen Pi | *Pericarpium Citri Reticulatae* | 3.75g | |
| Gan Jiang | *Rhizoma Zingiberis Officinalis* | 3.75g | (Sun-dried) |
| Shan Zha | *Fructus Crataegi* | 3.75g | |
| Sha Ren | *Fructus Amomi* | 3.75g | |
| Bai Dou Kou | *Fructus Amomi Rotundus* | 3.75g | |
| Sheng Jiang | *Rhizoma Zingiberis Recens* | 3 Slices | |
| Da Zao | *Fructus Jujubae* | 2 Pieces | |

### Jok Hasuoh Gwanjung Tang
*Lee Je-ma's Fleeceflower Smooth the Middle Decoction (Modified Kuan Zhong Tang)*

| | | | |
|---|---|---|---|
| Chi He Shou Wu | *Radix Polygoni Mult. Rubens* | 3.75g | |
| Bai He Shou Wu | *Radix Polygoni Multiflori Alba* | 3.75g | |
| Gao Liang Jiang | *Rhizoma Alpiniae Officinarum* | 3.75g | |
| Gan Jiang | *Rhizoma Zingiberis Officinalis* | 3.75g | (Sun-dried) |
| Qing Pi | *Pericarpium Citri Ret. Viridae* | 3.75g | |
| Chen Pi | *Pericarpium Citri Reticulatae* | 3.75g | |
| Xiang Fu Zi | *Rhizoma Cyperi* | 3.75g | |
| Yi Zhi Ren | *Fructus Alpiniae Oxyphyllae* | 3.75g | |
| Da Zao | *Fructus Jujubae* | 2 Pieces | |

This formula is prescribed for stiffness of the extremities, dysuria, erectile dysfunction, and occasional signs of superficial edema.

If 1.875g of Hou Po (*Cortex Magnoliae Officinalis*), Zhi Shi (*Fructus Aurantii Immaturus*), Mu Xiang (*Radix Aucklandiae*), and Da Fu Pi (*Pericarpium Arecae*) are added, they will enhance this formula's ability to promote the circulation of *Qi*. Even with edema, if one attempts to calm his/her mind and take two doses a day for 100 days, recovery is assured. When Ren Shen (*Radix Ginseng*) is used in place of Chi He Shou Wu (*Radix Polygoni Mult. Rubens*), this formula is known as *Insam Baek Hasuoh Gwanjung Tang* (Lee Je-ma's Ginseng and Fleeceflower Smooth the Middle Decoction). If Dang Gui (*Radix Angelicae Sinensis*) is used in place of Chi He Shou Wu (*Radix Polygoni Mult. Rubens*), then the formula is referred to as *Danggui Baek Hasuoh Gwanjung Tang* (Lee Je-ma's Angelica and Fleeceflower Smooth the Middle Decoction).

In ancient times, *Kuan Zhong Tang* (Smooth the Middle Decoction) consisted of equal amounts of Gan Jiang (*Rhizoma Zingiberis*), Gao Liang Jiang (*Rhizoma Alpiniae Officinarum*), Qing Pi (*Pericarpium Citri Ret. Viridae*), and Chen Pi (*Pericarpium Citri Reticulatae*), made into pills. In my experience, this formula is effective in treating a So Eum Individual with dysuria, erectile dysfunction, and/or stiffness and weakness of the extremities, and also produces miraculous effects when treating stomach pain if 3.75g of Wu Ling Zhi (*Faeces Trogopterorum*) and Yi Zhi Ren (*Fructus Alpiniae Oxyphyllae*) are added.

## Chong Mi Tang
*Lee Je-ma's Garlic and Honey Decoction*

| Bai He Shou Wu | *Radix Polygoni Multiflori Alba* | 3.75g |
| --- | --- | --- |
| Bai Zhu | *Radix Atractylodis Macrocephalae* | 3.75g |
| Bai Shao Yao | *Radix Paeoniae Lactiflorae* | 3.75g |
| Gui Zhi | *Ramulus Cinnamomi Cassiae* | 3.75g |
| Yin Chen Hao | *Herba Artemisiae Scopariae* | 3.75g |
| Yi Mu Cao | *Herba Leonuri* | 3.75g |
| Chi Shi Zhi | *Halloysitum Rubrum* | 3.75g |
| Ying Su Qiao | *Fructus Papaveris* | 3.75g |
| Garlic | | 5 Bulbs |
| Honey | | ½ Tablespoon |
| Sheng Jiang | *Rhizoma Zingiberis Recens* | 3 Slices |
| Da Zao | *Fructus Jujubae* | 2 Pieces |

This formula is prescribed for dysentery.

## Gye Sam Go
*Lee Je-ma's Chicken Ginseng Paste*

| Ren Shen | *Radix Ginseng* | 3.75g |
| --- | --- | --- |
| Gui Pi | *Cortex Cinnamomi* | 1.875g |
| Chicken | | 1 Chicken |

Boil ingredients until soft and then ingest as soup. Black pepper and/or honey may be added for enhanced flavor. This formula has traditionally been used for malaria and dysentery, with miraculous results. I once successfully treated long-term malaria by employing Ba Dou (*Semen Crotonis Pulveratum*) to promote sufficient bowel movement followed by *Gye Sam Go*

(Chicken Ginseng Paste) for two to three days. Gui Pi (*Cortex Cinnamomi*) can be replaced with Gui Shim (*Cinnamomum cassia Blume*).[84]

### Padu Dan
*Lee Je-ma's Croton Seed Pill*

| Ba Dou | Semen Crotonis Pulveratum | 1 Grain |
|---|---|---|

While boiling the accompanying[85] formula, remove 1 grain from Ba Dou (*Semen Crotonis Pulveratum*) husk and ingest (half to 1 grain) with warm water. Ba Dou is capable of descending the energy of the stomach and Intestines. Immediately after ingestion it will already have completed at least half the job of the accompanying formula. Once both the Ba Dou and accompanying formula are ingested, they will work together to promote the elimination of food in the stomach while raising the pure Yang energy. Ba Dou may be ingested a second time following a bowel movement and after the accompanying formula has been taken. A full grain of Ba Dou helps promote bowel movement, while a half grain melts away accumulation within the body.

### Insam Jinpi Tang
*Lee Je-ma's Ginseng and Tangerine Peel Decoction*

| Ren Shen | Radix Ginseng | 37.5g |
|---|---|---|
| Sheng Jiang | Rhizoma Zingiberis Recens | 3.75g |
| Sha Ren | Fructus Amomi | 3.75g |
| Chen Pi | Pericarpium Citri Reticulatae | 3.75g |
| Da Zao | Fructus Jujubae | 2 Pieces |

If Sheng Jiang (*Rhizoma Zingiberis Recens*) is replaced with Pao Gan Jiang (ginger that is sun-dried and fried until blackened), and 3.75g of Gui Pi (*Cortex Cinnamomi*) is added, this formula will have an even stronger effect on warming the stomach and chasing away the excessive Cold energy. I once treated a So Eum infant less than one year old who suffered from *Yin Duo Man Feng* syndrome.[86] He recovered after taking a little more than ten months of this herbal formula. Since his symptoms were improving, his parents discontinued administering his medicine, after which he later suffered from a relapse. At this point it was too late to save him.

---

84   The usage of Gui Shim (*Cinnamomum cassia Blume*) is unique to Korean Traditional Medicine. It is prepared by scraping off the outer, middle, and inner cortex layer of cinnamon bark, and has a warm nature, and a sweet and acrid taste. Gui Shim is indicated for heartburn, parasites, visual impairment, pain due to blood stagnation, cold and painful abdomen, and lower back/knee pain.

85   The ingestion of Ba Dou may precede the intake of other accompanying formulae in order to evacuate bowel and Cold toxin accumulation.

86   *Yin Duo Man Feng* (陰毒慢風) syndrome: Seizures due to the accumulation of *Yin Duo* (Yin toxin) within the body.

### Sam Yu Tang (aka Insam Ohsuyu Tang)
*Lee Je-ma's Ginseng and Evodia Fruit Decoction*

| | | |
|---|---|---|
| Ren Shen | *Radix Ginseng* | 37.5g |
| Wu Zhu Yu | *Fructus Evodiae* | 11.25g |
| Sheng Jiang | *Rhizoma Zingiberis Recens* | 11.25g |
| Bai Shao Yao | *Radix Paeoniae Lactiflorae* | 3.75g |
| Dang Gui | *Radix Angelicae Sinensis* | 3.75g |
| Gui Pi | *Cortex Cinnamomi* | 3.75g |

### Gwangye Buja Yijung Tang
*Lee Je-ma's Cinnamon and Aconite Regulate the Middle Decoction (Modified Li Zhong Tang)*

| | | | |
|---|---|---|---|
| Ren Shen | *Radix Ginseng* | 11.25g | |
| Bai Zhu | *Radix Atractylodis Macrocephalae* | 7.25g | |
| Pao Gan Jiang | *Rhizoma Zingiberis* | 7.25g | (Dry-fried until blackened) |
| Gui Pi | *Cortex Cinnamomi* | 7.25g | |
| Bai Shao Yao | *Radix Paeoniae Lactiflorae* | 3.75g | |
| Chen Pi | *Pericarpium Citri Reticulatae* | 3.75g | |
| Zhi Gan Cao | *Radix Glycrrhizae* | 3.75g | (Dry-fried with honey) |
| Pao Fu Zi | *Radix Aconiti Lateralis Praeparata* | 3.75–7.25g | (Dry-fried until blackened) |

### Ohsuyu Buja Yijung Tang
*Lee Je-ma's Evodia Fruit and Aconite Regulate the Middle Decoction (Modified Li Zhong Tang)*

| | | | |
|---|---|---|---|
| Ren Shen | *Radix Ginseng* | 7.25g | |
| Bai Zhu | *Radix Atractylodis Macrocephalae* | 7.25g | |
| Pao Gan Jiang | *Rhizoma Zingiberis* | 7.25g | (Dry-fried until blackened) |
| Gui Pi | *Cortex Cinnamomi* | 7.25g | |
| Bai Shao Yao | *Radix Paeoniae Lactiflorae* | 3.75g | |
| Chen Pi | *Pericarpium Citri Reticulatae* | 3.75g | |
| Zhi Gan Cao | *Radix Glycrrhizae* | 3.75g | (Dry-fried with honey) |
| Wu Zhu Yu | *Fructus Evodiae* | 3.75g | |

| Xiao Hui Xiang | Fructus Foeniculi | 3.75g | |
| Bu Gu Zhi | Fructus Psoraleae | 3.75g | |
| Pao Fu Zi | Radix Aconiti Lateralis Praeparata | 3.75–7.25g | (Dry-fried until blackened) |

## Baek Hasuoh Buja Yijung Tang

*Lee Je-ma's Fleeceflower and Aconite Regulate the Middle Decoction (Modified Fu Zi Li Zhong Tang)*

| Bai He Shou Wu | Radix Polygoni Multiflori Alba | 7.25g | |
| Bai Zhu | Radix Atractylodis Macrocephalae | 7.25g | |
| Bai Shao Yao | Radix Paeoniae Lactiflorae | 7.25g | |
| Gui Zhi | Ramulus Cinnamomi Cassiae | 7.25g | |
| Pao Gan Jiang | Rhizoma Zingiberis | 7.25g | (Dry-fried until blackened) |
| Chen Pi | Pericarpium Citri Reticulatae | 3.75g | |
| Zhi Gan Cao | Radix Glycrrhizae | 3.75g | (Dry-fried with honey) |
| Pao Fu Zi | Radix Aconiti Lateralis Praeparata | 3.75g | (Dry-fried until blackened) |

## Baek Hasuoh Yijung Tang

*Lee Je-ma's Fleeceflower Regulate the Middle Decoction (Modified Li Zhong Tang)*

| Bai He Shou Wu | Radix Polygoni Multiflori Alba | 7.25g | |
| Bai Zhu | Radix Atractylodis Macrocephalae | 7.25g | |
| Bai Shao Yao | Radix Paeoniae Lactiflorae | 7.25g | |
| Gui Zhi | Ramulus Cinnamomi Cassiae | 7.25g | |
| Pao Gan Jiang | Rhizoma Zingiberis | 7.25g | (Dry-fried until blackened) |
| Chen Pi | Pericarpium Citri Reticulatae | 3.75g | |
| Zhi Gan Cao | Radix Glycrrhizae | 3.75g | (Dry-fried with honey) |

Ren Shen (*Radix Ginseng*), if available, may be used in place of Bai He Shou Wu (*Radix Polygoni Multiflori Alba*). Ren Shen and Bai He Shou Wu are very similar but the former is slightly better at clearing [displaced Heat] and dispersing, while the latter is somewhat better at preserving the warmth of [the Middle *Jiao*]. In acute situations He Shou Wu should not be used, and at least 7.25g of Ren Shen is needed in its place. Due to a lack of reflection, the differences between Ren Shen and Bai He Shou Wu were rarely considered in the past.

Yet He Shou Wu's profound ability to preserve health was not completely ignored, since 18.75g was included in a formula called *He Ren Yin* (Polygonum Multiflorum Root and Ginseng Decoction), for treating malaria. When treating the So Eum Individual, Fu Zi (*Radix Aconiti*) should always be dry-fried until black,[87] Gan Cao (*Radix Glycyrrhizae*) should be dry-fried with honey,[88] Sheng Jiang (*Rhizoma Zingiberis Recens*) should be raw or dry-fried until black,[89] and Huang Qi (*Radix Astragali Membranacei*) should be either dry-fried with honey[90] or used raw.

In a secluded area where medicine is difficult to obtain, rather than waiting for an illness to worsen, it is better to have at least a few essential herbs on hand. For Yang Ming stage illness, Huang Qi (*Radix Astragali Membranacei*), Gui Zhi (*Ramulus Cinnamomi Cassiae*), Ren Shen (*Radix Ginseng*), and Bai Shao Yao (*Radix Paeoniae Lactiflorae*) are essential. For Shao Yin stage illness Fu Zi (*Radix Aconiti*), Bai Shao Yao (*Radix Paeoniae Lactiflorae*), Ren Shen (*Radix Ginseng*), and Gan Cao (*Radix Glycyrrhizae*) are essential. For Tai Yang stage illness Zi Su Ye (*Folium Perillae*), Cong Bai (*Radix Allii*), Huang Qi (*Radix Astragali Membranacei*), and Gui Zhi (*Ramulus Cinnamomi Cassiae*) are essential. For Tai Yin stage illness Bai Zhu (*Radix Atractylodis Macrocephalae*), Gan Jiang (*Rhizoma Zingiberis Officinalis*), Chen Pi (*Pericarpium Citri Reticulatae*), and Huo Xiang (*Herba Pogostemonis*) are essential. With just the above bare essentials, if an illness is caught before it advances, then recovery is possible. Even with various herbs at one's disposal, only those that are appropriate for the situation should be employed and those with no significance should be eliminated.

---

87   When dry-fried until black, Fu Zi is referred to as Pao Fu Zi.

88   When dry-fried with honey, Gan Cao is known as Zhi Gan Cao.

89   When dry-fried until black, Sheng Jiang is referred to as Pao Gan Jiang.

90   When dry-fried with honey, Huang Qi is known as Zhi Huang Qi.

Chapter 7 ─────────────────────────────

# The So Yang Individual's Illness

*Section 1*

## The So Yang Individual's Spleen Cold Causing Exterior Cold Syndrome[1]

### 少陽人脾受寒表寒病

張仲景이 曰太陽病에 脈浮緊하며 發熱 惡寒 身痛 不汗出而煩躁者는 大青龍湯을 主之니라.

According to Zhang Zhongjing, during a Tai Yang stage illness, if a floating, string-taut, and tense pulse, fever and chills, body aches, a lack of sweating, and vexation are present, then *Da Qing Long Tang* (Major Blue Green Dragon Decoction) should be administered.

論曰發熱 惡寒 脈浮緊하며 身痛 不汗出而煩躁者는 卽少陽人 脾受寒表寒病也니 此證에 不當用大青龍湯이오 當用荊防敗毒散이니라.

In my opinion, fever and chills, a floating and string-taut tense pulse, body aches, a lack of sweating, and vexation comprise nothing other than the So Yang Individual's

─────────────────────────────

1    The Exterior syndrome of the So Yang Individual isn't to be correlated directly with Shang Han Exterior disorders such as Tai Yang illness. The So Yang Individual has two major stages of Exterior illness: (a) Tai Yang, and (b) Shao Yang Shang Han. Keep in mind that External disorders of the So Yang Individual originate from the inability to regulate and harmonize their *Song* nature of anger, especially when they feel disrespected. This inhibits the downward flow of spleen energy and causes external vulnerability. Internal disorders, on the contrary, originate from the upward explosion of their *Jung* emotion of sorrow. Also worthy of note is that Exterior syndromes are not necessarily less threatening than Interior syndromes. The onset of diarrhea during the common cold of a Tai Yang stage illness of the So Yang Individual, for example, is already the first stage of *Mang Yin* syndrome—a life-threatening situation involving Yin depletion.

spleen Cold causing External Cold syndrome.[2] Instead of using *Da Qing Long Tang* (Major Blue Green Dragon Decoction), I suggest *Hyungbang Peidok San* (Lee Jema's Schizonepeta and Ledebouriella Powder to Overcome Pathogenic Influences).

**Table 7.1: The Tai Yang stage syndrome of the So Yang Individual**

| Syndrome | Due to | Symptoms | Treated with | Approach |
|----------|--------|----------|--------------|----------|
| Tai Yang stage | External Cold pathogen trapping spleen Yin | Fever and chills, a floating and string-taut tense pulse, body aches, no sweating, vexation, and headache* | *Hyungbang Peidok San* (Lee Je-ma's Schizonepeta and Ledebouriella Powder to Overcome Pathogenic Influences) | Encourage descent of spleen Yin |

*\* Headaches are a hallmark sign of Tai Yang stage illness of the So Yang Individual.*

張仲景이 曰少陽之爲病은 口苦 咽乾 目眩이니라. 眩而口苦 舌乾者는 屬少陽이니라. 口苦 耳聾 胸滿者는 少陽傷風證也니라. 口苦 咽乾 目眩 耳聾 胸脇滿하며 或往來寒熱而嘔는 屬少陽하니 忌吐下오 宜小柴胡湯으로 和之니라.

According to Zhang Zhongjing, Shao Yang stage illness is marked by a bitter taste in the mouth, dry throat, and an uncomfortable burning sensation in the eyes. The Shao Yang *Shang Feng* syndrome includes a bitter taste in the mouth, difficulty hearing, and fullness in the chest.

In general, Shao Yang stage syndrome consists of a bitter taste in the mouth, burning sensation in the eyes, difficulty hearing, chest and flank area fullness, alternating chills and fever, and dry heaves. During this stage of illness, Zhang Zhongjing states that the practitioner must refrain from promoting vomit or diarrhea. For this disorder, balance should be encouraged by prescribing *Xiao Chai Hu Tang* (Minor Bupleurum Decoction).

---

2   The External Pathogenic Heat entraps the Yin Cold within the So Yang Individual's stronger spleen. With Yin entrapped inside the spleen, the Exterior Heat energy will produce typical externally related Tai Yang stage symptoms such as rhinitis, fever, chills, and general body aches. Yet with a stronger spleen and its association with Yang Heat energy, the So Yang's Cold Exterior syndrome quickly transforms into Internal Heat via the Shao Yang Stage.

張仲景所論 少陽病에 口苦 咽乾 目眩 耳聾 胸脇滿 或往來寒熱之證은 卽
少陽人 腎局陰氣가 爲熱邪所陷하고 而脾局陰氣가 爲熱邪所壅하야 不
能下降連接於腎局而凝聚膂間하야 膠固囚滯之病이니 此證에 嘔者는 外
寒이 包裡熱而挾疾하야 上逆也오 寒熱往來者는 脾局陰氣가 欲降하나
未降而或降인 故로 寒熱이 或往或來也오 口苦 咽乾 目眩 耳聾者는 陰
氣가 囚滯膂間하야 欲降하나 未降인 故로 但寒無熱而至於耳聾也니 口
苦 咽乾 目眩者는 例證也오 耳聾者는 重證也며 胸脇滿者는 結胸之漸
也니 脇滿者는 猶輕也어니와 胸滿者는 重證也니라.

From my perspective, the prescription of *Hyungbang Peidok San* (Lee Je-ma's Schizonepeta and Ledebouriella Powder to Overcome Pathogenic Influences) or *Hyungbang Dojok San* (Lee Je-ma's Schizonepeta and Ledebouriella Guide the Red Powder) are more suitable than *Xiao Chai Hu Tang* (Minor Bupleurum Decoction) in the above situation. Zhang Zhongjing's description of a bitter taste in the mouth, dry mouth, chest and flank area fullness, and alternative fever and chills pertains to pathogenic Heat entrapping the So Yang Individual's kidney Yin, causing it to sink downwards [rather than flow upwards to nourish the upper body]. Pathogenic Heat will also entrap the spleen Yin, inhibiting its ability to descend and communicate with the kidneys. Yin then gets stuck in the thoracic area and becomes sticky like glue. Dry heaves are caused by the influence of accumulating Yin Cold [in the thoracic area] as it compresses the Internal [stomach] Heat, causing it to rebel upwards. The alternation of fever and chills is due to the inability, or only occasional ability, of spleen Yin to descend. The bitter taste in the mouth, dry throat, burning eyes, and inability to hear well is due to the stagnation and failure of Yin to descend from the thoracic area. Consistent Cold influence and a lack of fever will lead to the inability to hear. A bitter taste in the mouth and burning eyes are relatively moderate symptoms. Loss of hearing is more serious. Chest and flank fullness is a sign that *Jie Xiong*[3] syndrome is worsening, with flank area less severe than chest fullness.

---

3   *Jie Xiong* (結胸), as mentioned previously, translated literally as "blockage in the chest," is marked by a hardening of the epigastric from fluid accumulation in the thoracic cavity as a result of Exterior Yin stagnation and accumulation. According to Lee Je-ma, this syndrome is unique to the So Yang, and not the So Eum, Individual. If, in rare cases, the So Eum does experience *Jie Xiong*, it is referred to as *Zhang Jie*, a life-threatening situation.

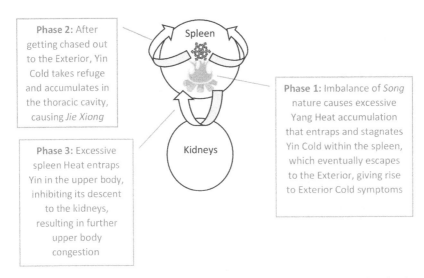

**Phase 2:** After getting chased out to the Exterior, Yin Cold takes refuge and accumulates in the thoracic cavity, causing *Jie Xiong*

**Phase 3:** Excessive spleen Heat entraps Yin in the upper body, inhibiting its descent to the kidneys, resulting in further upper body congestion

**Phase 1:** Imbalance of *Song* nature causes excessive Yang Heat accumulation that entraps and stagnates Yin Cold within the spleen, which eventually escapes to the Exterior, giving rise to Exterior Cold symptoms

*Figure 7.1: The Shao Yang Shang Feng syndrome of the So Yang Individual*

古人之於此證에 用汗 吐 下 三法則其病이 輒生譫語壞證하야 病益危險인 故로 仲景이 變通之而用小柴胡湯하야 淸痰燥痰하며 溫冷相雜하야 平均和解하야 欲其病으로 不傳變而自愈하니 此法은 以汗吐下三法으로 論之면 則可謂近善而巧矣나 然이나 此小柴胡湯이 亦非平均和解病不傳變之藥則從古斯今에 得此病者가 眞是寒心矣로다. 耳聾 胸滿 傷風之病을 豈可以小柴胡湯으로 擬之乎아

In ancient times, vomiting and diarrhea were induced to treat *Jie Xiong* syndrome, which leading to incoherent and frantic speech, only made matters worse. Zhang Zhongjing recognized this tendency and therefore focused on clearing and drying phlegm with *Xiao Chai Hu Tang* (Minor Bupleurum Decoction). At first glance, this formula appears to promote balance between Heat and Cold, and prevent the Shao Yang stage illness from spreading further by promoting sweat, diarrhea, and emesis. Yet, [such aggressive methods prove that] *Xiao Chai Hu Tang* doesn't promote balance and encourage the body to recover. It is hard to imagine how many unfortunate patients have received this pathetic method of treatment. How can a lack of hearing and chest fullness due to a Shao Yang *Shang Feng* illness be treated with *Xiao Chai Hu Tang*?

噫라 後來龔信所製 荊防敗毒散이 豈非少陽人表寒病에 三神山不死藥
乎아 此證에 清裡熱而降表陰則痰飲이 自散而結胸之證도 預防不成
也어니와 清痰而燥痰則無益於陰降痰散이오 延拖하야 結胸이 將成而或
別生奇證也니라.

How can Gong Xin's *Jing Fang Bai Du San* (Schizonepeta and Saposhnikoviae Powder to Overcome Pathogenic Influences) be anything but a savior for the So Yang Individual with External Cold syndrome for generations to come? This formula clears Internal Heat and descends External Yin,[4] naturally clearing phlegm accumulation coming from food stagnation and preventing the occurrence of *Jie Xiong* syndrome. It is useless to dry or disperse phlegm[5] in order to descend Yin. [If a doctor wastes several days in such pursuits] then *Jie Xiong* or other serious illness may occur.

朱肱曰凡發汗에 腰以上이 雖淋漓而腰以下로 至足에 微潤則病終不解
也라.

According to Zhu Gong, if after the promotion of sweat the upper extremities sweat copiously, with clammy lower extremities, then the illness is incurable.

論曰少陽人病은 無論表裏病하고 手足掌心에 有汗則病解하고 手足掌
心에 不汗則雖全體에 皆汗而病不解니라. 少陽人 傷寒病에 有再痛三
痛 發汗而愈者하니 此病은 非再三感風寒而再痛發汗三痛發汗也라 少陽
人이 頭痛 腦强 寒熱往來 耳聾 胸滿하야 尤甚之病은 元來如此하니 表
邪가 深結하야 至於三痛然後에 方解也니 無論初痛再痛三痛하고 用荊
防敗毒散 或荊防導赤散 荊防瀉白散하되 每日二貼式하야 至病解而用
之하며 病解後에 又用十餘貼이니 如此則自無後病而完健이니라.

As I see it, in both External and Internal illness, sweating of the palms and soles is a sign of recovery. If there is profuse sweat throughout the body except for the palms or soles, the illness cannot be cured.[6]

In most cases, if the So Yang Individual begins to sweat after two or three bouts of Shang Han Exterior Cold, it is a sign of recovery. However, when the Exterior Cold pathogen becomes lodged in both the Exterior and Interior, no more sweating will occur after the third bout of Shang Han Exterior Cold syndrome, indicating

---

4    Internal Heat refers to stomach Heat and External Yin refers to spleen Yin.

5    In traditional Chinese medicine, herbs used to clear phlegm often have a drying and warm nature. If the So Yang Individual ingests medicine with this nature, further dryness and congestion of Yin in the chest will follow, resulting in the accumulation of sticky phlegm.

6    Excessive sweating during an illness of the So Yang Individual indicates exhaustion and loss of Yin, or *Mang Yin* syndrome. Excessive sweating during an illness of the So Eum Individual, on the contrary, indicates exhaustion of Yang, or *Mang Yang* syndrome. For the So Yang Individual, sweating from the palms indicates the release of excessive Heat from the stomach, a sign of recovery.

that the situation is getting worse. In severe cases, this situation will be accompanied by occipital headache, alternating fever and chills, loss of hearing, and fullness in the chest. It will take three bouts of this illness to recover if the Exterior Cold pathogen makes its way deep into the body. Depending on whether it is the first, second, or third bout from onset, two packs of *Hyungbang Peidok San* (Lee Je-ma's Schizonepeta and Ledebouriella Powder to Overcome Pathogenic Influences), *Hyungbang Dojok San* (Lee Je-ma's Schizonepeta and Ledebouriella Guide the Red Powder), or *Hyungbang Sabaek San* (Lee Je-ma's Schizonepeta and Ledebouriella Clear the White Powder) should be administered daily until recovery. Afterwards, ten more packs will prevent the return of illness and facilitate a complete return to health.

張仲景이 曰少陽證에 ㄷㄷ汗出하며 心下痞硬滿하며 引脇下痛하며 乾嘔 短氣 不惡寒은 表解나 裡未和也니 宜十棗湯이니 若合下인데 不下면 令 人脹滿하야 遍身浮腫이니라.

According to Zhang Zhongjing, if a Shao Yang stage syndrome is accompanied by clammy sweating, fullness and hardness in the epigastric area,[7] a pulling and uncomfortable feeling underneath the ribs, incoherent speech, shortness of breath, but there is an absence of chills, it is a sign that the Exterior Cold has been dispersed, but the pathogen has transferred to the Interior. In this case, *Shi Zao Tang* (Ten Jujube Decoction) is called for. If the promotion of diarrhea is advisable[8] but not heeded, fullness of the abdomen and superficial edema will occur.

傷寒 表未解에 醫反下之면 膈內拒痛하야 手不可近하며 心下滿而硬 痛하나니 此爲結胸이니 宜大陷胸湯이니라. 渴欲飮水하나 水入卽吐를 名 曰水逆이니 五苓散을 主之니라

[According to Zhang Zhongjing,] if diarrhea is promoted prematurely [before the recovery of External illness], and there is pain due to stagnation in the chest and flank area with aversion even to the slightest pressure, and subjective fullness and hardness [to touch] in the epigastric area, *Jie Xiong* syndrome is present; in which case *Da Xian Xiong Tang* (Major Sinking into the Chest Decoction) should be prescribed. Thirst but an inability to swallow water without vomiting it up again indicates *Sui Ni*.[9]

---

7    Hardness of the epigastrium is a reference to *Jie Xiong* syndrome.

8    This sentence refers to the situation in which there is no longer an External pathogenic influence, but stagnation of the Interior calls for laxative treatment.

9    *Sui Ni* (水逆) syndrome, or "water reversal," is a reflection of acute *Jie Xiong* syndrome occurrence, indicated by the vomiting of fluids directly after ingestion.

杜壬이 曰裏未和者는 蓋痰與燥氣가 壅於中焦인 故로 頭痛┌乾嘔하며 汗
出은 痰隔也니 非十棗湯이면 不治니라.

According to Du Ren,[10] internal imbalance is usually due to the accumulation
and stagnation of phlegm and dryness in the Middle *Jiao*, a syndrome usually
accompanied by headaches, incoherent speech, sweating, and congestion of phlegm.
For this, he maintained that *Shi Zao Tang* (Ten Jujube Decoction) is the only cure.

龔信이 曰心下硬痛하야 手不可近하며 燥渴譫語하며 大便實하며 脈沈實
有力은 爲大結胸이니 大陷胸湯으로 下之오 反加煩躁者는 死니라. 小結
胸은 正在心下하야 按之則痛이니 宜小陷胸湯이라.

According to Gong Xin, *Da Jie Xiong*[11] syndrome is marked by severe pain causing
an aversion to even the slightest pressure, hardness of the epigastric area, dry mouth
and thirst, incoherent speech, excessive bowel movement, and a full pulse felt at
the deep level.[12] For this, he recommended the use of *Da Xian Xiong Tang* (Major
Sinking into the Chest Decoction). He claimed that death is inescapable if vexation
and anxiety accompany this syndrome. The *Xiao Jie Xiong*[13] syndrome is marked by
a lack of hardness and less pain with pressure in the epigastric area, which in this
case *Xiao Xian Xiong Tang* (Minor Sinking into the Chest Decoction) should be
prescribed.

論曰右張仲景所論三證은 皆結胸病而膈內拒痛하야 手不可近하며 燥渴
譫語者는 結胸之最尤甚證也오 飮水하면 水入卽吐하며 心下痞硬滿하며
乾嘔短氣者는 次證也라 凡結胸病에 皆藥湯入口면 輒還吐하되 惟甘遂
末을 入口하야 口涎含下하고 因以溫水로 漱口而下則藥不還吐니라.

From my perspective, the above three syndromes described by Zhang Zhongjing all
fall under the category of *Jie Xiong* syndrome. If severe, *Jie Xiong* will include pain
in the epigastric and flank area causing an aversion to even the slightest amount of
pressure. In even worse cases, these symptoms will be accompanied by vomiting
water after ingestion, hardness and fullness in the epigastric area, incoherent speech,
and shortness of breath. In most cases, the patient suffering from this illness will
be unable to ingest medicine without vomiting. Yet if Gan Sui (*Radix Euphorbiae
Kansui*) powder is placed in the mouth and swallowed without water, or swallowed
after gargling with warm water, it will be retained.

---

10  There is little known about Du Ren except for the fact that he was a physician of the Song Dynasty and
authored a book entitled *Du Ren Yi Zhun* (*Du Ren's Model of Oriental Medicine*), no longer in print.

11  *Da Jie Xiong* (大結胸) translates as "greater *Jie Xiong*" syndrome, indicating an acute form of *Jie Xiong*
syndrome.

12  "Deep level" indicates the third, or "organ," level of the pulse. This level is deeper than the other two levels:
the first, or "Qi," level, and the second, or "blood," level.

13  *Xiao Jie Xiong* (小結胸) translates as "lesser *Jie Xiong*" syndrome, a less acute form of *Jie Xiong* syndrome
compared to *Da Jie Xiong* syndrome.

嘗治結胸할새 用甘遂散하야 溫水調下한대 五次輒還吐하나 至六次하야
不還吐而下利一度하고 其翌日에 又水還吐어늘 又用甘遂하니 一次快通
利而病愈니라. 凡結胸은 無非險證이니 當先用甘遂하고 仍煎荊防導赤散
以壓之오 乾嘔 短氣而藥不還吐者는 不用甘遂하고 但用荊防導赤散 加
茯苓 澤瀉 各一錢하야 二三服하고 又連日服而亦病愈하니라. 燥渴 譫
語者는 尤極險證也니 急用甘遂하고 仍煎地黃白虎湯 三四貼으로 以壓
之하며 又連日服地黃白虎湯이니라.

I once prescribed Gan Sui (*Radix Euphorbiae Kansui*) powder with warm water for a patient with *Jie Xiong* syndrome who vomited the medicine the first three times and was able to ingest it the fourth time. Shortly after ingestion, the patient experienced one bout of diarrhea. After two more days, he started to vomit again after drinking water. Following one more dose of Gan Sui (*Radix Euphorbiae Kansui*), the patient experienced another bout of diarrhea[14] and then recovered.

[From its onset] *Jie Xiong* is considered a severe syndrome and should therefore be addressed immediately with the administration of Gan Sui (*Radix Euphorbiae Kansui*), then followed by *Hyungbang Dojok San* (Lee Je-ma's Schizonepeta and Ledebouriella Guide the Red Powder) for further support. If the patient suffers from incoherent speech, shortness of breath, and shows no symptoms of vomiting, then Gan Sui (*Radix Euphorbiae Kansui*) is inadvisable. Instead, *Hyungbang Dojok San* (Lee Je-ma's Schizonepeta and Ledebouriella Guide the Red Powder) with 3.75g of Fu Ling (*Poria Alba*) and Ze Xie (*Rhizoma Alismatis*) should be administered. The patient will recover after at least three doses of this medication. Yet if this syndrome is accompanied by thirst and talking in one's sleep, it is considered more severe, and should be treated immediately with Gan Sui (*Radix Euphorbiae Kansui*), followed by *Jihwang Baekho Tang* (Lee Je-ma's White Tiger Decoction with Rhemannia). This method should be administered at least three to four times for the patient to recover, with *Jihwang Baekho Tang* (Lee Je-ma's White Tiger Decoction with Rhemannia) prescribed continuously until full recovery.

14    The occurrence of diarrhea after administration of Gan Sui (*Radix Euphorbiae Kansui*) indicates the release of water retention from the chest and epigastric area through the stools.

**Table 7.2: The Shao Yang stage external syndrome of the So Yang Individual**

| Syndrome | Due to | Common symptoms | Additional symptoms | Treated with |
|---|---|---|---|---|
| Tai Yang/Shao Yang Stage<br><br>Beginning onset | External Cold pathogen entrapping spleen and kidney Yin, spleen Yin Cold entraps stomach Heat | | Early stage onset of common symptoms (see column on the left) with body aches and a floating and string-taut pulse | *Hyungbang Peidok San* (Lee Je-ma's Schizonepeta and Ledebouriella Powder to Overcome Pathogenic Influences)* |
| Shao Yang stage<br><br>(*Jie Xiong* syndrome)<br><br>Moderate to severe condition | Ongoing battle with External Cold pathogen leads to severe Yin stagnation and fluid retention in chest and epigastrium and spleen Yin Cold entrapment of stomach Heat | Bitter taste in the mouth, dry mouth, chest and flank area fullness, and alternative fever and chills | Hardening and acute pain of the epigastric area with aversion to Cold and pressure, difficult passage of bowel and urine, vomiting | Gan Sui (*Radix Euphorbiae Kansui*)**<br><br>*Hyungbang Dojok San* (Lee Je-ma's Schizonepeta and Ledebouriella Guide the Red Powder) with 3.75g of Fu Ling (*Poria Alba*) and Ze Xie (*Rhizoma Alismatis*)*** |
| Shao Yang stage<br><br>(*Jie Xiong* syndrome)<br><br>Severe condition | | | Same as above with lack of sweating, occipital headache, alternating fever and chills, loss of hearing, and fullness in the chest | Gan Sui (*Radix Euphorbiae Kansui*)**<br><br>*Hyungbang Sabaek San* (Lee Je-ma's Schizonepeta and Ledebouriella Clear the White Powder)**** |
| Shao Yang stage<br><br>(*Jie Xiong* syndrome)<br><br>Critical condition | | | Same as above with thirst and talking in one's sleep, possible vomiting of water after ingestion, incoherent speech, shortness of breath | Gan Sui (*Radix Euphorbiae Kansui*)<br><br>*Jihwang Baekho Tang* (Lee Je-ma's White Tiger Decoction with Rhemannia) |

* *This formula should also be prescribed if there is sudden vomiting with no other signs or symptoms. Sudden vomiting indicates Heat accumulation within the stomach, a common signal of further health-related issues to come for the So Yang Individual.*

** *Lee Je-ma contraindicates the use of Gan Sui (Radix Euphorbiae Kansui) in situations without the occurrence of vomiting.*

*** *This formula is prescribed after two bouts of Shang Han illness.*

**** *This formula is prescribed after three bouts of Shang Han illness.*

張仲景이 曰傷寒 表未解에 醫反下之云者는 以大承氣湯으로 下之之謂
也오 非十棗와 陷胸으로 下之之謂也라. 然이나 十棗와 陷胸은 不如單
用甘遂오 或用甘遂天一丸이니 結胸에는 甘遂末을 例用三分이오 大結
胸에는 用五分이니라. 龔信所論 燥渴 譫語 煩躁死者라도 若十棗湯으로
下後에 因以譫語證으로 治之하야 連用白虎湯則煩躁者도 必無不治之
理니라.

Zhang Zhongjing was referring to the use of *Da Cheng Qi Tang* (Major Guide
the Qi Decoction)[15] when he wrote of how doctors in the past would mistakenly
promote diarrhea even though the External Cold pathogen still lingers. Here he
is not referring to the use of *Shi Zao Tang* (Ten Jujube Decoction) or *Xian Xiong
Tang* (Sinking into the Chest Decoction). Yet the effect of these formulae cannot be
compared to even one dose of Gan Sui (*Radix Euphorbiae Kansui*) or *Kamsu Chonil
Wan* (Lee Je-ma's Divine Gan Sui Pill). In the case of *Xiao Jie Xiong* syndrome, 1.13g
of Gan Sui (*Radix Euphorbiae Kansui*) should be prescribed, and 1.9g for the *Xiao Jie
Xiong* syndrome. I disagree with Gong Xin's statement that *Jie Xiong* is not curable
if the patient experiences excessive thirst, incoherent speech, vexation, and anxiety.
Even after diarrhea is promoted with *Shi Zao Tang* (Ten Jujube Decoction), the
patient is capable of recovering from incoherent speech. Yet this formula falls short
of addressing fear and anxiety, for which *Bai Hu Tang* (White Tiger Decoction) is
continuously prescribed until the patient fully recovers.

甘遂는 表寒病에 破水結之藥也오 石膏는 裡熱病에 通大便之藥也니
表病에 可用甘遂而不用石膏하며 裡病에 可用石膏而不可用甘遂니라.
然이나 揚手擲足하고 引飮泄瀉證에는 用石膏오 痺風膝寒하고 大便不通
證에는 用甘遂니라.

Gan Sui (*Radix Euphorbiae Kansui*) disperses water accumulation caused by External
Cold syndrome. Shi Gao (*Gypsum Fibrosum*) promotes the movement of bowel in
the case of Internal Heat syndrome. Gan Sui (*Radix Euphorbiae Kansui*) can be used
for External syndromes, but Shi Gao (*Gypsum Fibrosum*) cannot be administered
in such cases. Shi Gao (*Gypsum Fibrosum*) can be used for Internal syndromes, but
not Gan Sui (*Radix Euphorbiae Kansui*) in such cases. If there is uncontrollable
movement of the hands and feet, excessive thirst, and diarrhea then Shi Gao (*Gypsum
Fibrosum*) is indicated.[16] If the knees feel numb and cold, with a lack of bowel flow,
then Gan Sui (*Radix Euphorbiae Kansui*) is called for.[17]

---

15    Please refer to the So Eum Individual's 23 Formulae from Zhang Zhongjing's *Shang Han Lun*.

16    Despite the fact that diarrhea is often a result of Exterior Cold syndrome of the So Yang Individual, if it is
      accompanied by Internal Heat-related symptoms, such as uncontrollable movement of the hands and feet,
      and excessive thirst, then Shi Gao, rather than Gan Sui, should be used to clear Internal Heat.

17    Despite the fact that constipation is often a result of Internal Heat syndrome of the So Yang Individual, if it is
      accompanied by External Cold-related symptoms, such as numbness and coldness of the feet, then Gan Sui,
      rather than Shi Gao, should be used to clear External Cold, eliminate water retention, and promote diarrhea.

少陰人이 傷寒病에 有小腹硬滿之證하고 少陽人이 傷寒病에 有心下結胸
之證하니 此二證은 俱是表氣陰陽이 虛弱하야 正邪相爭하야 累日不決之
中에 裡氣가 亦秘澁不和而變生此證也라.

In the case of Cold-related syndromes, the So Eum Individual may exhibit
excessive hardness of the lower abdomen, whereas the So Yang Individual may
exhibit excessive hardness in the epigastric area. Both conditions are caused
by the weakening of exterior Yin and Yang due to several days of constant battle
between the pathogen and the *Zheng Qi*, with no winner in sight. They occur when
the Internal energy stagnates, leading to difficulty with elimination of bowel and urine.

李子建의 傷寒十勸論에 曰傷寒腹痛이 亦有熱證하니 不可輕服溫煖
藥하라 又曰傷寒自利를 當觀陰陽證이오 不可例服溫煖及止瀉藥이니라

According to Li Zijian's[18] *Shang Han Shi Quan* (*The Ten Teachings of the Shang Han
Lun*), Heat may be the culprit behind abdominal pain due to External pathogenic
influence. Hence warming and hot-natured herbs should not be administered in
haste. Moreover, the relationship between Yin and Yang must be carefully observed
with urgent diarrhea, since in such cases, warm/hot-natured herbs and anti-diarrheal
herbs are always contraindicated.

朱震亨이 曰傷寒陽證에 身熱 脈數하며 煩渴引飲하며 大便自利어든 宜
柴苓湯이니라.

According to Zhu Zhenheng, *Chai Ling Tang* (Bupleurum and Poria Decoction)[19] is
prescribed for the Yang Pattern Shang Han syndrome[20] marked by fever, rapid pulse,
excessive thirst, and compulsive eating followed by urgent diarrhea.

---

18   Li Zijian (李子建) was a medical doctor and scholar of the Song Dynasty.

19   Lee Je-ma doesn't give reference to *Chai Ling Tang* elsewhere in this text and so its ingredients are mentioned
     here: Chai Hu (*Radix Bupleuri*) 3–12g, Zhi Ban Xia (*Rhizoma Pinelliae Preparatum*) 3–14g, Huang Qin
     (*Radix Scutellariae*) 3–18g, Ren Shen (*Radix Ginseng*) 1–9g, Gan Cao (*Radix Glycyrrhizae*) 1.5–14g, Bai
     Zhu (*Radix Atractylodis Macrocephalae*) 3–15g, Zhu Ling (*Polyporus*) 5–18g, Fu Ling (*Poria Alba*) 9–18g, Ze
     Xie (*Rhizoma Alismatis*) 4.5–16g, Gui Zhi (*Ramulus Cinnamomi*) 3–10g, Da Zao (*Fructus Zizyphi Jujubae*)
     3–6g, and Sheng Jiang (*Rhizoma Zingiberis Recens*) 3–6g. Source: *Shen Shi and Zun Sheng Shu* (沈氏尊生書),
     written by Shen Jin-Ao (1773).

20   The Yang Pattern Shang Han syndrome is a Heat-related syndrome affecting all three of the Yang stages (Tai
     Yang, Yang Ming, Shao Yang). It is the result of a Shang Han (External Cold) pathogenic influence with
     Internal Heat accumulation. This syndrome contrasts with the Yin Pattern Shang Han syndrome, in which
     an Exterior Cold pathogenic influence affects all three Yin stages (Tai Yin, Shao Yin, Jue Yin) due to Internal
     Cold accumulation. The former syndrome is more often a disorder of the So Yang Individual, while the latter
     is most often a So Eum disorder.

盤龍山老人이 論曰少陽人의 身熱 頭痛 泄瀉에 當用猪苓車前子湯 荊防
瀉白散이오 身寒 腹痛 泄瀉에 當用滑石苦參湯 荊防地黃湯이니 此病을
名謂之亡陰病이니라.

The Elder at Mt. Panlong[21] states that *Joryong Chajonja Tang* (Lee Je-ma's Polyporus and Plantago Seed Decoction)[22] or *Hyungbang Sabaek San* (Lee Je-ma's Schizonepeta and Ledebouriella Clear the White Powder) should be prescribed when the So Yang Individual experiences fever, headache, and diarrhea. If he or she experiences chills, abdominal pain, and diarrhea then *Hwalsok Gosam Tang* (Lee Je-ma's Talcum and Sophora Decoction) or *Hyungbang Jihwang Tang* (Lee Je-ma's Schizonepeta, Ledebouriella, and Rhemannia Decoction) are called for. These syndromes are all referred to as *Mang Yin*.[23]

少陽人이 身熱 頭痛 泄瀉라가 一二日 或 三四日에 而泄瀉가 無故로 自
止하고 身熱┌頭痛이 不愈하며 大便이 反秘者는 此는 危證也니 距譫語가
不遠이니라.

If a So Yang Individual experiences fever, headache, and diarrhea lasting one to two days, or after the third or fourth day diarrhea, fever, and headache suddenly cease and constipation ensues, it is a sign of a severe illness. If this illness is not addressed, incoherent speech will develop.

泄瀉後에 大便이 一晝夜間에 艱辛一次滑利하며 或三四五次小小滑
利하고 身熱┌頭痛이 因存者는 此는 便秘之兆也ㅣ니 譫語前에 有此證則
譫語가 當在數日이오 譫語後에 有此證則動風이 必在咫尺이니라.

If after experiencing diarrhea, there is only one bout, or three to five smaller bouts, of difficult-to-pass watery stool within a 24-hour period, along with continuous fever and headache, constipation will ensue. If these symptoms are not addressed within a few days then incoherent speech follows, and if so, it is a sign of Internal Wind stirring.

---

21   Lee Je-ma refers to himself as the Elder at Mt. Panlong (盤龍山老人) to emphasize his fluency in the subject and offer crucial advice.

22   Lee Je-ma doesn't give reference to *Joryong Chajonja Tang* elsewhere in this text and so its ingredients are mentioned here: Ze Xie (*Rhizoma Alismatis*) 7.5g, Fu Ling (*Poria Alba*) 7.5g, Zhu Ling (*Polyporus*) 5.625g, Che Qian Zi (*Semen Plantaginis*) 5.625g, Zhi Mu (*Rhizoma Anemarrhenae*) 3.75g, Shi Gao (*Gypsum Fibrosum*) 3.75g, Qian Huo (*Rhizoma seu Radix Notopterygii*) 3.75g, Du Huo (*Radix Angelicae Pubescentis*) 3.75g, Jing Jie (*Herba Schizonepetae*) 3.75g, and Fang Feng (*Radix Saposhnikoviae*) 3.75g. Source: *Sasang Jinryo Euijon* (*The Collection of Medical Prescription in Sasang Medicine*).

23   *Mang Yin* (亡陰病), or Collapse of Yin syndrome, is marked by excessive watery diarrhea that occurs after the onset of a Shang Han illness of the So Yang Individual. This syndrome occurs as a result of significant Yin deficiency that is instigated by the onset of external disease, which leads to leakage of remaining Yin through the stools. Both *Mang Yang* of the So Eum Individual and *Mang Yin* of the So Yang Individual are life-threatening situations that, if not addressed immediately, may lead to complete separation of Yin and Yang, and ultimately death.

少陽人이 忽然有吐者는 必生奇證也니 當用荊防敗毒散하야 以觀動
靜하되 而身熱 頭痛 泄瀉者는 用石膏無疑오 身寒 腹痛 泄瀉者는 用黃連
苦參이 無疑니라.

When the So Yang Individual suddenly vomits, it is a sure sign of unusual symptoms to come. In this case, *Hyungbang Peidok San* (Lee Je-ma's Schizonepeta and Ledebouriella Powder to Overcome Pathogenic Influences) should be prescribed without hesitation, with careful monitoring. If fever, headaches, and diarrhea appear, then Shi Gao (*Gypsum Fibrosum*) should be prescribed without a doubt. If chills, abdominal pain, and diarrhea begin to occur then Huang Lian (*Rhizoma Coptidis*) and Ku Shen (*Radix Sophorae*) are necessary.

嘗見少陽人兒 生未一周年에 忽先一吐而後에 泄瀉하더니 身熱ㄱ頭痛하며
揚手擲足하며 轉輾其身하며 引飲泄瀉를 四五六次하야 無度數者할새 用
荊防瀉白散 日三貼하야 兩日六貼然後에 泄瀉方止하고 身熱頭痛이 淸
淨이러니 又五六貼而安이니라.

I once treated a So Yang infant who, after sudden vomiting, experienced diarrhea, fever, headache, uncontrollable waving of the hands and feet, and prancing this way and that. After drinking water, he would have four to six bouts of diarrhea, which suddenly came to a halt. After three packs per day for two days of *Hyungbang Sabaek San* (Lee Je-ma's Schizonepeta and Ledebouriella Clear the White Powder), his diarrhea, fever, and headache subsided. I continued to prescribe about six more packs, resulting in full recovery.

少陽人이 身熱頭痛하며 揚手擲足하며 引飲者는 此는 險證也니 雖泄
瀉라도 必用石膏니라. 無論泄瀉有無하고 當用荊防瀉白散에 加黃連 瓜蔞
各一錢 或地黃白虎湯이니라.

If a So Yang Individual experiences fever, uncontrollable waving of the hands and feet, and excessive thirst, it is considered a severe illness. Shi Gao (*Gypsum Fibrosum*) should be used even if diarrhea is the only additional symptom. Depending on the continuation or cessation of diarrhea, either *Hyungbang Sabaek San* (Lee Je-ma's Schizonepeta and Ledebouriella Clear the White Powder) with 3.75g of Huang Lian (*Rhizoma Coptidis*) and 3.75g of Gua Lou (*Semen Trichosanthis*) or *Jihwang Baekho Tang* (Lee Je-ma's White Tiger Decoction with Rhemannia) should be prescribed.

凡少陽人이 有身熱頭痛則已非輕證而兼有泄瀉則危險證也니 必用荊防瀉
白散을 日二三服 又連日服하야 身熱頭痛이 淸淨然後에 可免危險이니라.

A fever with headache is already considered a serious condition for the So Yang Individual. Yet if diarrhea is added to the picture, it is considered life threatening, in which case, two to three packs per day of *Hyungbang Sabaek San* (Lee Je-ma's Schizonepeta and Ledebouriella Clear the White Powder) should be prescribed. This should be continued if the above symptoms persist. Only when fever and headache are resolved can the situation be considered less serious.

少陽人이 身寒 腹痛 泄瀉하야 一晝夜間에 三四五次者는 當用滑石苦蔘湯이오 身寒腹痛하며 二三晝夜間에 無泄瀉이거나 或艱辛一次泄瀉者는 當用滑石苦蔘湯이오 或用熟地黃苦蔘湯이니라.

If a So Yang Individual experiences chills, abdominal pain, and three to five bouts of diarrhea within a 24-hour period, then *Hwalsok Gosam Tang* (Lee Je-ma's Talcum and Sophora Decoction) should be prescribed. If there are chills, abdominal pain, and two to three days without or only sporadic bouts of diarrhea, then *Hwalsok Gosam Tang* (Lee Je-ma's Talcum and Sophora Decoction) or *Sukjihwang Gosam Tang* (Lee Je-ma's Processed Rhemannia and Sophora Decoction) should be prescribed.

嘗見少陽人이 恒有腹痛患苦者할새 用六味地黃湯 六十貼而病愈하고 又見少陽人이 十餘年腹痛患苦하야 一次起痛則或五六個月 或三四個月一二個月 呌苦者하니 每起痛臨時에 急用滑石苦蔘湯 十餘貼하며 不痛時에 平心靜慮하야 恒戒哀心怒心하니 如此로 延拖一周年而病愈하고

I once cured a So Yang Individual with severe abdominal pain with 60 packs of *Liu Wei Di Huang Tang* (Six Ingredient Decoction with Rhemannia). There was another case in which a So Yang Individual suffered for ten years from abdominal pain that would continue in the acute phase for one to six months after an initial episode. Whenever symptoms started, I would immediately prescribe ten packs of *Hwalsok Gosam Tang* (Lee Je-ma's Talcum and Sophora Decoction) to eliminate her pain. Without pain, she made a sincere effort to calm her mind and spirit and rid herself of excessive anger. She completely recovered after one year.

又見少陽人小兒가 恒有滯證痞滿하며 間有腹痛 腰痛하며 又有口眼喎斜初證者하니 用獨活地黃湯하야 一百日內에 二百貼을 服하고 使之平心靜慮하야 恒戒哀心怒心하니 一百日而身健病愈하니라.

I once treated a boy who suffered continuously from food stagnation that caused abdominal fullness with occasional stomach and lower back pain, and the beginning signs and symptoms of Bell's palsy, with 200 packs of *Dokhwal Jihwang Tang* (Lee Je-ma's Angelica Pubescens and Rehmannia Decoction) for 100 days. Afterwards, he fully overcame his illness by calming his mind and spirit and controlling his sorrow and anger.

古醫有言하되 頭無冷痛이오 腹無熱痛이라하니 此言은 非也라. 何謂然
耶아 少陰人이 元來冷勝則其頭痛이 亦自非熱痛而即冷痛也오
少陽人이 元來熱勝則其腹痛이 亦自非冷痛而即熱痛也니라.

The ancient doctors wrongly believed that pain and illness will not occur if the head is cool and the stomach is warm. In actuality, Cold rather than Heat is the cause of the So Eum Individual's headaches because they are prone to Cold-induced disorders. Heat, rather than Cold, is the cause of the So Yang Individual's abdomen pain because they are prone to Heat-induced disorders.

古醫又言하되 汗多는 亡陽이오 下多는 亡陰이라하니 此言은 是也라. 何
謂然耶아 少陰人이 雖則冷勝한즉 然하여 陰盛格陽하야 敗陽이 外逼則
煩熱而汗多也니 此之謂亡陽病也며少陽人이 雖則熱勝한즉 然하여 陽盛
格陰하야 敗陰이 內逼則畏寒而泄下也니 此之謂亡陰病也라 亡陽과 亡陰
病은 非用藥이면 必死也오 不急治면 必死也니라.

The ancient doctors correctly believed that excessive sweating leads to *Mang Yang* syndrome, while excessive diarrhea leads to *Mang Yin* syndrome. Accordingly, the So Eum Individual's dominance of Cold and abundance of Yin quarrels with Yang, provoking it to escape outwards. This eventually leads to *Mang Yang* syndrome, characterized by vexation, deficient Heat, and excessive sweating. The So Yang Individual's dominance of Heat and abundance of Yang quarrels with Yin, causing it to escape inwards. This eventually leads to *Mang Yin* syndrome, which is characterized by an aversion to Cold, and diarrhea due to the escape of Yin. Both *Mang Yang* and *Mang Yin* syndromes are life threatening and need to be addressed immediately with the appropriate medicine. If medicine is delayed or not prescribed at all, death will be imminent.

亡陽者는 陽不上升而反爲下降則亡陽也오
亡陰者는 陰不下降而反爲上升則亡陰也라.

*Mang Yang* syndrome results from the inability of Yang to ascend, instead sinking downwards. *Mang Yin* syndrome is due to the inability of Yin to descend, which instead rises upwards.

陰盛格陽於上則陽爲陰抑하야 不能上升於胸膈하고 下陷大腸而外遁膀
胱인 故로 背表煩熱而汗出也니 煩熱而汗出者는 非陽盛也라. 此所謂內氷
外炭이니 陽將亡之兆也 오
陽盛格陰於下則陰爲陽壅하야 不能下降於膀胱하고 上逆背膂而內遁膈
裡인 故로 腸胃畏寒而泄下也니 畏寒而泄下者는 非陰盛也라 此所謂內炭
外氷이니 陰將亡之兆也니라.

When Yin becomes excessive, it will embattle Yang.[24] In this situation, excessive heavy Yin will eventually compress Yang, making it unable to ascend to the chest and diaphragm. Yang will therefore descend to the large intestine and then escape outwards through the urinary bladder, leading to vexation and Heat in the thoracic area and sweating. These symptoms are by no means due to excessive Yang Heat, because further observation will reveal that the inside of the body is as cold as ice while the outside is as hot as charcoal, a sign that Yang is about to be extinguished.

When Yang becomes excessive, it will embattle Yin.[25] Here, excessively [agitated] Yang will eventually entrap Yin, making it unable to descend to the sacrum/urinary bladder. It will therefore ascend and escape inwards to the diaphragm,[26] leading to aversion to Cold in the stomach area and diarrhea. These symptoms are by no means due to excessive Yin Cold, because further observation will reveal that the inside of the body will be as hot as charcoal while the outside is as cold as ice, a sign that Yin is about to be extinguished.

少陰人病이 一日發汗하고 陽氣上升하야 人中穴에 先汗則病必愈也而二
日三日에 汗不止 病不愈則陽不上升而亡陽이 無疑也오
少陽人病이 一日滑利하고 陰氣下降하야 手足掌心에 先汗則病必愈也而
二日三日에 泄不止 病不愈則陰不下降而亡陰이 無疑也라.

If the So Eum Individual begins to sweat below the nose on the first day of illness, it means that Yang energy is capable of ascending to the upper body and recovery[27] is imminent. If there is continuous sweating for two to three days without recovery from illness, it is a sign that Yang is incapable of ascending and is in danger of collapsing.

---

24  This situation, also referred to as Yin overwhelming Yang, or *Yin Sheng Ge Yang* (陰盛格陽), is the basis of the So Eum Individual's *Mang Yang* illness. If it progresses into *Mang Yang* syndrome, Yang will not only escape from the urinary bladder and produce slight sweating, but also from the exterior portion of the entire body via profuse sweating.

25  This situation, also referred to as Yang overwhelming Yin, or *Yang Sheng Ge Yin* (陽盛格陰), is the basis of the So Yang Individual's *Mang Yin* illness. If it progresses into *Mang Yin* syndrome, Yin will not only escape to the stomach and diaphragm and cause slight diarrhea, but also from the large intestine via acute diarrhea.

26  The sacrum and urinary bladder correlate with the So Yang Individual's weaker organ, the kidneys. Yet the diaphragm correlates with the spleen, the So Yang Individual's stronger organ. Hence in this situation, the So Yang Individual's Yang energy will escape to where it feels safe, the stronger diaphragm. Balance and health are dependent on the smooth, unobstructed descent of Yin from the Yang organs and the smooth ascent of Yang from the Yin organs.

27  The So Eum Individual's health is dependent on the smooth flow of Yang energy from the kidneys to the spleen. This flow is easily obstructed due to the tendency towards kidney Yang stagnation and spleen deficiency.

If the So Yang Individual experiences diarrhea on the first day of illness, it is a sign of recovery since Yin energy is capable of descending,[28] which also leads to sweating of the hands and feet. Continuous diarrhea for two to three days without recovery from illness is a sign that Yin is incapable of descending and is in danger of collapsing.

凡亡陽과 亡陰證은 明知醫理者는 得病前에 可以預執證也려니와 得病 一二日에는 明白易見也오 至于三日則雖愚者라도 執證이 亦明若觀火 矣리니 用藥을 必無過二三日矣니 四日則晚矣오 五日則臨危也니라.

The majority of *Mang Yang* and *Mang Yin* syndromes can be detected in advance by a skilled doctor. In all cases, however, there will be obvious signs after one to two days, and after three days, no matter how ignorant a doctor may be, he will see it clearly as if staring at fire.

If *Mang Yang* or *Mang Yin* syndrome occurs, medicine should be prescribed within two to three days. Addressing the situation after four days is often too late. A delay of five days renders the situation critical.

少陰人이 平居에 裡煩 汗多者가 得病則必成亡陽也오 少陽人이 平居에 表寒 下多者가 得病則必成亡陰也니 亡陽과 亡陰人은 平居에 預治補陰 補陽이 可也오 不可至於亡陽亡陰하야 得病臨危然後에 救病也니라.

If a So Eum Individual is often plagued by vexation and excessive sweating, then illness will inevitably lead to *Mang Yang* syndrome. If a So Yang Individual is often plagued by chills and excessive diarrhea, then illness will inevitably lead to *Mang Yin* syndrome. For those who are prone to *Mang Yang* or *Mang Yin*, the situation should be remedied in advance by supporting Yang or Yin. A doctor should not wait until critical symptoms manifest to treat these syndromes.

少陰人의 病愈之汗은 人中에 先汗而一次發汗에 胸膈이 壯快而活潑하며 亡陽之汗은 人中에 或汗 或不汗하고 屢次發汗하되 胸膈이 悶燥而下陷 也오
少陽人의 病愈之泄은 手足掌心에 先汗而一次滑泄에 表氣淸寧而精神이 爽明하며 亡陰之泄은 手足掌心에 不汗하고 屢次泄利하되 表氣溯寒而精 神이 鬱冒니라.

When a So Eum Individual recovers from illness, he or she will experience sweating underneath the nose, and then a release of chest distress and an increase of energy.

---

28   The So Yang Individual's health depends on the smooth flow of Yin energy from the spleen to the kidneys. This flow is easily obstructed because of the tendency towards spleen Yin stagnation and kidney deficiency.

With *Mang Yang* syndrome, there may be only a hint of sweat beneath the nose, occurring again and again with chest discomfort, vexation, and a sinking of energy.[29]

When a So Yang Individual recovers from illness, he or she will first experience sweating of the hands and feet, and then one bout of diarrhea, which is followed by the cessation of chills, and clarity of the mind. In the case of *Mang Yin* syndrome, there will be an absence of hand and foot sweating, and several bouts of diarrhea will be followed by chills, vertigo, and a lack of clear thinking.

少陰人의 胃家實病과 少陽人의 結胸病은 正邪陰陽이 相敵而相格인
故로 日久而後에 危證이 始見也오 少陰人의 亡陽病과 少陽人의 亡陰
病은 正邪陰陽이 不敵而相格인 故로 初證에 已爲險證하야 繼而因爲危
證矣니라.

If the *Zheng Qi* and pathogenic influence are engaged in battle, as seen in the So Eum Individual's *Wei Jia Shi* syndrome and the So Yang Individual's *Jie Xiong* syndrome, it would take a longer time for illness to become life threatening. When *Mang Yin* or *Mang Yang* syndromes occur, there is no longer any energy to fight the lingering battle between the *Zheng Qi*, the pathogenic influence, and Yin and Yang. Hence from the outset, these syndromes are considered critical and life threatening if not addressed in a timely fashion.

譬如用兵컨대 合戰交鋒할새 初一日合戰에 正兵이 爲邪兵所敗하야 折正
兵幾許兵數하고 二日에 又戰又敗하야 又折幾許數하고 三日에 又戰又
敗하야 又折幾許數하니 以三日交鋒으로 觀之則將愈益戰而愈益敗 愈益
折矣리라. 若四日復戰하며 五日復戰則正兵之全軍이 覆沒을 可知矣니 所
以用藥을 必無過三日也니라.

The above situation can be compared to a major war fought by the "Righteous" army directly after troop deployment. On the first day of war against the "Pathogenic" army, the "Righteous" loses numerous soldiers. After the second day of battle, the "Righteous" army suffers even more casualties. After three days, it dwindles further. After four and then five days of battle, it becomes clear that the "Righteous" army has lost. Therefore, it is crucial that medicine be administered for *Mang Yang* and *Mang Yin* syndromes within three days.

---

29    In this sentence, "a sinking of energy" is a translation of *Hasa* (下陷), or "sinking downwards." It can be interpreted in two ways: "extreme fatigue," and "sinking of Yin." The latter interpretation helps illustrate how the So Eum Individual's abundant and heavy Yin sinks downwards while deficient Yang hovers above, causing vexation.

盤龍山老人者는 李翁所居地에 有盤龍山인 故로 李翁이 自謂盤龍山老人
也니 此書中에 論曰二字는 無非盤龍山老人之論而此章에 特擧盤龍山老
人者는 蓋亡陽과 亡陰이 最是險病而人必尋常視之하야 易於例治인 故로
別以盤龍山老人으로 提擧驚呼而警覺之也라.

The Elder at Mt. Panlong refers to an elderly man residing in Mt. Panlong. The words "From my perspective" mentioned above are nothing but the words of the Panlong Elder, and are of my own making. I chose this name to claim seniority and proclaim the extreme danger behind *Mang Yang* and *Mang Yin* syndrome. Most doctors think lightly of these disorders, claiming that they are easy to treat, and approach them like other common illnesses. I hope when I use this name, doctors will take my admonition seriously.

亡陰證은 古醫에 別無經驗用藥頭話而李子建과 朱震亨書中에 若干論
及之나 然이나 自無明的快驗하니 蓋此病이 從古以來로 殺人이 孟浪甚
速하야 未暇經驗獵得裡許故也니라.

The doctors of the past made little mention of *Mang Yang* or *Mang Yin*-related treatment. Lee Shijian and Zhu Zhenheng gave light attention to these syndromes, accumulating no significant experience in addressing them. Since ancient times, doctors didn't believe that [early signs of] *Mang Yang* and *Mang Yin* syndrome could lead to death. Urgent treatment was implemented after it was too late, giving no time to record their progression.

**Table 7.3: The Yang Pattern Shang Han syndrome of the So Yang Individual**

| Syndrome | Due to | Common symptoms | Additional symptoms | Treated with |
|---|---|---|---|---|
| Combined Tai Yang, Shao Yang, and Yang Ming stage syndrome (*Mang Yin* syndrome) | Spleen Yang Heat chases out spleen Yin cold and entraps stomach Heat | Continuous diarrhea | Fever, headache, and diarrhea | *Joryong Chajonja Tang* (Lee Je-ma's Polyporus and Plantago Seed Decoction) *Hyungbang Sabaek San* (Lee Je-ma's Schizonepeta and Ledebouriella Clear the White Powder) |
| | | | Same as above with addition of constipation after several continuous bouts of diarrhea, excessive thirst and uncontrolled waving of the hands and feet, malaria-like symptoms of alternative bouts of excessive fever and minor chills, minute pulse, red complexion, itchy skin, little to no sweating | *Hyungbang Sabaek San* (Lee Je-ma's Schizonepeta and Ledebouriella Clear the White Powder) with 3.75g of Huang Lian (*Rhizoma Coptidis*) and 3.75g of Gua Lou (*Semen Trichosanthis*)* *Jihwang Baekho Tang* (Lee Je-ma's White Tiger Decoction with Rhemannia)** |
| | | | Chills, abdomen pain, 3–5 bouts of diarrhea within a week | *Hwalsok Gosam Tang* (Lee Je-ma's Talcum and Sophora Decoction)*** *Sukjihwang Gosam Tang* (Lee Je-ma's Processed Rhemannia and Sophora Decoction)**** |
| | | | Psychosis, incoherent speech, insomnia, thirst, dysuria, edema, chronic food stagnation | *Hyungbang Jihwang Tang* (Lee Je-ma's Schizonepeta, Ledebouriella, and Rhemannia Decoction) |

*Prescribed if there is a bowel movement in less than 24 hours.*

**Prescribed if there is no bowel movement for 24 hours or more.*

***This formula is prescribed if there are 3–5 bouts of diarrhea within a 24-hour period or if only sporadic bouts of diarrhea with chills and abdomen pain occur.*

****Also used when there are only sporadic bouts of or no diarrhea with accompanying symptoms.*

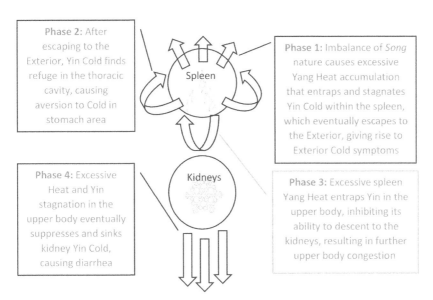

*Figure 7.2: The Mang Yin syndrome of the So Yang Individual*

張仲景이 曰太陽病이 不解하야 轉入少陽者는 脇下硬滿하고 乾嘔 不能食하며 往來寒熱者이니 尚未吐下하고 脈沈緊者는 與小柴胡湯이오 若已吐下 發汗에 譫語하고 柴胡證이 證罷하면 此爲壞病이니 依壞法으로 治之라.

According to Zhang Zhongjing, a lingering Tai Yang stage illness will eventually enter the Shao Yang stage, manifesting in fullness and hardness below the ribs, dry heaves and a lack of appetite, and alternating fever and chills. If vomit or diarrhea has not yet been promoted in this situation and the pulse is deep and tight, then *Xiao Chai Hu Tang* (Minor Bupleurum Decoction) should be prescribed. If, after the promotion of vomiting or diarrhea, there are signs of incoherent speech and excessive sweating, serious illness is present and beyond the capacity of *Xiao Chai Hu Tang* (Minor Bupleurum Decoction) treatment. In this case, the situation must be treated according to its severity.

傷寒에 脈弦細하며 頭痛發熱者는 屬少陽하니 不可發汗이니 發汗하면 則譫語니라

[From my perspective,] a headache and fever with a narrow and minute pulse during a Shang Han invasion is a signal of Shao Yang stage illness, and therefore sweating should not be induced. If it is during the Shao Yang stage, symptoms of delirium will inevitably occur.

嘗治少陽人이 傷寒에 發狂 譫語證할새 時則乙亥年淸明節候也라. 少陽人 一人이 得傷寒하야 寒多熱少之病하야 四五日後 午未辰刻에 喘促短氣어늘 伊時에 經驗이 未熟하야 但知少陽人應用藥으로 六味湯이 最好之理인 故로 不敢用他藥하고 而祇用六味湯 一貼호니 病人喘促이 卽時頓定이러니

I once treated a So Yang Individual suffering from psychosis and delirium due to a Shang Han stage illness in April of 1874. This person experienced Greater Cold and Lesser Heat syndrome[30] after four to five days of onset, characterized by difficult and rapid breathing between the hours of 11am and 3pm. Since this occurred earlier in my career as a doctor, I was simply attuned to the fact that *Liu Wei Di Huang Tang* (Six Ingredient Decoction with Rhemannia) was suitable for the So Yang Individual, and was not aware of any other type of medicine for this constitution. However, after just one pack of *Liu Wei Di Huang Tang*, the patient recovered from shortness of breath.

又數日後에 病人이 發狂譫語하며 喘促又發이어늘 又用六味湯 一貼則喘促이 雖少定而不如前日之頓定矣오 病人이 發狂連三日하고 午後에 喘促이 又發이어늘 又用六味湯한데 喘促이 略不少定이라가 有頃에 舌卷動風하야 口噤不語하니

A few days later, the patient began to experience another bout of psychosis and delirium with shortness of breath, for which I then prescribed the same formula for a second time. Although the patient's breathing improved slightly, the results were not nearly as good as the first time.

For three more days, this patient was continuously psychotic and had difficulty breathing in the evening. I prescribed *Liu Wei Di Huang Tang* (Six Ingredient Decoction with Rhemannia) for a third time, but with no relief from shortness of breath. Instead, shortly afterwards, the patient's tongue began to dry out and Internal Wind accumulation occurred, causing lockjaw.

於是而始知六味湯之無能爲也라. 急煎白虎湯一貼하야 以竹管으로 吹入病人鼻中하야 下咽而察其動靜則舌卷口噤之證은 不解而病人腹中이 微鳴이라 仍以兩爐煎藥하야 荏苒灌鼻한데 數三貼後에 病人이 腹中大鳴하며 放氣出焉이어늘 三人이 扶持病人하고 竹管으로 吹鼻灌藥而病人氣力이 益屈强하야 三人扶持之力이 幾不能支當矣호라 又荏苒灌鼻하야 自未申時로 至亥子時까지 凡用石膏八兩하니 末境에 病人腹中이 大脹하고 角弓反張之證이 出焉하더니 角弓反張後 少頃에 得汗而

---

睡하고 翌日平明에 病人이 又服白虎湯一貼하니 日出後에 滑便一次而病
快愈하니라.

At this point, I finally realized that *Liu Wei Di Huang Tang* (Six Ingredient Decoction with Rhemannia) is not the appropriate formula, so I immediately prescribed one pack of *Bai Hu Tang* (White Tiger Decoction) by blowing it through a bamboo straw placed inside her nostril, in order to get it down her throat. I then proceeded to observe her condition and noticed that there was no symptomatic improvement, but there was a gentle gurgling sound coming from her stomach.

Therefore, I boiled two more pots of medicine over two fire pits and continued to administer two to three packs of these herbs. Shortly afterwards, the gurgling sounds became louder and resulted in flatulence. As the formula also helped increase energy, it took three people to anchor the patient down as I administered the herbs a second time through the nose. Even three people were barely successful.

After continuous administration of herbs during the hours of 1pm to 1am, totaling 300g of Shi Gao (*Gypsum Fibrosum*), the patient's abdomen began to swell acutely and she began to experience opisthotones. Shortly afterwards, she started to sweat and then enter a deep sleep.

On the second day, the patient ingested one more pack of *Bai Hu Tang* (White Tiger Decoction), and that evening she had one bout of diarrhea, recovering soon afterwards.

愈後에 有眼病이어늘 用石膏 黃栢末 各一錢하야 日再服하니 七八日
後에 眼病이 亦愈니라. 伊時에 未知大便驗法인 故로 不察大便之秘閉幾
日이나 然이나 想必此病人이 先自表寒病으로 得病後에 有大便秘閉而發
此證矣리라.

After recovering from her illness, the patient began to experience visual problems. In response, I prescribed 3.75g of Shi Gao (*Gypsum Fibrosum*) powder and 3.75g of Huang Bai (*Cortex Phellodendri*) powder. After she ingested this formula twice per day for seven to eight days, her visual problems completely disappeared.

At that time I was unaware of the need to observe her bowel flow to decipher the stage of illness. In retrospect, I see that I overlooked the fact that she had experienced several days of constipation at the onset of her illness. It was likely that this situation was due to the occurrence of constipation after an External Cold attack.

其後에 又有少陽人 一人이 得傷寒에 熱多寒少之病하니 有人이 敎服雉
肉湯하야 仍成陽毒發斑이어늘 余가 敎服白虎湯 連三貼而其人이 只服半
貼하더니 數日後에 譫語而病重하니 病家에서 愍急이어늘 顚倒往觀則病
人 外證이 昏憒하야 已有動風之漸而耳聾 譫語하며 舌上白胎라.

Following this experience, I had another chance to treat a So Yang Individual who contracted Greater Heat and Lesser Cold[31] syndrome with red skin eruptions due to the accumulation of Yang toxin[32] after another doctor prescribed soup made from pheasant.[33] Even though I prescribed three packs of *Bai Hu Tang* (White Tiger Decoction), the patient became delirious, and the illness appeared to get worse after a few days and ingesting only half a pack of herbs. A family member then rushed to my home to relay the news of his condition and I left immediately to assist him. I noticed that the patient was drifting in and out of consciousness and had lost his hearing. His tongue was also thickly white coated and he was delirious, indicating that Wind had already made its way towards the Interior.

藥囊에 祇有石膏一斤 滑石一兩而無他藥인 故로 急煎石膏一兩 滑石一
錢을 頓服而其翌日에 又服石膏一兩 滑石一錢하니 此兩日則大便秘閉가
皆不過一晝夜라. 至于第三日하야 病家에서 以過用石膏를 歸咎인 故로
一日不用石膏矣호니 至于第四日하야 病家에서 愍急이어늘 顚倒往觀則
病人大便秘閉가 兩夜一晝而語韻이 不分明하고 牙關緊急하야 水飮不
入이어늘 急煎石膏二兩하야 艱辛下咽而半吐半下咽하니 少頃에 牙關開
而語韻則不分明如前이라. 又連用石膏 一兩하고 其翌日則以午後動風에
藥不下咽之慮인 故로 預爲午前用藥하야 以備動風而又五六日 用之하니
前後用石膏를 凡十四兩而末境에 發狂數日하고 語韻이 宏壯而病愈하야
數月然後에 方出門庭하니라.

After reaching into my herb bag, I realized that only 600g of Shi Gao (*Gypsum Fibrosum*) and 37.5g of Hua Shi (*Talcum*) remained. So I prescribed 37.5g of Shi Gao (*Gypsum Fibrosum*) and 3.75g of Hua Shi (*Talcum*) as a single dose as tea. Fortunately, the patient was able to have a bowel movement each day for two days while continuing with the same dosage. However, on the third day, his family was greatly concerned about such a high amount of Shi Gao (*Gypsum Fibrosum*) and refused to give him another dose. On the fourth day, a family member rushed to my home to report his urgent condition, upon which I immediately rushed to his side. I

---

31  Greater Heat and Lesser Cold (熱多寒少之病) syndrome refers to an Exterior Cold influence advancing towards the Interior and transforming into a Heat-dominant syndrome with the addition of minor lingering External Cold-related symptoms, indicating that the pathogen has not made its way completely into the Interior.

32  Yang toxin, or *Yang Duo* (陽毒), occurs after long-term, or acute, Yang Heat accumulation within the body and often manifests as red elevated skin eruptions.

33  Pheasant meat is hot-natured and can intensify the already hot nature of the So Yang Individual's stronger spleen. It is recommended for the So Eum Individual, who can use the hot nature of pheasant meat to warm his/her deficient spleen.

noticed that for two nights and a day he had no bowel movement. Lockjaw rendered his speech unclear, which also made it impossible to drink fluids.

I immediately prescribed 75g of Shi Gao (*Gypsum Fibrosum*) and was barely able to get it down his throat as he vomited half of it up again. He could open his mouth again shortly afterwards, but his speech remained unclear.

I continued by prescribing another 37.5g of Shi Gao (*Gypsum Fibrosum*) the following day. On the following day, I feared the return of Internal Wind, making it difficult to swallow the medicine, so I came back early in the morning to administer another dose of preventive herbs. I continued with this dosage for another five to six days, accumulating a total of 525g of Shi Gao (*Gypsum Fibrosum*). Afterwards, he experienced an episode of psychosis followed by an increasingly loud voice. He was able to leave the house a few months later, and completely recovered from his illness.

其後에 又有少陽人 一人이 初得頭痛 身熱表寒病하야 八九日이라 其間에 用黃連 瓜蔞 羌活 防風等屬하니 病勢少愈而永不快祛矣하니 仍爲發狂三 日이어늘 病家에서 以尋常例證으로 視之而祇用黃連 瓜蔞等屬하고 又譫 語數日에 始用地黃白虎湯一貼하니 其翌日午後에 動風이어늘 急煎地黃 白虎湯 連三貼하야 救急而艱辛下咽하고 其翌日則白虎湯 加石膏一兩을 午前用之하야 以備動風而連三日用之하니 病人이 自起坐立하야 能大小 便하며 病勢를 比前하면 快蘇快壯矣니라. 不幸히 病加於少愈에 慮不周 於完治하야 此人을 竟不救하니 恨不午前에 祇用白虎湯二貼하야 以備動 風而午後에 全不用藥以繼之也로다.

Afterwards, another So Yang Individual began to experience fever and then headaches following an eight to nine day onset of Exterior Cold syndrome. For this, I prescribed herbs such as Huang Lian (*Rhizoma Coptidis*), Gua Lou (*Semen Trichosanthis*), Qiang Huo (*Rhizoma seu Radix Notopterygii*), and Fang Feng (*Radix Saposhnikoviae*), and even though the condition improved slightly, for the most part, it lingered. She then became delirious, which according to her family was not unusual. I decided to continue with Huang Lian (*Rhizoma Coptidis*), Guo Lou (*Semen Trichosanthis*), and other similar herbs, but her symptoms persisted, so I prescribed one pack of *Jihwang Baekho Tang* (Lee Je-ma's White Tiger Decoction with Rhemannia). On the second evening, she contracted Internal Wind, for which I immediately prescribed another three doses of *Jihwang Baekho Tang*, which, because of her tight jaw, she was unable to swallow. I was able to prevent further advancement of Internal Wind with 37.5g of Shi Gao (*Gypsum Fibrosum*) in *Bai Hu Tang* (White Tiger Decoction) on the morning of the onset's second day. On the third day, she showed significant signs of improvement and was able to sit and stand on her own and have normal bowel function and urination. Unfortunately, however, I didn't think carefully enough about continuing treatment until her full recovery, and was not able to save her. In retrospect, I should not have stopped at preventing the Internal stirring of Wind with two packs of *Bai Hu Tang* (White Tiger Decoction) without prescribing medicine to take during the evening before I left.

以此三人病으로 觀之則發狂譫語證에 白虎湯을 非但午前用藥하야 以備 動風而已矣오. 日用五六貼 七八貼 十餘貼하야 以晝繼夜則好矣하며 不必 待譫語後而藥이오 發狂時에 當用藥이 可也며 不必待發狂後而用藥이오 發狂前에 早察發狂之漸이 可也니라.

The aforementioned three cases all suffered from Psychosis and Delirium[34] syndrome, and were thus treated with *Bai Hu Tang* (White Tiger Decoction). This formula should be prescribed not only in the morning, but also later in the day, to prevent the Internal advancement of Wind. I recommend five to six, seven to eight, or even ten packs of this formula throughout the day. One should never wait for delirium to occur before administering medicine. Moreover, with any sign of psychosis, this formula should be prescribed immediately. I am not, however, advocating the administration of *Bai Hu Tang* (White Tiger Decoction) after the onset of psychosis, since it is best to begin treatment when the first signs of Exterior Cold progression are detected.

其後에 又有少陽人 十七歲 女兒가 素證이 間有悖氣┌食滯┌腹痛矣하니 忽一日에 頭痛 寒熱 食滯어늘 有醫가 用蘇合元 三箇하야 薑湯에 調 下하니 仍爲泄瀉하야 日數十行 十餘日不止하고 引飮不眠하며 間有譫語 證하니 時則乙亥年 冬十一月 二十三日也ㅣ라 卽夜에 用生地黃 石膏 各 六兩 知母 三兩하니 其夜에 泄瀉度數가 減半하고 其翌日에는 用荊防地 黃湯 加石膏四錢하야 二貼連服하니 安睡而能通小便하니 荊防地黃湯 二 貼藥力이 十倍於知母白虎湯을 可知矣니라.

Subsequently, there was another 17-year-old So Yang Individual who often suffered from hiccups, food stagnation, and stomach pain. One day, she suddenly had a headache with chills and fever, followed by a bout of food stagnation. Another doctor prescribed three pills of *Su He Xiang Wan* (Liquid Styrax Pill) with ginger[35] tea. Shortly afterwards she experienced more than 20 bouts of diarrhea per day over a period of ten days. She was constantly given water and couldn't sleep at night due to continuous diarrhea after fluid ingestion, and she was also occasionally delirious. It was at this time, November 23, 1839, that I first arrived to assist her.

---

34  Psychosis and Delirium syndrome is a translation of the Chinese term *Fa Kuang Zhan Yu* (發狂譫語), which literally translates as "insanity" (發狂) and "talking nonsense" (譫語) and it occurs as a result of an explosive upward movement of Yang.

35  Ginger is one of the most beneficial herbs for the So Eum Individual because of its Hot-natured and spleen-supporting functions. Contrarily it is one of the most contraindicated herbs for the So Yang Individual, born with a larger (stronger) spleen and a tendency towards excessive spleen Heat.

That evening, after ingesting 225g of Sheng Di Huang (*Radix Rehmanniae*) and Shi Gao (*Gypsum Fibrosum*), and 112g of Zhi Mu (*Rhizoma Anemarrhenae*), her diarrhea was only half as frequent as before. On the second day, I prescribed two packs of *Hyungbang Jihwang Tang* (Lee Je-ma's Schizonepeta, Ledebouriella, and Rhemannia Decoction) with 150g of Shi Gao (*Gypsum Fibrosum*). She slept very well that night and was finally able to urinate. This helped me realize that two packs of *Hyungbang Jihwang Tang* (Lee Je-ma's Schizonepeta, Ledebouriella, and Rhemannia Decoction) works ten or more times better than *Zhi Mu Bai Hu Tang* (White Tiger Decoction with Added Anemarrhena) for this situation.

於是에 每日用此藥 四貼하되 晝에 二貼連服하며 夜에 二貼連服하야 數日用之하니 泄瀉永止하고 頭部兩鬢에 有汗而病兒 譫語證이 變爲發狂證이어늘 病家에서 驚惑하야 二晝夜를 疑不用藥하니 病勢逾危하야 頭汗이 不出하고 小便이 秘結하며 口ㄷ氷片하고 不省人事하니 爻象이 可惡矣라 勢無奈何하야 以不得已之計로 一夜間에 用荊防地黃湯 加石膏一兩하야 連十貼灌口한데 其夜에 小便이 通三碗하고 狂證은 不止나 然이나 知人看面하며 稍有知覺이라. 其翌日에 又用六貼하고 連五日을 日用四五六貼하니 發狂이 始止하고 夜間에 或霎時就睡나 然이나 不能久睡便覺이어늘 又用三四貼하야 連五日하니 頭頂兩鬢에 有汗而能半時刻을 就睡하며 稍進粥飮少許라

After a few more days of two packs of this formula in the morning and two packs in the evening, her diarrhea ceased. Her illness took a sudden negative turn, and she began to sweat along her scalp and behind both ears.[36] Even worse, she also fell into psychosis and then became delirious. Her family was completely surprised and didn't know what to do, so in the midst of doubt, they prevented her from taking medicine for two weeks. Needless to say, her condition became critical, as she no longer sweated on her scalp, had difficulty urinating, and drifted in and out of consciousness. [In order to cool things off,] she was also constantly sucking on an ice cube.

Not knowing how to approach such a critical situation, I could do nothing but continue with my original plan. That evening, I prescribed another ten packs of *Hyungbang Jihwang Tang* (Lee Je-ma's Schizonepeta, Ledebouriella, and Rhemannia Decoction), continually pouring it into her mouth. Shortly afterwards, although still somewhat delirious, she produced three bowls of urine, and started to recognize others and gather her senses.

I continued to prescribe six packs of this formula the following day. Over the next five days, I prescribed between four and six packs, and she was no longer delirious for the first time. At this point, she was also able to sleep for very short

---

36   This type of sweating is a sign of Yin depletion, as it gets pushed out by excessive Yang through the skin pores of the upper body.

periods of time, so I reduced her dosage from ten to three, and occasionally four, packs a day. On the fifth day, she started to sweat on her scalp, forehead, and behind the ears, and slept for one hour straight. She was also able to eat small amounts of rice porridge.

其後에 每日 荊防地黃湯 加石膏一錢하야 日二貼用之하되 大便이 過一日 則加四錢하야 至于十二月 二十三日하니 始得免危하야 能起立房中하니 一朔內에 凡用石膏 四十五兩이러라. 新年正月十五日에 能行步一里地 而來見我하고 其後에 又連用荊防地黃湯 加石膏一錢하야 至于新年三 月하니라.

From the sixth day onwards, I continued to prescribe two packs a day of *Hyungbang Jihwang Tang* (Lee Je-ma's Schizonepeta, Ledebouriella, and Rhemannia Decoction) with 3.75g of Shi Gao (*Gypsum Fibrosum*), or 15g of Shi Gao (*Gypsum Fibrosum*) if she skipped a day of bowel movement. For the first time, on December 23, 1839, she was no longer in a critical stage of illness, and was able to stand up in her bedroom for short periods of time.

During the entire month since I had begun treating her, she ingested a total of 1688g of Shi Gao (*Gypsum Fibrosum*). On January 15 of the following year, she walked a distance of one quarter mile to my home. On that day I prescribed two and a half months of *Hyungbang Jihwang Tang* (Lee Je-ma's Schizonepeta, Ledebouriella, and Rhemannia Decoction) with 3.75g of Shi Gao (*Gypsum Fibrosum*).

論曰少陽人病은 以火熱爲證인 故로 變動이 甚速하니 初證에 不可輕易 視之也니라. 凡少陽人은 表病에 有頭痛하며 裏病에 有便秘則已爲重病 也니 重病에 不當用之藥을 一二三貼 誤投則必殺人이오 險病危證에 當 用之藥을 一二三貼 不及則亦不救命이니라.

From my perspective, the So Yang Individual has a propensity towards Fire and Heat-related illnesses, which tend to advance rapidly. Therefore, even the first stage of illness should be observed carefully. If a So Yang Individual experiences a headache with Exterior-related symptoms or constipation with Interior-related symptoms, it is already classified as a serious situation in which one to three packs of the wrong prescription can be lethal. In the case of life-threatening, critical-stage illness, there is little chance of recovery if one to three packs of the correct formula is indicated but not prescribed.

Section 2

# The So Yang Individual's Stomach Heat Causing Interior Heat Syndrome[1]

少陽人胃受熱裏熱病

張仲景이 曰太陽病 八九日에 如瘧狀하야 發熱惡寒하며 熱多寒少하며
脈微而惡寒者는 此는 陰陽이 俱虛니 不可更發汗 更下 更吐오 面色이
反有熱色者는 未欲解也라 不能得小汗出이면 身必痒이니 宜桂麻各半
湯이니라.

According to Zhang Zhongjing, if after eight to nine days of Tai Yang stage illness, there are malaria-like symptoms of alternative bouts of excessive fever and minor chills[2] with a minute pulse, it is a sign of both Yin and Yang deficiency. At this point, the practitioner must refrain from promoting sweat, bowel movement, or vomiting. A reddish complexion indicates that the pathogen is still lodged within the body. With limited sweating, the body will definitely feel itchy.[3] In this case, *Gui Ma Ge Ban Tang* (Combined Cinnamon Twig and Ephedra Decoction)[4] should be prescribed.

太陽病이 似瘧하야 發熱惡寒하며 熱多寒少하며 脈微弱者는 此는 亡陽
也ㅣ니 身不痒이면 不可發汗이니 宜桂婢各半湯이니라.

[According to Zhang Zhongjing,] during a Tai Yang stage illness, malaria-like symptoms of alternate bouts of excessive fever and minor chills with a minute pulse signify *Mang Yin* syndrome. If the body is not itchy, then sweat shouldn't be promoted, and *Gui Bi Ge Ban Tang* (Combined Cinnamon Twig and Gypsum Decoction)[5] is what's called for.

---

1   The So Yang Individual's stomach Heat causing Interior Heat syndrome is due to the upward explosion of his/her *Jung* emotion of sadness and the belief that others are not acknowledging or harboring secrets about them, a sign of imbalanced *Chon Shi*.

2   In this section, Zhang Zhongjing also refers to this condition as greater Heat and Lesser Cold syndrome, indicating an Interior Heat situation with lingering Exterior influence. The Greater Cold and Lesser Heat syndrome of the So Yang Individual indicates an Exterior Cold situation and is marked by excessive chills and minor or no fever. Hence, increased fever and decreased chills mean that the pathogen is entering the Interior.

3   Itchiness is a sign of Internal Heat stagnation that has not been released due to a lack of sweating. Internal Heat is released through sweating, bowel movement, and urination.

4   Lee Je-ma doesn't give reference to the ingredients of *Gui Ma Ge Ban Tang* elsewhere, so here they are: Gui Zhi (*Ramulus Cinnamomi*) 5g, Bai Shao Yao (*Radix Paeoniae Lactiflorae*) 3g, Sheng Jiang (*Rhizoma Zingiberis Recens*) 3g, Gan Cao (*Radix Glycyrrhizae*) 3g, Ma Huang (*Herba Ephedrae*) 3g, Da Zao (*Fructus Zizyphi Jujubae*) 4 Pieces, and Xing Ren (*Semen Armeniacae Amarae*) 3g. Source: Zhang Zhongjing's *Shang Han Lun*.

5   Lee Je-ma doesn't give reference to the ingredients of *Gui Bi Ge Ban Tang* elsewhere, so here they are: Shi Gao (*Gypsum Fibrosum*) 8g, Gui Zhi (*Ramulus Cinnamomi*) 4g, Bai Shao Yao (*Radix Paeoniae Lactiflorae*) 4g, Ma Huang (*Herba Ephedrae*) 4g, Gan Cao (*Radix Glycyrrhizae*) 1.2g, Sheng Jiang (*Rhizoma Zingiberis Recens*) 3g, and Da Zao (*Fructus Zizyphi Jujubae*) 2 Pieces. Source: Zhang Zhongjing's *Shang Han Lun*.

論曰此證에 大便 不過一晝夜而通者는 當用荊防瀉白散이오 大便이 過一晝夜而不通者는 當用地黃白虎湯이니라.

As I see it, if this illness includes less than 24 hours with no bowel movement, *Hyungbang Sabaek San* (Lee Je-ma's Schizonepeta and Ledebouriella Clear the White Powder) should be prescribed. If more than 24 hours pass without a bowel movement, then *Jihwang Baekho Tang* (Lee Je-ma's White Tiger Decoction with Rhemannia) should be prescribed.

張仲景이 曰陽明證에 小便不利하며 脈浮而渴이어든 猪苓湯을 主之니라. 三陽合病하야 頭痛 面垢하며 譫語 遺尿는 中外俱熱이니 自汗煩渴하며 腹痛身重이어든 白虎湯을 主之니라.

According to Zhang Zhongjing, if there is dysuria, a floating pulse, and thirst accompanying an episode of Yang Ming stage illness, then *Zhu Ling Tang* (Polyporus Decoction) should be prescribed. When all three Yang stages are involved, there will be headaches, delirium, enuresis, spontaneous sweating, thirst, abdominal pain, and a feeling of heaviness throughout the body. The face will appear soiled, and there will be Heat signs of both the Exterior and Interior. In this case, Zhang Zhongjing suggests *Bai Hu Tang* (White Tiger Decoction).

論曰陽明證者는 但熱無寒之謂也오 三陽合病者는 太陽 少陽 陽明證이 俱有之謂也라 此證에 當用猪苓湯 白虎湯이나 然이나 古方猪苓湯이 不如新方猪苓車前子湯之具備오 古方白虎湯이 不如新方地黃白虎湯之全美矣니 若陽明證에 小便不利者가 兼大便秘燥則當用地黃白虎湯이니라.

From my perspective, Yang Ming stage illness is characterized by fever without chills. Moreover, the Three Yang stage illness described above is due to a combination of Tai Yang, Shao Yang, and Yang Ming stage illnesses, and should therefore be treated with *Zhu Ling Tang* (Polyporus Decoction) or *Bai Hu Tang* (White Tiger Decoction). However, the effects of *Zhu Ling Tang* (Polyporus Decoction) cannot compare with *Joryong Chajonja Tang* (Lee Je-ma's Polyporus and Plantago Seed Decoction), nor can *Bai Hu Tang* (White Tiger Decoction) be compared with *Jihwang Baekho Tang* (Lee Je-ma's White Tiger Decoction with Rhemannia).[6] If there is difficulty with urination and defecation, then *Jihwang Baekho Tang* (Lee Je-ma's White Tiger Decoction with Rhemannia) is needed.

---

6    In this sentence Lee Je-ma exclaims how the classic formulae of *Zhu Ling Tang* and *Bai Hu Tang* each contain several herbal ingredients that are not suitable for the So Yang Individual. The two formulae, *Joryong Chajonja Tang* and *Jihwang Baekho Tang*, are modifications of *Zhu Ling Tang* and *Bai Hu Tang* respectively. To modify these formulae, Lee Je-ma added and omitted certain herbs, making them appropriate for the So Yang Individual.

朱肱이 曰陽厥者는 初得病에 必身熱頭痛하야 外有陽證하다가 至四五
日에 方發厥하며 厥至半日하야 却身熱이니 蓋熱氣深하야 方能發厥이라.
若微厥 却發熱者는 熱甚故也니 其脈이 雖伏이나 按之滑者는 爲裏
熱이오 或飮水하며 或揚手擲足하며 或煩躁 不得眠하며 大便秘하며 小
便赤하며 外證이 多昏憒하면 用白虎湯이니라.

Zhu Gong once stated that Exterior Yang-related symptoms such as headaches and fever are the first signs of *Yang Jue* syndrome,[7] which after four to five days result in the occurrence of icy-cold hands and feet. However, on the first half day of these symptoms, the rest of the body will feel hot rather than cold. In general, if fever is severe, it will eventually lead to *Yang Jue* syndrome. If fever occurs with frigid hands and feet syndrome, it is a sign of severe Heat,[8] and there will be a full and slippery pulse, indicating Internal Heat. If there is thirst, frigid hands and feet, vexation, anxiety, insomnia, dry stools, reddish urine, and an unclear consciousness, then *Bai Hu Tang* (White Tiger Decoction) should be prescribed.

論曰少陽人裡熱病에 地黃白虎湯이 爲聖藥而用之者는 必觀於大便之
通不通也니 大便이 一晝夜有餘而不通則可用也오 二晝夜不通則必用
也니라. 凡少陽人 大便이 一晝夜不通則胃熱이 已結也오 二晝夜不通則熱
重也며 三晝夜不通則危險也니 一晝夜 八九辰刻과 二晝夜에 恰好用之오
無至三晝夜之危險하고 若譫語證에 便秘則不可過一晝夜니라.

From my perspective, if the So Yang Individual experiences an Internal Heat-related illness, then *Jihwang Baekho Tang* (Lee Je-ma's White Tiger Decoction with Rhemannia) is most appropriate. While this formula is administered, it is crucial to observe the frequency of bowel movement. If 24 hours go by without a bowel movement, then this is the appropriate formula. If 48 hours or more go by, then the administration of this formula is critical. If 24 hours elapse without a bowel movement, it is a sign that Heat has already caused a blockage in the stomach of the So Yang Individual. If 48 hours pass, it is a sign of acute Heat accumulation, and after 72 hours, the situation becomes critical. If the above medicine is administered within 42 hours or even 48 hours of bowel movement, there is a greater chance of recovery. The practitioner should not let 72 hours elapse and the illness become critical without providing this formula. Constipation with delirium calls for medicine within 24 hours.

---

7    *Yang Jue* syndrome is the result of extreme accumulation of Heat and Yang within the body, which pushes Cold energy out to the extremities, causing frigid hands and feet. Yet there will also be Heat-related symptoms such as a high fever, red complexion and facial heat, dryness of the lips and throat, reddish and difficult-to-pass urine, dry stools, and fading consciousness.

8    Fever with frigid extremities during *Jue* syndrome indicates severe Heat accumulation because not only has it resulted in elevated body temperature, but it has also chased the remaining Cold energy outwards to the extremities.

少陽人이 胃受熱則大便이 燥也오 脾受寒則泄瀉也니 故로 亡陰證은 泄瀉二三日而大便秘一晝夜則淸陰이 將亡而危境也오 胃熱證은 大便이 三晝夜不通而汗出則淸陽이 將渴而危境也니라.

If a So Yang Individual suffers from Heat in the stomach, there will be dry stools [and/or constipation]. Cold in the spleen results in diarrhea. If, during the occurrence of *Mang Yin* syndrome, one day of constipation follows two to three days of diarrhea, it is a sign of diminishing *Clear Yin*,[9] a critical situation. If stomach Heat occurs and 72 hours go by without a bowel movement, there will be sweating, an indication of a critical situation in which *Clear Yang*[10] is diminishing.

少陽人 大便不通病에 用白虎湯 三四服하여도 當日大便不通者는 將爲融會貫通하리니 大吉之兆也라 不必疑惑而翌日에 又服二三貼則必無不通이니라.

There is nothing to fear, even if, after prescribing three to four packs of *Bai Hu Tang* (White Tiger Decoction) for the So Yang Individual with constipation, there is still no bowel movement on the first day. A lack of bowel movement within 24 hours is due to the fact that the stools may take an extra day to melt [from the effects of *Bai Hu Tang*]. If two or three packs are prescribed on the second day, a bowel movement will doubtlessly occur.

少陽人 表裏病의 結解는 必觀於大便而少陽人大便이 頭燥尾滑하야 體大而疏通者는 平時無病者之大便也오 其次는 大滑便 一二次 快滑泄하고 廣多而止者는 有病者之病이 快解之大便也오其次는 一二次 尋常滑便者는 有病者의 病勢가 不加之大便也오 其次는 或過一晝夜有餘不通커나 或一晝夜間 三四五次 小小滑利者는 將澁之候也ㅣ오 非好便也니 宜預防이니라.

The bowels must be observed in order to determine if a So Yang Individual is still suffering from, or is in the process of overcoming, an External or Internal illness. If the stools of a So Yang Individual are ample in size, dry at first but towards the end becoming looser, it is a sign of health. If one to two bouts of abundant and loose stool, which feels completely evacuated, are followed by normal bowel movement, it shows complete recovery from illness. If the So Yang Individual experiences one to two bouts of loose stools a day, it is a sign of [a less acute] illness that has not

---

9   *Clear Yin* (淸陰) describes the state in which Yin can easily and smoothly descend within the body without obstruction or accumulation. It contrasts with *Turbid Yin* (濁陰), which signifies obstructed and inhibited Yin, which cannot flow smoothly downward, leading to toxic accumulation within the body and sinking/evacuation of *Clear Yin*, in the form of diarrhea.

10   *Clear Yang* (淸陽) describes the state in which Yang can easily and smoothly rise within the body without obstruction or accumulation. It contrasts with *Turbid Yang* (濁陽), which signifies obstructed and inhibited Yang, which cannot flow smoothly upwards, leading to toxic Heat accumulation. *Clear Yang* is also associated with the unobstructed flow of *Wei* (Protective) *Qi* and healthy *Qi* and blood circulation to the skin, muscles, and tendons of the extremities. Sweating, in the above situation, indicates a leakage of *Clear Yang*.

advanced further. If there are only three to five smaller/incomplete loose bowel movements, or none at all for an entire week, then it is a sign of constipation, and precautionary medicinal steps should be taken.

少陰人 裏寒病에 臍腹冷證은 受病之初에 已有腹鳴泄瀉之機驗而其機가 甚顯則其病은 執證易見而用藥을 可早也어니와 少陽人 裏熱病에 胸膈熱 證은 受病之初에 雖有胸煩悶燥之機驗而其機가 不甚顯則執證이 難見而 用藥이 太晚也니라. 若使少陽人病으로 胸煩悶燥之驗이 顯然露出하야 使 人可覺則其病은 已險而難爲措手矣리라.

If the So Eum Individual is afflicted with a Cold-induced illness and the umbilical area feels cold to the touch, or if during the first stage of illness they experience borborygmos, diarrhea is sure to occur. These symptoms are helpful in the early detection of disease, as they indicate the use of preventive herbal medicine. If *Xiong Ge Re* syndrome[11] occurs in the early stage of the So Yang Individual's Internal Heat syndrome, marked by fullness in the chest and vexation, it is already too late to avoid danger, even with the use of herbal medicine. Moreover, these symptoms are not clearly detectable at first, often leading to extreme delay in treatment.

凡少陽人表病에 有頭痛則自是表病이 明白易見之初證也니 若復引 飮하며 小便赤則可畏也오 泄瀉하며 揚手擲足則大畏也니라. 少陽人裏 病에 大便이 過一晝夜有餘而不通則自是裏病이 明白易見之初證也니 若 復大便이 過三晝夜不通則危險矣니라.

Headaches are a classic symptom of the So Yang Individual's first stage of External illness. If headaches are accompanied by thirst and reddish urine, the situation becomes worrisome. If headaches are accompanied by uncontrollable movement of the hands and feet, the situation is even more worrisome. The So Yang Individual's constipation for one day or more is a tell-tale indication of first-stage Internal Heat-related illness, which becomes life threatening after three or more days of no bowel movement.

背癰 腦疽 脣瘇 纏喉風 咽喉等病은 受病之日에 已爲危險證也오 陽毒發 斑 流注丹毒 黃疸等病은 受病之日에 已爲險證也오 面目口鼻牙齒之病은 成病之日에 皆爲重證也니라 凡少陽人 表病에 有頭痛證則必用荊防敗毒 散이오 裏病에 有大便過一晝夜不通證則用白虎湯이니라.

The occurrence of spinal tumor(s), occipital area tumor(s), severe swelling of the throat, or other throat disorder indicates that the situation has already reached

---

11   *Xiong Ge Re* (胸膈熱證) syndrome, translated directly as "Chest and Diaphragm Heat syndrome," occurs as a result of excessive Heat accumulation within the stomach of the So Yang Individual. It is marked by vexation and chest fullness due to the rebellion of pressurized stomach Heat upwards into the diaphragm and chest.

the critical stage.[12] Otherwise stated, if there is illness of the face, eyes, mouth, or nose of the So Yang Individual, then the situation is already in the critical stage. [To avoid such acute situations, action should be taken without delay, and] if the So Yang Individual experiences a headache due to an External illness, then *Hyungbang Peidok San* (Lee Je-ma's Schizonepeta and Ledebouriella Powder to Overcome Pathogenic Influences) should be prescribed. If there is a lack of bowel movement for one day or more during an Internal illness, then *Bai Hu Tang* (White Tiger Decoction) should be prescribed.

王好古가 曰渴病有三하니 曰消渴이오 曰消中이오 曰消腎이니라.

Wang Hao Gu once stated that there are three types of thirst syndromes:[13] *Xiao Ge*,[14] *Xiao Zhong*[15] (diabetes of the center), and *Xiao Shen*.[16]

**Table 7.4: Yang Ming and three Yang stage syndromes of the So Yang Individual**

| Syndrome | General information | Symptoms | Treated with |
|---|---|---|---|
| Yang Ming stage syndrome (Internal Heat) | Lingering Tai Yang stage illness transfers to the Yang Ming stage (spleen Cold pressurizes stomach Heat) | One or more days of constipation* | *Jihwang Baekho Tang* (Lee Je-ma's White Tiger Decoction with Rhemannia)** |
| Combined three Yang stage illness (acute Internal Heat) | Lingering Tai Yang stage illness with accumulated Heat within the stomach (spleen Cold further pressurizes stomach Heat further) | Headaches, delirium, enuresis, spontaneous sweating, thirst, abdominal pain, a feeling of heaviness throughout the body, soiled face, External and Internal Heat symptoms | *Joryong Chajonja Tang* (Lee Je-ma's Polyporus and Plantago Seed Decoction)*** *Jihwang Baekho Tang* (Lee Je-ma's White Tiger Decoction with Rhemannia) |

*\* Constipation is a hallmark symptom of the So Yang Individual's Internal Heat illness.*

*\*\* Prescribed if there is difficulty with defecation or both urination and defecation.*

*\*\*\* Prescribed if there is difficulty with urination only.*

熱氣上騰하면 胸中이 煩躁하며 舌赤脣紅하니 此渴은 引飲常多하고 小便이 數而少하나니 病屬上焦니 謂之消渴이오 熱蓄於中하면 消穀善飢하며 飲食이 倍常이로되 不生肌肉하니 此渴은 亦不甚煩하고 小便이 數而舌甘하나니 病屬中焦니 謂之消中이오 熱伏於下하면 腿膝이 枯細하며 骨

---

12  The occurrence of spinal tumor(s), occipital area tumor(s), severe swelling of the throat, or other throat disorder is the result of long-term or acute stomach Yang Heat stagnation and rebellion towards the upper body, leading to toxic accumulation.

13  The term "thirst syndromes" is a direct translation of *Ge Bing* (渴病), also interpreted as "wasting and thirsting disorder" or, more commonly, diabetes.

14  *Xiao Ge* (消渴) translates as "diabetes with thirst" or "wasting and thirsting disorder."

15  *Xiao Zhong* (消中) translates as "diabetes of the center" or "wasting of the center."

16  *Xiao Shen* (消腎) translates as "diabetes of the kidneys" or "wasting of the kidneys."

節이 ﹁疼하며 飮水不多호대 隨卽尿下하야 小便이 多而濁하나니 病屬下
焦니 謂之消腎이니라.

[Wang Hao Gu continued by stating that] *Xiao Ge* syndrome causes Heat to rise upwards, resulting in vexation, anxiety, a red tongue, red lips, and excessive thirst, with frequent urge to urinate with only limited output. It is referred to as "*Xiao Ge*" (diabetes with thirst) because it occurs in the Upper *Jiao*.

*Xiao Zhong* syndrome is characterized by the accumulation of Heat in the Middle *Jiao*, which leads to excessive appetite and digestive capacity, several times the individual's common food intake, without an increase in weight. This type of thirst syndrome is not accompanied by vexation or anxiety; however, there will be frequent desire to urinate. The urine of *Xiao Zhong* syndrome tastes sweet. This illness is referred to as "*Xiao Zhong*" (diabetes of the middle) because it primarily affects the stomach of the Middle *Jiao*.

*Xiao Shen* syndrome is characterized by the accumulation of Heat in the lower body, leading to thinning of the thighs, legs, and knees, pain, and pins-and-needles sensation in the joints. [Even though this is also referred to as a thirst syndrome,] there will be little thirst but abundant turbid urine. This illness is referred to as "*Xiao Shen*" (diabetes of the kidneys) because it occurs in the Lower *Jiao*.

又有五石過度之人이 眞氣既盡이나 石勢獨留하야 陽道興强하며 不
交精泄을 謂之强中이니 消渴은 輕也오 消中은 甚焉하고 消腎은 尤甚
焉하나니 若强中則其斃를 可立而待也니라.

[Wang Hao Gu continued by stating that] if an individual with deficient *Zhen Qi*[17] ingests too many minerals, which eventually become the only source of energy in his body, then the Yin channels may become overstimulated, leading to a constant erection and frequent ejaculation, even without sexual intercourse.

*Xiao Ge* syndrome is considered a light illness, while *Xiao Zhong* is considered serious and *Xiao Shen* is considered even more serious. If *Xiao Shen* is accompanied by a continuous erection and frequent ejaculation even without intercourse, a grave situation is evident.

朱震亨이 曰上消者는 舌上이 赤裂하며 大渴引飮이니 白虎湯을 主
之오中消者는 善食而瘦하며 自汗하며 大便硬하며 小便數이니 黃連猪肚
丸을 主之오 下消者는 煩躁引飮하며 小便이 如膏하며 腿膝이 枯細하니
六味地黃湯을 主之니라.

Zhu Zhenheng once stated that a red tongue indicates *Shang Xiao*.[18] The tongue may also be cracked, indicating severe thirst, for which he recommended *Bai Hu Tang*

---

17 *Zhen Qi* (眞氣), or True *Qi*, consists of *Ying Qi* (Nutritive *Qi*) and *Wei Qi* (Protective *Qi*). It circulates throughout the body via the energy meridians, nourishing and protecting the organs.

18 *Shang Xiao* (上消) is translated as "Upper [*Jiao*] diabetes," or "Upper [*Jiao*] wasting and thirsting disorder."

(White Tiger Decoction). *Zhong Xiao*[19] is characterized by excessive eating without weight gain, spontaneous sweating, dry stools, and frequent urination. For this, he recommended *Huang Lian Jie Du Tang* (Coptis Decoction to Relieve Toxicity).[20] *Xia Xiao*[21] is characterized by vexation and fullness in the chest, thirst, oily urine, and thinning of the thighs and legs. He recommended that *Liu Wei Di Huang Tang* (Six Ingredient Decoction with Rhemannia) be prescribed for this.

醫學綱目에 曰渴而多飲이 爲上消오 消穀善飢가 爲中消오 渴而尿數하며 有膏油는 爲下消니라.

The *Yixue Gangmu* contains the statement that excessive thirst and fluid intake indicates *Shang Xiao*; excessive appetite with abundant food intake is a sign of *Zhong Xiao*; and thirst, a frequent desire to urinate, and oily urine signify *Xia Xiao*.

危亦林이 曰因耽嗜色慾하야 或服丹石하고 眞氣旣脫하되 熱邪獨盛하야 飲食이 如湯消雪하고 肌膚日削하며 小便이 如膏油하며 陽强興盛하야 不交精洩하나니 三消之中에 最爲難治니라.

Wei Yilin states that excessive indulgence in sexual activity, or excessive intake of minerals, deplete *Zheng Qi,* and the accumulation of pathogenic Heat will linger. Day by day, the skin will dry out and shrivel like snow melting inside of boiling water, while urine will appear oily, and the penis will be constantly erect, even without sexual arousal, often accompanied by spontaneous ejaculation. The latter situation is the most difficult to treat.

論曰消渴者는 病人胸次가 不能寬遠「達而陋固膠小하야 所見者는 淺하고 所欲者는 速하며 計策이 鷓突하며 意思가 艱乏則大腸淸陽上升 之氣가 自不快足하야 日月耗困而生此病也니라. 胃局淸陽이 上升而不快 足於頭面四肢則成上消病하고 大腸局淸陽이 上升而不快足於胃局則成中 消病하나니 消는 自爲重證而中消는 倍重於上消오 中消는 自爲險證而下 消는 倍險於中消니라.

From my perspective, diabetes is a result of the inability to broaden one's mind, focus on the big picture, and look beyond trifling matters, inhibiting the ability to be generous and tolerant. It is due to narrow-mindedness and lack of self-cultivation, versatility, and a tendency towards a frivolous and hasty character. If the So Yang Individual gets fully absorbed in their plans without a clue of how to pursue them, then the *Clear Yang* energy of the intestines will not be able to carry out its natural

---

19    *Zhong Xiao* (中消) is translated as "Middle [*Jiao*] diabetes," or "Middle [*Jiao*] wasting and thirsting disorder."

20    Lee Je-Ma doesn't mention *Huang Lian Jie Du Tang* elsewhere in this text, so the ingredients are listed here: Huang Lian (*Rhizoma Coptidis*) 9g, Huang Qin (*Radix Scutellaria*) 6g, Huang Bai (*Cortex Phellodendri*) 6g, and Zhi Zi (*Fructus Gardeniae Jasminoidis*) 6–12g. Source: *Wai Tai Bi Yao* (*Arcane Essentials from the Imperial Library*).

21    *Xia Xiao* (下消) is translated as "Lower [*Jiao*] diabetes," or "Lower [*Jiao*] wasting and thirsting disorder."

ability to gather and flow upwards. As the days and months go by, it will start to exhaust and waste away. This is precisely how diabetes occurs.

*Shang Xiao* results from the inability of *Clear Yang* to rise upwards and nourish the head, face, and four extremities. If the *Clear Yang* rises [up to the Middle *Jiao*] but is incapable of gathering in the upper body, then *Zhong Xiao* will occur. Although *Shang Xiao* is a serious illness, *Zhong Xiao* is several times more severe. Even though *Zhong Xiao* is several times more severe, *Xia Xiao* is the most critical of the three.

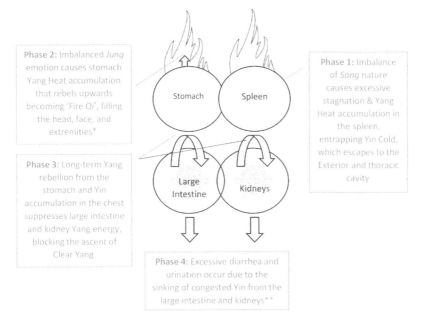

*Figure 7.3: Shang Xiao, Zhong Xiao, and Xia Xiao syndromes of the So Yang Individual*

\* *Phase 3 will result in excessive thirst, the hallmark sign of Shang Xiao. As the situation advances, it will transform into Zhong Xiao, marked by excessive appetite.*

\*\* *Phase 5 will result in excessive diarrhea and urination, the hallmark sign of Xia Xiao.*

上消에 宜用涼膈散火湯이오 中消에 宜用忍冬藤地骨皮湯이오 下消에 宜用熟地黃苦參湯이로되 尤宜寬闊其心이오 不宜膠小其心이니 寬闊則 所欲이 必緩하야 淸陽이 上達하고 膠小則所欲이 必速하야 淸陽이 下 耗니라.

[From my perspective] *Yanggyuk Sanhwa Tang* (Lee Je-ma's Cool the Diaphragm and Disperse Heat Decoction) should be prescribed for *Shang Xiao*; *Indongdeng Jigolpi Tang* (Lee Je-ma's Honeysuckle and Lycium Decoction) should be prescribed for *Zhong Xiao*; and *Sukjihwang Gosam Tang* (Lee Je-ma's Processed Rhemannia and Sophora Decoction) should be prescribed for *Xia Xiao*. In order to overcome diabetes, it is crucial for the So Yang Individual to broaden their mind and refrain from being rigid in their ways.

If the So Yang Individual opens their mind, or at least makes an effort in this direction, then *Clear Yang* will naturally gather, rise, and then spread out. If they remain narrow minded or even make an attempt to disengage an open mind, then hastiness will cause the *Clear Yang* to sink downwards and waste away.

平心靜思則陽氣가 上升하야 輕淸而充足於頭面四肢也니 此는 元氣也며 淸陽也오 勞心焦思則陽氣가 下陷하야 重濁而鬱熱於頭面四肢也니 此는 火氣也며 耗陽也니라.

If the mind is quiet and at ease, then the *Clear Yang* will rise and cleanse the channels along its way upward, gathering in the head, face, and four extremities. Hence, *Clear Yang* is also referred to as Source *Qi*[22] [because it distributes essence, *Qi*, and blood throughout the body]. The *Clear Yang* of a morally tainted or angry So Yang Individual will sink downwards, becoming heavy and turbid, while stagnant Heat remains in the head, face, and extremities. This energy is referred to as both the Fire *Qi*[23] and Wasted Yang *Qi*.[24]

危亦林이 曰消渴은 須防發癰疽니 忍冬藤을 不拘多少하고 根莖花葉을 皆可服이니라.

Wei Yilin stated that it is necessary at all costs to avoid the occurrence of tumors and carbuncles as a result of diabetic onset. In order to accomplish this, not only should Ren Dong Teng (*Caulis Lonicerae*)[25] be prescribed, but also the root, flowers, and leaves of Japanese Honeysuckle (*Lonicera Japonica*).

李杲가 曰消渴之疾에 能食者는 末傳必發腦疽 背瘡이오 不能食者는 必 傳中滿 鼓脹이니라.

Li Gao stated that excessive eating related to the onset of diabetes will eventually lead to occipital tumor or spinal tumor if left to fate. A lack of appetite related to diabetes will eventually lead to severe abdominal distension and bloating.[26]

東醫醫方類聚에 曰消渴之病은 變成癰疽오 或成水病하며 或雙目이 失 明이니라.

The *Dongyi Fangleiju* (*Classified Prescriptions*) includes the statement that diabetes may lead to the formation of tumors and carbuncles, edema, and/or loss of eyesight.

---

22  The term "Source *Qi*" is a translation of *Yuan Qi* (元氣), which rises from the kidneys and spreads throughout the body, giving life to the organs and extremities.

23  "Fire *Qi*" is the result of Yang Heat stagnation and accumulation in the stomach, leading to acute Heat-related symptoms.

24  "Wasted Yang *Qi*" refers to the consumption and withering away of Yang *Qi* as it burns itself out.

25  Ren Dong Teng (*Caulis Lonicerae*) is the stem of Japanese Honeysuckle (*Lonicera Japonica*).

26  "Acute distension and bloating" is a translation of the term *Gu Zhang* (鼓脹), which is a combination of the words "drum" and "swelling." During an episode of *Gu Zhang* syndrome, the abdomen is acutely swollen, and when percussed, sounds like a hollow drum.

論曰癰疽 眼病은 皆是中消之變證也오 中消는 自爲險證則上消에 當早治
也오 中消에 必急治也며 下消則濱死니라.

From my perspective, tumors, carbuncles, and loss of eyesight are all related to *Zhong Xiao*,[27] which is a life-threatening illness. When it comes to treatment, *Shang Xiao* should be addressed in the early stages, *Zhong Xiao* should be attended immediately, and even *with* treatment, *Xia Xiao* is a grave illness.

王好古가 曰一童子가 自嬰至童에 盜汗이 七年이라 諸藥이 不效러니 服
凉膈散 三日에 病已니라.

Wang Hao Gu recalled an episode in which, no matter how much he tried, he could not cure a young boy who suffered since infancy from night sweats, over a period of seven years. It wasn't until he administered *Liang Ge San* (Cool the Diaphragm Powder) that, after three days, the boy's night sweats completely ceased.

論曰少陽人 大腸淸陽이 快足於胃하야 充溢於頭面四肢則汗必不出也니
少陽人 汗者는 自是陽弱也而服凉膈散하야 病已則此病은 卽上消而其
病은 輕也니라.

From my perspective, if the intestinal *Clear Yang* of the So Yang Individual flows smoothly upward and outward, filling up the head and extremities, then sweating will not be an issue. The night sweat of a So Yang Individual is the result of Yang weakness [and leakage]. Since the boy mentioned above recovered after taking *Liang Ge San* (Cool the Diaphragm Powder), it means he suffered from a light case of *Shang Xiao*.

東醫 醫方類聚에 曰夫渴者는 數飮水하며 其人이 必頭面이 眩하며 背寒
而嘔니 因虛故也니라.

The *Dongyi Fangleiju* (*Classified Prescriptions*) states that thirsting syndrome is marked by a constant desire to drink fluids, dizziness, a Cold sensation of the spine, and dry heaves. These symptoms are all caused by deficiency.

龔信이 曰凡陰虛證은 每日午後에 惡寒發熱하다가 至晚하야 亦得微汗而
解니 誤作瘧治하야 多致不救니라.

Gong Xin said that in the case of Yin deficiency, if there is an aversion to Cold in the evening with sudden feverish feelings and sweating after dusk, then recovery is certain. If this is treated as malaria,[28] however, recovery would be impossible.

---

27  Lee Je-ma correlates tumors, carbuncles, and loss of eyesight with *Zhong Xiao* because, in the So Yang Individual's case, excessive Heat rises primarily from the stomach in the *Zhong*, or Middle *Jiao*.

28  Alternate fever and chills are symptoms of both malaria and Yin deficiency. The occurrence of fever after dusk, however, is a sign of Yin deficiency rather than malaria. Hence Gong Xin warns against misdiagnosis and faulty treatment.

孫思邈 千金方書에 曰消渴에 宜愼者가 有三하니 一飮酒오 二房勞오 三ᄀ
食及麵이니 能愼此三者면 雖不服藥이라도 亦可自愈니라.

Sun Si Miao once stated in his text entitled, *Qianjin Fang* (*One Thousand Golden Formulae*) that diabetics must avoid three things: drinking alcohol, having intercourse, and eating salty food or food made from wheat flour. If these three things are avoided, then recovery from diabetes is possible even without the help of herbal medicine.

論曰上消와 中消는 裡陽升氣가 雖則虛損이나 表陰降氣가 猶恃完壯인
故로 其病이 雖險이나 猶能歲月支撑者가 以此也어니와 若夫陰虛午
熱하며 飮水하며 背寒而嘔者는 表裏陰陽이 俱爲虛損이니 所以爲病이
尤險하야 與下消로 略相輕重이라, 然이나 善攝身心服藥則十之六七은 尙
可生也오 不善攝身心服藥則百之百이 必死也니 此證에 當用獨活地黃湯
十二味地黃湯이니라.

From my perspective, *Shang Xiao* and *Zhong Xiao* are both due to the excessive descent of abundant External Yin, which suppresses and depreciates Internal Yang, making it impossible for Yang energy to ascend. Despite the fact that diabetes is a critical disease, since the Yin energy remains intact, it can be endured for a significant amount of time. If there is Yin deficiency-related fever in the late afternoon, excessive thirst, a cold sensation in the thoracic spine, and dry heaves, it is a sign of both Exterior and Interior Yang and Yin deficiency. This indicates the progression of diabetes into the Lower *Jiao*, leading to *Xia Xiao*, the most critical stage of diabetes. On the whole, both light and critical forms of diabetes have similar aspects, making it crucial to scrupulously examine both the mind and body of the patient. If carefully examined and treated, six to seven out of ten people will survive. If the mind and body are not carefully examined and the medicine itself is inappropriately prescribed, then not even one person can survive. For the treatment of *Xia Jiao*, I suggest prescribing *Dokhwal Jihwang Tang* (Lee Je-ma's Angelica Pubescens and Rehmannia Decoction) or *Shipimi Jihwang Tang* (Lee Je-ma's Twelve Ingredient Rehmannia Decoction).

易之需九三爻辭에 曰需于泥니 致寇至리라하고 象曰需于泥는 災在外
也새라 自我致寇니 敬愼이면 不敗也리라하니 以此意而倣之曰陰虛午
熱하며 背寒而嘔는 其病이 雖險이나 然이나 死尙在外也니 能齋戒其
心하며 恭敬其身하고 又服好藥이면 不死也니라.

The third line of the fifth *I Ching* hexagram[29] states: "Waiting in the muddy swamp, one suffers from theft." The Confucian commentary on the fifth hexagram states that "waiting in the muddy swamp refers to the occurrence of an external calamity.

---

29   The fifth hexagram of the *I Ching* is entitled "*Xu*," or "Needing" (as translated by Alfred Huang in his book *The Complete I Ching*). It is depicted by the trigram for Water above and the trigram for Heaven below. Water above represents approaching danger, and Heaven below signifies strength and resolve. As a whole, this hexagram represents sincerity, faithfulness, righteousness, and being steadfast.

The responsibility of theft, in this case, lies not in the hands of the thief, but in one's own actions. Respect and restraint are the only ways to avoid defeat." When viewed in the context of the human body, this concept illustrates how if one purifies his mind and respects his body, and also takes the appropriate medicine when needed, then even if Yin is deficient, with daytime fever, a cold sensation of the spine, and dry heaves, one is still capable of avoiding death.

**Table 7.5: The thirsting disorder syndromes of the Shao Yang Individual**

| Syndrome | Due to | Common energetic source | Common emotional source | Additional symptoms | Treated with |
|---|---|---|---|---|---|
| *Shang Xiao* (diabetes of the Upper *Jiao*) | Yang deficiency with External Yin sinking | Clear Yang cannot ascend towards the head and spreads out to the extremities while stagnant Yang Heat remains in head, face, and extremities | Inability to broaden one's mind, focus on the big picture, and look beyond trifling matters, lack of generosity, tolerance, self-cultivation, and versatility, a tendency towards a frivolous and hasty character | Red and cracked in the tongue with excessive thirst, night sweating, throat swelling | *Yanggyuk Sanhwa Tang* (Lee Je-ma's Cool the Diaphragm and Disperse Heat Decoction) |
| *Zhong Xiao* (diabetes of the Middle *Jiao*) | | | | Excessive eating without weight gain, spontaneous sweating, dry stools, and frequent urination **Acute stage:** Tumors, carbuncles, and loss of eyesight | *Indongdeng Jigolpi Tang* (Lee Je-ma's Honeysuckle and Lycium Decoction) |
| *Xia Xiao* (diabetes of the Lower *Jiao*) | Exterior and Interior Yin and Yang deficiency | | | Excessive thirst, a frequent desire to urinate, oily urine, vexation and fullness in the chest, thinning of the thighs and legs, fever during the day, cold sensation of the spine, and dry heaves | *Sukjihwang Gosam Tang* (Lee Je-ma's Processed Rhemannia and Sophora Decoction) *Dokhwal Jihwang Tang* (Lee Je-ma's Angelica Pubescens and Rehmannia Decoction)* *Shipimi Jihwang Tang* (Lee Je-ma's Twelve Ingredient Rehmannia Decoction)** |

* *This formula is also used after the occurrence of a stroke.*

** *This formula is also used when there is vomiting of blood.*

# A Synopsis of So Yang Illness

# 泛論

少陽人病에 中風 吐血 嘔吐 腹痛 食滯痞滿 五證은 同出一屬而自有輕
重하며 浮腫 喘促 結胸 痢疾 寒熱往來 胸脇滿 五證은 同出一屬而自有輕
重이니라.

The So Yang Individual's stroke, vomiting of blood, dry heaves, abdominal pain, food stagnation, and abdominal fullness are all associated with one another[30] and each is categorized according to its own lighter and critical stages. The So Yang Individual's edema, wheezing, *Jie Xiong*, dysentery, alternating chills and fever, and fullness in the epigastric and flank area are all associated with one another[31] and each has both lighter and critical stages.

少陽人의 中風에 半身不遂와 一臂不遂는 未如何之疾也라 重者는 必
死하고 輕者는 猶生이나 間以服藥하며 安而復之하야 待其自愈而不可期
必治法之疾也니라.

If a So Yang Individual suffers from hemiplegia due to stroke, no intervention can be claimed as a definite cure. If one suffers a critical stroke, then death is imminent, but if a minor stroke occurs and the individual is periodically treated with medicine while keeping his/her mind at ease, waiting for a slight chance of recovery is the only option.

少陽人 吐血者는 必蕩滌剛愎偏急與人幷驅爭塗之하고 淡食服藥하되 修
養如釋道하면 一百日則可以少愈오 二百日則可以大愈오 一周年則可以
快愈오 三周年則可保其壽라.

Vomiting blood [is a clear and urgent signal for the So Yang Individual to] reflect on their behavior, avoid the tendency towards a rough and vulgar nature, attempt to be less one-sided and stubborn, and temper an over-competitive disposition. If the So Yang Individual eats lightly, takes herbal medicine, cultivates the mind, and discovers their *Dao*,[32] then after 100 days, he/she will feel slightly better, and after 200 days, significantly better, and after 300 days, live a normal life.

---

30   The So Yang Individual's stroke, vomiting of blood, dry heaves, abdominal pain, food stagnation, and abdominal fullness are all associated with Internal Heat syndrome.

31   The So Yang Individual's edema, wheezing, *Jie Xiong*, dysentery, alternating chills and fever, and fullness in the epigastric and flank area are all associated with External Cold syndrome.

32   The *Dao* (道) is often translated as the "way." To discover the *Dao* is to understand the nature of all things and realize one's unique mission in life. According to Confucius, this is carried out through the process of *Sugishin* (修己身) or self-cultivation.

凡吐血은 調養을 失道則必再發이오 再發則前功이 皆歸於虛地하나니
若再發者則又自再發日計數하야 一百日이면 少愈하며 一周年이면 快
愈하니 若十年 二十年을 調養則必得高壽니라.

Vomiting of blood will recur if the So Yang Individual doesn't focus on balancing the mind and preserving his or her health despite the amount of effort made to overcome it the first time. Every time such vomiting recurs, it will take 100 days to recover slightly and one year to recover fully. If the So Yang Individual makes it a priority to balance their mind and preserve their health for 10 or 20 years, then he or she will live a long and healthy life.

凡少陽人이 間有鼻血少許하며 或口鼻間痰涎中에 有血은 雖細微라도 皆
吐血之屬也오 又口中에 暗有冷涎逆上者는 雖不嘔吐라도 亦嘔吐之屬
也니라 少年에 有此證者는 多致夭折하나니 以其等閒任置故也니라. 此二
證은 必在重病險病之例니
不可不豫防服藥하야 永除病根然後에 可保無虞니라.

Even if the So Yang Individual experiences infrequent cases of light nose bleeds, or blood mixed with phlegm or saliva discharged from the nose and/or throat, it is still in the same category as vomiting blood. Even if the So Yang Individual experiences otherwise undetectable signs of cool temperature sputum rising up from the stomach, it belongs to the same category as vomiting blood. If the So Yang Individual who experiences the above symptoms dies at a young age, it is because these signs went unheeded. Since these are serious and not to be thought of lightly, their cause must be clearly addressed and medicine administered. Only after these steps are taken can one feel at ease.

中風은 受病이 太重인 故로 治法을 不可期必이오 吐血은 受病이 猶輕인
故로 治法을 可以期必이니 中風과 吐血에는 調養이 爲主오 服藥이 次
之며 嘔吐以下 腹痛 食滯 痞滿은 服藥調養則其病이 易愈니라.

Although there is no certainty that even with the administration of herbs one can recover from an illness as critical as a stroke, lighter illnesses such as vomiting blood often have a better prognosis. If either of the above situations occurs, balancing the mind and preserving one's health are the first priority, while the administration of herbal medicine is second. In the case of food stagnation, abdominal pain, and/or abdominal distension, administering herbs, balancing the mind, and preserving health can easily lead to recovery.

中風과 嘔吐에 宜用獨活地黃湯이오 吐血에 宜用十二味地黃湯이니라.

For the occurrence of stroke, I recommend the use of *Dokhwal Jihwang Tang* (Lee Je-ma's Angelica Pubescens and Rehmannia Decoction). For vomiting of blood, *Shipimi Jihwang Tang* (Lee Je-ma's Twelve Ingredient Rehmannia Decoction) should be prescribed.

浮腫爲病은 急治則生하고 不急治則危하며 用藥이 早則容易愈也오 用
藥이 不早則孟浪死也라. 此病은 外勢平緩하야 似不速死인 故로 人必易
之나 此病은 實是急證이니 四五日內에 必治之疾이오 謾不可以十日論之
也니라.

If a So Yang Individual with edema is treated without delay, they will likely
survive. If treatment for edema is delayed, it can then become critical. This
illness is relatively easy to cure when addressed immediately, but if neglected,
the patient will die an unnecessary death. Since there are very few acute external
signs, doctors often dismiss it as a lighter illness, thinking that there is no
possibility of internal damage. Yet they ignore the fact that edema is a sign of
serious illness[33] that must be treated within four to five days, even though some
sources say that it can be treated within ten days.

浮腫初發에는 當用木通大安湯 或荊防地黃湯 加木通하야 日再服則六
七日內에 浮腫이 必解하고 浮腫解後에는 百日內에 必用荊防地黃湯 加
木通 二三錢하야 每日 一二貼用之하야 以淸小便하야 以防再發이니 再
發하면 難治니라. 浮腫初解에 飮食을 尤宜忍飢而小食이니 若如平人大食
則必不免再發이오. 大畏小便赤也니 小便이 淸則浮腫이 解하고 小便이
赤則浮腫이 結이라.

During the beginning stages of edema, *Moktong Daean Tang* (Lee Je-ma's Akebia
Great Relief Decoction) or *Hyungbang Jihwang Tang* (Lee Je-ma's Schizonepeta,
Ledebouriella, and Rhemannia Decoction) with added Mu Tong (*Caulis Akebiae*)
should be prescribed. If two packs a day of either formula is prescribed, edema
will undoubtedly cease within six to seven days. Two packs a day of *Hyungbang
Jihwang Tang* (Lee Je-ma's Schizonepeta, Ledebouriella, and Rhemannia Decoction)
with 7.5g to 11.25g of Mu Tong (*Caulis Akebiae*) should be prescribed for another
100 days after edema ceases. During this time, urine should remain clear and
edema should be prevented [with consistent use of herbs]. If edema recurs, it will be
difficult to cure. As edema begins to improve, the patient will experience an increase
in appetite. While recovering, the So Yang Individual must refrain from increasing
food intake and continue to eat lightly. If they choose to eat as much as an average
healthy person does, then edema will return and be difficult to cure. Reddish urine
should be a cause for concern. Clear urine is a sign that edema is improving, while
reddish urine is an indication that it is lingering.

---

33  Edema of the So Yang Individual is a result of spleen Cold syndrome, which in serious cases leads to chronic
*Jie Xiong*. With edema, the body has difficulty eliminating excess fluid accumulation due to Cold pathogenic
influence and Yin fluid stagnation in the chest.

少陽人 中消者가 腹脹則必成鼓脹하니 鼓脹은 不治라. 少陽人 鼓脹病이
如少陰人 藏結病하야 皆經歷五六七八月하며 或周年而竟死하니 蓋少陰
人 藏結은 表陽溫氣가 雖在幾絶이나 裡陰溫氣가 猶恃完壯이오 少陽人
鼓脹은 裡陽淸氣가 雖在幾絶이나 表陰淸氣가 猶恃完壯인 故로 皆經歷
久遠而死也니라.

If the So Yang Individual with *Zhong Xiao* experiences abdominal distension, it indicates the onset of tympanites, which cannot be cured. The So Yang Individual's tympanites correlates with the So Eum Individual's *Zhang Jie* illness.[34] If either of these syndromes occurs, then the patient will die after five to eight months or one year of illness. It is easy to overlook the severity of the So Eum Individual's *Zhang Jie* illness because even though the Warm Yang *Qi* of the Exterior is on the verge of depletion, the Warm Yin *Qi* of the Interior is intact and robust. It is also easy to overlook the severity of the So Yang Individual's tympanites because even though the Clear Yang *Qi* of the Internal is on the verge of depletion, the Clear Yang *Qi* of the External is intact and robust. Hence, after a long period of suffering, death will be imminent.

少陽人 傷寒에 喘促이어늘 宜先用靈砂一分하야 溫水로 調下하고 因煎
荊防 瓜蔞等藥을 用之則必無煎藥時刻遲滯하여 救病이라.

If a So Yang Individual experiences shortness of breath and wheezing, .375g of Ling Sha (*Mercury Sulfate*)[35] should be ingested with warm water. If other herbs such as Jing Jie (*Herba Schizonepetae*), Fang Feng (*Radix Saposhnikoviae*), and Gua Lou (*Semen Trichosanthis*) are decocted and taken with this formula, then as long as the patient can endure the time it takes to prepare the medicine, recovery is certain.

靈砂는 藥力이 急迫하니 可以一再用而不可屢用이니라.
蓋救急之藥은 敏於救急而已오 藥必湯服然後에 充滿腸胃하야 能爲補陰
補陽이니라.

Since Ling Sha (*Mercury Sulfate*) is a quick and effective medicine, it should be used only once or twice, rather than continuously. Acute measures need to be taken in acute situations. When this medicine is prescribed in such situations, results can soon be seen. [To reduce toxicity,] Ling Sha (*Mercury Sulfate*) must be decocted before ingestion. It supports the function of the stomach and tonifies both Yin and Yang.

---

34  As mentioned in Chapter 6, *Zhang Jie* (臟結), literally translated as "hardening of the organs," is a life-threatening syndrome marked by a hardening of the epigastric area during a Yin stage illness of the So Eum Individual. It occurs as a result of waning Yang energy and a severe blockage of Cold toxin within the stomach and epigastrium.

35  Since Ling Sha (*Mercury Sulfate*) is extremely toxic, it is no longer utilized in Sasang medicine.

痢疾之比結胸則痢疾이 爲順證也而痢疾之謂重證者는 其浮腫相近
也일새오. 嘔吐之比腹痛則嘔吐는 爲逆證也而嘔吐之謂惡證者는 以其距
中風이 不遠也일새라 少陽人 痢疾에 宜用黃連淸腸湯이니라.

Dysentery is considered mild compared to *Jie Xiong* syndrome, which is still considered a serious illness because it may progress into edema [, a life-threatening illness]. Abdominal pain is considered mild compared to vomiting. This is because vomiting may lead to stroke. For dysentery of the So Yang Individual, *Hwangyon Chongjang Tang* (Lee Je-ma's Coptis Clear the Intestine Decoction) should be prescribed.

少陽人 瘧病이 有間兩日發者하니 即勞瘧也ㅣ라 可以緩治오 不可急治니
此證은 瘧不發日에 用獨活地黃湯 二貼하야 朝暮服하고 瘧發日에 預煎
荊防敗毒散 二貼하야 待惡寒發作時하야 二貼連服하라 一月之內에 以獨
活地黃湯 四十貼과 荊防敗毒散 二十貼으로 爲準的則其瘧이 必無不退之
理리라.

Malaria that occurs for two or more days is referred to as *Lao Nue*.[36] This type of malaria should be treated slowly and cannot be cured through hasty action. When symptoms do not manifest, two packs of *Dokhwal Jihwang Tang* (Lee Je-ma's Angelica Pubescens and Rehmannia Decoction) should be administered, one pack in the morning and the other in the evening. When symptoms manifest, two packs of *Hyungbang Peidok San* (Lee Je-ma's Schizonepeta and Ledebouriella Powder to Overcome Pathogenic Influences), boiled beforehand, should be prescribed. This approach should be repeated as soon as chills occur. If 40 packs of *Dokhwal Jihwang Tang* (Lee Je-ma's Angelica Pubescens and Rehmannia Decoction) and 20 packs of *Hyungbang Peidok San* (Lee Je-ma's Schizonepeta and Ledebouriella Powder to Overcome Pathogenic Influences) are prescribed for up to one month, then malaria will have no chance to linger.

少陽人이 內發咽喉하며 外腫項頰者를 謂之纏喉風이니 二三日內에 殺
人이 最急하고 又上唇人中穴瘇을 謂之唇瘇이니 凡人中左右 逼近處一指
許에 發瘇하면 雖微如栗粒이라도 亦危證也니라.

If a So Yang Individual suffers from Internal illness marked by a throat disorder and External illness marked by swollen cheeks, it is referred to as *Chan Hou Feng*.[37]

---

36    *Lao Nue* (勞瘧) syndrome is literally translated as "tormenting malaria." This type of malaria isn't acute but instead its symptoms linger on for a prolonged period of time. It is characterized by non-acute alternate fever and chills, and excessive sweating with even the slightest body movement. *Lao Nue*, also accompanied by a lack of appetite, is due to extensive *Zhen Qi* and Yin deficiency.

37    *Chan Hou Feng* (纏喉風) syndrome, literally translated as "Entangled Wind syndrome," is marked in the initial stages by sore throat, swelling, and dryness accompanied by a feeling of Heat in the neck. It may also progress into swelling of the lips, cheeks, and breasts, stiffness and itchiness of the neck, asthma, lockjaw, tight chest, dysphagia, and sudden chills and fever.

This is one of the So Yang Individual's most acute illnesses, which can lead to death within a few days. Moreover, if swelling of the upper lip reaches the *renzhong* (GV 26)[38] acupuncture point, it is referred to as *Chun Zhong*.[39] If, in addition to these symptoms, a cyst or even a small rice-sized pimple appears, on either side of the *renzhong* (GV 26) acupuncture point, the situation is critical.

此二證이 始發而輕者는 當用涼膈散火湯 陽毒白虎湯이오 重者는 當用水銀熏鼻方하야 一炷熏鼻而項頰에 汗出則愈니라. 若倉卒에 無熏鼻藥則輕粉末 一分五里와 乳香 沒藥 甘遂末 各五分을 和勻糊丸하야 一服盡하라.

The initial stages of both of the above conditions are not serious and could be treated with *Yanggyuk Sanhwa Tang* (Lee Je-ma's Cool the Diaphragm and Disperse Heat Decoction) or *Yangdok Baekho Tang* (Lee Je-ma's White Tiger Decoction to Eliminate Yang Toxin). If the situation gets worse, then *Shuiyin Xunbi Fang* (Inhaled Mercury Formula) should be administered by wrapping its ingredients in paper, igniting, and directing the accompanying smoke towards the nose (see formula section for preparation details). Recovery is detected by the onset of sweat from the neck and cheeks. If this condition occurs suddenly and *Shuiyin Xunbi Fang* (Inhaled Mercury Formula) is not readily available, then thoroughly blend together .56g of Qing Fen (*Calomelas*) with 1.875g of Ru Xiang (*Resina Olibani*), Mo Yao (*Myrrhae*), and Gan Sui (*Radix Euphorbiae Kansui*), until the mixture becomes a paste, evenly mixing each portion. Then roll into a single pill and administer in one dose.

少陽人 小兒의 食多肌瘦에는 宜用蘆┌肥兒丸 忍冬藤地骨皮湯이니라.

If a So Yang infant has a voracious appetite but doesn't gain weight, then administer *Lu Hui Fei Er Wan* (Fat Baby Pill) or *Indongdeng Jigolpi Tang* (Lee Je-ma's Honeysuckle and Lycium Decoction).

嘗見少陽人의 肩上에 有毒瘇이어늘 火熬香油를 灌瘡하니 肌肉이 焦爛而不知其熱이라. 有醫가 敎以牛角片을 置火炭上하고 燒而熏之한대 煙入瘡口하니 毒汁이 自流하고 其瘇이 立愈하니라.

I once treated a So Yang Individual's neck tumor with heated sesame seed oil placed directly on the skin above the tumor. The patient felt no pain from the procedure and recovered quickly. A doctor once treated the same situation with a bull horn that was placed in burning charcoal and then applied directly to the skin. After smoke from the burning horn entered the tumor, toxic fluid oozed out and his patient recovered soon afterwards.

---

38   The *renzhong* (GV 26) acupuncture point is located above the upper lip on the midline, at the junction of the upper third and lower two thirds of the philtrum.

39   *Chun Zhong* (脣瘇), or edema of the lip, is a symptom of *Chan Hou Feng* (Entangled Wind).

嘗見少陽人 七十老人이 發腦疽어늘 有醫가 敎以河豚卵을 作末傅之하니
其疽가 立愈라. 河豚卵은 至毒하야 牛犬이 食之則立死하고 掛於林木
間하니 烏鵲이 不敢食하더라.

There was once a 70-year-old So Yang Individual with a cyst on the nape of his
neck. When his doctor applied powdered blowfish eggs directly to the cyst, it
instantly disappeared. Blowfish eggs are so toxic that they immediately cause death
if consumed by a cow or pig. Even if they were hung between trees to dry, the
seagulls and crows wouldn't dare to eat them.

嘗治少陽人의 蛇頭瘡할새 河豚卵을 作末少許하야 點으로 膏藥上傅之
而一日一次하야 易以新末하니 傅藥五六日에 病效而新肉이 急生而有妬
肉이어늘 因以磨刀砥末하야 傅之한대 妬肉이 立消而病愈하고 又用之於
連珠痰하야 多日傅之者는 必效하고 用之於爲炭火所傷與狗咬蟲咬하니
無不得效니라.

I once treated a So Yang Individual's acutely swollen finger by sprinkling it with
powdered blowfish eggs. The swelling reduced after I applied fresh powder once
a day for five to six days. However, a layer of flabby superficial skin formed, so
instead I applied whetstone shavings from a sharpening stone and it disappeared
as the patient completely recovered. Whetstone shavings can also be applied for
several days to completely resolve pus-emitting scrofula sores. It can also be applied
to dog or insect bites and to areas of the skin that have been burned from contact
with charcoal.

嘗治少陽人 六十老人이 中風一臂不遂病할새 用輕粉 五里하니 其病이
輒加하고 又少陽人 二十歲 少年이 一脚微不仁痺風할새 用輕粉甘遂龍虎
丹하야 二三次用之하니 得效하니라.

I once cured a 60-year-old So Yang Individual suffering from stroke-related
hemiplegia with .187g of Qing Fen (*Calomelas*). Another time I treated a 20-year-
old So Yang Individual who suffered from Wind *Bi* syndrome causing immobility
of one of his legs with *Kyungbun Kamsu Yongho Dan* (Lee Je-ma's Calomel and Kan
Sui Root Dragon Tiger Pill). He fully recovered after ingesting two doses.

嘗治少陽人이 咽喉할새 水醬不入하고 大便不通三日하고 病至危
境이어늘 用甘遂天一丸하니 卽效니라.

A So Yang Individual who was inflicted with a throat disorder could not ingest water
or rice porridge,[40] and went without a bowel movement for three days. Despite the
severity of the situation, the patient immediately recovered after I treated him with
*Kamsu Chonil Wan* (Lee Je-ma's Divine Gan Sui Pill).

---

40  Lee Je-ma often prescribed rice porridge, regardless of his patient's constitution, in order to nurture the
digestion system back to health.

嘗治少陽人 七十老人이 大便四五日不通하고 或六七日不通하며 飲食如
常하며 兩脚이 膝寒無力하니 用輕粉甘遂龍虎丹하니 大便이 即通하고
後數日에 大便이 又秘則又用하야 屢次用之하니 竟以大便이 一日一度로
爲準而病愈하야 此老가 竟得八十壽하니라.

I once treated a 70-year-old So Yang Individual who had no bowel movement for
seven days. His appetite didn't change but his knees were aching and cold, with no
strength in his legs. His bowels started to flow soon after he took *Kyungbun Kamsu
Yongho Dan* (Lee Je-ma's Calomel and Kan Sui Root Dragon Tiger Pill). A few days
after he ingested this formula, his constipation returned, so I prescribed it again
and his bowels started to flow. This pattern continued on several occasions until he
finally achieved consistent bowel movements once a day, and lived for another ten
healthy years.

嘗見少陽人이 當門二齒齦縫에 血出하야 頃刻間에 數碗하고 將至危
境이어늘 有醫가 敎以熬香油하야 以新綿點油하야 乘熱로 灼齒縫하니
仍爲止血하니라.

I once witnessed a So Yang Individual who had received treatment for severe gum
bleeding that gushed out of her mouth, filling two rice bowls shortly after it started.
Recognizing the critical nature of this illness, her doctor thereupon placed heated
sesame oil dabbed with cotton directly on her gums, scorching the skin. Her bleeding
stopped immediately.

嘗見少陽人 一人이 每日一次梳頭하야 數月後에 得口眼ㄏ斜病하고 其
後에 又見少陽人이 日梳라가 得ㄏ斜病者가 凡三人이니 蓋日梳는 少陽
人의 禁忌也니라

I once witnessed a So Yang Individual who contracted Bell's palsy after combing
her hair every day for several months. Afterwards, I noticed three other So Yang
Individuals who were stricken with Bell's palsy after brushing their hair every day. I
counsel against everyday hair brushing for the So Yang Individual.[41] There was once
an 80-year-old Tae Eum Individual, however, who brushed his hair every day for
40 years [without suffering health issues] because he "liked the feeling."

---

41   In the past, the process of hair brushing in Korea was much more involved than in the present day due to
the fact that cutting hair, or altering the body in any way, was considered unfilial. Hence, both males and
females let their hair grow continuously. To keep hair from getting out of control, it was often braided, placed
in a topknot, and/or covered with a hat. Brushing and detangling the hair was therefore a laborious process.
Although Lee Je-ma doesn't elaborate, it is likely that daily and/or rigorous hair brushing could aggravate the
already excessive upper body Yang Heat energy of the So Yang Individual, causing Wind to stir in the head
and face.

## The So Yang Individual's Ten Formulae from Zhang Zhongjing's *Shang Han Lun*

### Bai Hu Tang
*White Tiger Decoction*

| Shi Gao | Gypsum Fibrosum | 18.75g |
|---------|-----------------|--------|
| Geng Mi | Semen Oryzae Sativae | 9.375g |
| Zhi Mu | Rhizoma Anemarrhenae | 7.5g |
| Gan Cao | Radix Glycyrrhizae | 2.625g |

### Zhu Ling Tang
*Polyporus Decoction*

| Zhu Ling | Polyporus | 3.75g |
|----------|-----------|-------|
| Chi Fu Ling | Poria Rubra | 3.75g |
| Ze Xie | Rhizoma Alismatis | 3.75g |
| Hua Shi | Talcum | 3.75g |
| E Jiao | Colla Corii Asini | 3.75g |

### Wu Ling San
*Five Ingredients Powder with Poria*

| Ze Xie | Rhizoma Alismatis | 9.375g |
|--------|-------------------|--------|
| Chi Fu Ling | Poria Rubra | 5.625g |
| Zhu Ling | Polyporus | 5.625g |
| Bai Zhu | Rhizoma Actractylodis | 5.625g |
| Rou Gui | Cortex Cinnamomi | 1.875g |

### Xiao Chai Hu Tang
*Minor Bupleurum Decoction*

| Chai Hu | Radix Bupleuri | 11.25g |
|---------|----------------|--------|
| Huang Qin | Radix Scutellariae | 7.5g |
| Ren Shen | Radix Ginseng | 5.625g |
| Ban Xia | Rhizoma Pinelliae | 5.625g |
| Gan Cao | Radix Glycyrrhizae | 1.875g |

### Da Qing Long Tang
*Major Blue Green Dragon Decoction*

| Shi Gao | Gypsum Fibrosum | 18.75g |
|---|---|---|
| Ma Huang | Herba Ephedrae | 11.25g |
| Gui Zhi | Ramulus Cinnamomi | 7.5g |
| Xing Ren | Semen Armeniaecae Amarum | 3.75g |
| Gan Cao | Radix Glycyrrhizae | 1.875g |
| Sheng Jiang | Radix Ziniberis Recens | 3 Slices |
| Da Zao | Fructus Jujubae | 2 Pieces |

### Gui Bi Ge Ban Tang
*Combined Cinnamon Twig and Gypsum Decoction*

| Shi Gao | Gypsum Fibrosum | 7.5g |
|---|---|---|
| Ma Huang | Herba Ephedrae | 3.75g |
| Gui Zhi | Ramulus Cinnamomi | 3.75g |
| Bai Shao Yao | Radix Paeoniae Alba | 3.75g |
| Gan Cao | Radix Glycyrrhizae | 1.125g |
| Sheng Jiang | Radix Ziniberis Recens | 3 Slices |
| Da Zao | Fructus Jujubae | 2 Pieces |

### Xiao Xian Xiong Tang
*Minor Sinking into the Chest Decoction*

| Ban Xia | Rhizoma Pinelliae | 18.75g |
|---|---|---|
| Huan Lian | Rhizoma Coptidis | 9.375g |
| Gua Lou | Fructus Trichosanthis | ¼ Large fruit |

### Da Xian Xiong Tang
*Major Sinking into the Chest Decoction*

| Da Huang | Radix et Rhizoma Rhei | 11.25g |
|---|---|---|
| Mang Xiao | Natrii Sulfas | 7.5g |
| Gan Sui | Radix Euphorbiae Kansui | 1.875g |

### *Shi Zao Tang*
*Ten Jujube Decoction*

| Yuan Hua | *Flos Genkwa* | (Dry-fried until dry) |
| Gan Sui | *Radix Euphorbiae Kansui* | |
| Da Ji | *Radix Euphorbiae Pekinensis* | (Dry-fried) |

For this formula, grind an equal amount of each ingredient into powder. Place ten pieces of Da Zao (*Fructus Jujubae*) in one cup of boiling water. Boil until only half a cup of water remains and then remove the Da Zao (*Fructus Jujubae*). Cook the powdered herbs with the remaining water after removing Da Zao (*Fructus Jujubae*). For the individual with a stronger constitution, 3.75g of powder can be added. For an individual with a weaker constitution only 1.875g should be added to the Da Zao (*Fructus Jujubae*) tea. Rice porridge should be ingested to regain strength after a smooth bowel movement and reduction of fluid retention is noticed.

### *Jin Gui Shen Qi Wan*
*Kidney Qi Pill from the Golden Cabinet*

| Shu Di Huang | *Radix Rehmanniae Preparata* | 6g |
| Shan Zhu Yu | *Fructus Corni Officinalis* | 3.75g |
| Shan Yao | *Radix Dioscoreae Oppositae* | 3.75g |
| Fu Ling | *Poria Alba* | 3.75g |
| Mu Dan Pi | *Cortex Moutan* | 3.75g |
| Ze Xie | *Rhizoma Alismatis* | 3.75g |
| Wu Wei Zi | *Fructus Shizandrae* | 3.75g |

## The So Yang Individual's Nine Formulae Presented by Doctors of the Yuan and Ming Dynasties

### *Liang Ge San*
*Cool the Diaphragm Powder*

| Lian Qiao | *Fructus Forsythiae* | 7.5g |
| Da Huang | *Radix et Rhizoma Rhei* | 3.75g |
| Mang Xiao | *Natrii Sulfas* | 3.75g |
| Gan Cao | *Radix Glycyrrhizae* | 3.75g |
| Bo He | *Herba Menthae* | 1.875g |
| Huang Qin | *Radix Scutellariae* | 1.875g |
| Zhi Zi | *Fructus Gardenia* | 1.875g |

This formula, mentioned in the *Ju Fang* (*Formularies of the Bureau of People's Welfare Pharmacies*), is indicated for *Ji Re*[42] syndrome accompanied by an unsettled feeling in the chest, canker sores of the mouth and tongue, redness of the eyes, and vertigo/dizziness.

From my experience it is necessary to omit Da Huang (*Radix et Rhizoma Rhei*) and Huang Qin (*Radix Scutellariae*) [because they are herbs prescribed for the Tae Eum constitution] and Gan Cao (*Radix Glycyrrhizae*) [because it is a herb prescribed for the So Eum constitution] from the above formula.

### Huang Lian Jie Du Wan
*Coptis Decoction to Relieve Toxicity*

| Male pig stomach | | 1 Stomach | |
|---|---|---|---|
| Huang Lian | *Rhizoma Coptidis* | 187.5g | |
| Wheat flour | | 187.5g | (Dry-fried) |
| Tian Hua Fen | *Radix Trichosanthis* | 150g | |
| Fu Ling | *Poria Alba* | 150g | |
| Mai Men Dong | *Tuber Ophiopogonis* | 75g | |

Grind the above herbs (expect for the pig stomach) into a thin powder and then place inside the pig stomach. Stitch the stomach together with the herbs inside and then prepare as a standard herbal decoction. Afterwards, strain the excess water and shape the herbs into empress tree seed-sized herbal pills.

This formula, mentioned in Wei Yi-lin's text entitled *Dexiaofang* (*Collection of Effective Prescriptions*), is prescribed for *Jiang Zhong*[43] syndrome.

In my experience, Mai Men Dong (*Tuber Ophiopogonis*) is the only herb in this formula affiliated with the lungs, which have the function of descending *Qi* while the kidneys ascend *Qi*. The remaining five herbs have an affinity for the kidneys. Since there is only one herb for the lungs [which is the Tae Eum's weaker organ], and all others go to the kidneys [which is the So Yang's weaker organ], the former will have no significantly negative impact, so there is no need to be overly concerned.

---

42  *Ji Re* (積熱) is an acute syndrome marked by swelling of the cheeks, thirst, oral infections, constipation, and fullness of the chest. It later develops into general body swelling in advanced stages.

43  *Jiang Zhong* (强中證) syndrome, first described in Zhang Zhongjing's *Shang Han Lun*, is marked by excessive weight loss, spermatorrhea, and frothy urination as a result of excessive sexual activity and/or excessive intake of mineral-based herbs.

### Liu Wei Di Huang Wan

*Six Ingredient Decoction with Rhemannia*

| | | |
|---|---|---|
| Shu Di Huang | *Radix Rehmanniae Preparata* | 15g |
| Shan Yao | *Radix Dioscoreae Oppositae* | 7.5g |
| Shan Zhu Yu | *Fructus Corni Officinalis* | 7.5g |
| Ze Xie | *Rhizoma Alismatis* | 5.625g |
| Mu Dan Pi | *Cortex Moutan* | 5.625g |
| Fu Ling | *Poria Alba* | 5.625g |

This formula, mentioned in Yu Tuan's *Yi Xue Zheng Zhuan* (*True Lineage of Medicine*), is prescribed for deficiency caused by overwork.

From my perspective, Shan Yao (*Radix Dioscoreae Oppositae*), which has an affinity for the lungs [which is the Tae Eum's weakest organ], should be omitted.

### Sheng Shu Di Huang Wan

*Combined Raw and Prepared Rehmannia Decoction*

| | | | |
|---|---|---|---|
| Sheng Di Huang | *Radix Rehmanniae* | 37.5g | (Dried) |
| Shu Di Huang | *Radix Rehmanniae Preparata* | 37.5g | |
| Xuan Shen | *Radix Scrophulariae* | 37.5g | |
| Shi Gao | *Gypsum Fibrosum* | 37.5g | |

Grind the above ingredients into fine powder, make into a paste, and then into empress tree seed-sized pills. Ingest 50–70 pills on an empty stomach with a cup of green tea.

This formula, in Li Chan's *Yixue Rumen* (*Introduction to Medicine*), is for weakened vision.

### Dao Chi San

*Guide the Red Powder*

| | | |
|---|---|---|
| Mu Tong | *Caulis Akebiae* | 3.75g |
| Hua Shi | *Talcum* | 3.75g |
| Huang Bai | *Cortex Phellodendri* | 3.75g |
| Chi Fu Ling | *Poria Rubra* | 3.75g |
| Sheng Di Huang | *Radix Rehmanniae* | 3.75g |
| Zhi Zi | *Fructus Gardenia* | 3.75g |
| Gan Cao | *Radix Glycyrrhizae* | 3.75g |
| Zhi Ke | *Fructus Aurantii* | 1.875g |
| Bai Zhu | *Radix Atractylodis Macrocephalae* | 1.875g |

This formula, which Gong Xin mentions in his text *Wan Bing Hui Chun* (*Restoring Health from Tens of Thousands of Diseases*), is indicated for cloudy white urine. Recovery will occur after just two doses.

In my system, Zhi Ke (*Fructus Aurantii*), Bai Zhu (*Radix Atractylodis Macrocephalae*), and Gan Cao (*Radix Glycyrrhizae*) should definitely be removed from this formula [because they are for the So Eum constitution].

### Jing Fang Bai Du San
*Schizonepeta and Saposhnikoviae Powder to Overcome Pathogenic Influences*

| | | |
|---|---|---|
| Qiang Huo | *Rhizoma seu Radix Notopterygii* | 3.75g |
| Du Huo | *Radix Angelicae Pubescentis* | 3.75g |
| Chai Hu | *Radix Bupleuri* | 3.75g |
| Qian Hu | *Radix Peucedani* | 3.75g |
| Chi Fu Ling | *Poria Rubra* | 3.75g |
| Jing Jie | *Herba Schizonepetae* | 3.75g |
| Fang Feng | *Radix Saposhnikoviae* | 3.75g |
| Zhi Ke | *Fructus Aurantii* | 3.75g |
| Jie Geng | *Radix Platycodi* | 3.75g |
| Chuan Xiong | *Radix Ligustici Chuanxiong* | 3.75g |
| Ren Shen | *Radix Ginseng* | 3.75g |
| Gan Cao | *Radix Glycyrrhizae* | 3.75g |
| Bo He | *Herba Menthae* | Small amount |

This formula, given in Gong Xin's work entitled *Yijianshu* (*Mirror of Eastern Medicine*), is prescribed as a remedy for Shang Han disorders or epidemic diseases marked by fever, headaches, stiffening of the neck and shoulders, and pain, burning, and restlessness of the extremities.

From my perspective, Zhi Ke (*Fructus Aurantii*), Chuan Xiong (*Radix Ligustici Chuanxiong*), Ren Shen (*Radix Ginseng*), and Gan Cao (*Radix Glycyrrhizae*) [which are for the So Eum constitution] and Jie Geng (*Radix Platycodi*) [prescribed for the Tae Eum constitution] should be omitted.

### Lu Hui Fei Er Wan/Fei Er Wan
*Fat Baby Pill*

| | | |
|---|---|---|
| Hu Huang Lian | *Rhizoma Picrorhizae* | 18.75g |
| Shi Jun Zi | *Fructus Quisqualis* | 16.875g |
| Ren Shen | *Radix Ginseng* | 13.125g |
| Huang Lian | *Rhizoma Coptidis* | 13.125g |

| Shen Qu | *Massa Fermentata Medicinalis* | 13.125g | |
| Mai Ye | *Fructus Hordei Germiniatus* | 13.125g | |
| Shan Zha | *Fructus Crataegi* | 13.125g | |
| Fu Ling | *Poria Alba* | 11.25g | |
| Bai Zhu | *Radix Atractylodis Macrocephalae* | 11.25g | |
| Zhi Gan Cao | *Radix Glycyrrhizae* | 11.25g | (Dry-fried with honey) |
| Lu Hui | *Aloe* | 9.375g | |

Grind the above into fine powder and mix with glutinous millet paste to form pills the size of a green pea. Ingest 20–30 pills with rice porridge.

This formula, mentioned in Gong Xin's work *Yijianshu* (*Mirror of Eastern Medicine*), is used as a remedy for infantile malnutrition.

From my perspective, Ren Shen (*Radix Ginseng*), Bai Zhu (*Radix Atractylodis Macrocephalae*), Shan Zha (*Fructus Crataegi*), and Gan Cao (*Radix Glycyrrhizae*) [for the So Eum Individual] should be omitted. I have yet to thoroughly examine the effects of Shi Jun Zi (*Fructus Quisqualis*) and as a result cannot determine whether or not it is appropriate in the formula or for use with the So Yang Individual.

### Xiao Du Yin

*Decoction to Eliminate Toxins*

| Niu Bang Zi | *Fructus Arctii* | 7.5g |
| Jing Jie | *Herba Schizonepetae* | 3.75g |
| Gan Cao | *Radix Glycyrrhizae* | 1.875g |
| Fang Feng | *Radix Saposhnikoviae* | 1.875g |

This formula, which Gong Xin mentioned in his *Yijianshu* (*Mirror of Eastern Medicine*), is prescribed as a remedy for pea-size skin sores which do not fully erupt and are concentrated within the chest area during a smallpox outbreak. If three or four packs of this formula are administered without delay, it will have a remarkable effect on detoxifying and venting smallpox-related skin sores.

I recommend that Gan Cao (*Radix Glycyrrhizae*) [which is specific to the So Eum Individual] should be omitted.

### *Shuiyin Xunbi Fang*
*Inhaled Mercury Formula*

| Hei Yan | *Graphite* | 3.75g |
|---|---|---|
| Shui Yin | *Hydrargyrum* | 3.75g |
| Zhu Sha[44] | *Cinnabaris* | 1.875g |
| Ru Xiang | *Resina Olibani* | 1.875g |
| Mo Yao | *Myrrhae* | 1.875g |
| Xue Xie | *Sanguis Draconis* | 1.125g |
| Xiong Huang | *Realgar* | 1.125g |
| Chen Xiang | *Lignum Aquilariae Resinatum* | 1.125g |

Grind the above ingredients into a powder and mix thoroughly. Roll into seven herbal cigarettes. Dip the tip into sesame oil and ignite. Fix the herbal cigarette to the top of a chair and let the smoke spread throughout the room. Have the patient lie in a fetal position while covering his or her whole body with a blanket. Keep mouth filled with cold water to prevent drying of the gums, while rinsing repeatedly. Repeat this process with three herbal cigarettes on the first day and one herbal cigarette a day thereafter. This formula, mentioned in Zhu Zhenheng's book entitled *Danxi Xinfa* (*The Teachings of Danxi*), is prescribed for pemphigus and skin lesions due to sexually transmitted disease.

From my perspective, Shui Yin (*Hydrargyrum*) is effective in treating Heat accumulation and clearing the eyes and head. It is the most effective medicine for regulating the Yang and returning Yin to the Lower *Jiao* of the So Yang Individual. However, this medicine should be used only in acute situations and not used continuously to nurture Yin because it is so strong. Just one application can address the root of an illness, but if administered a second time, it can damage the *Zheng Qi*. This can be likened to a military tactic, making an initial attack on the enemy with tremendous force, inflicting as much damage as possible. If a second attack with such caliber is implemented on an already scattered enemy, energy would be wasted and retaliation would ensue. Shui Yin (*Hydrargyrum*) should always be prescribed in cases of diphtheria.

If the So Yang Individual experiences paralysis of one or both legs, 0.1875–.375g of Qing Fen (*Calomelas*) powder should be prescribed. Even if they do not recover after three days, it is important to discontinue intake [due to fear of excessive toxicity]. It is also crucial to stay within the above dosage range per day of intake. During the recovery period, cold air or drafts should be avoided while making every attempt to preserve one's health. Qing Fen (*Calomelas*) is contraindicated and can lead to death if administered in cases of monoplegia of the upper limb, hemiplegia, and facial palsy.

Whereas acute illness should be addressed immediately, chronic illness should be given careful attention and provided scrupulous care. Qing Fen (*Calomelas*) is capable of addressing major illness but should not be prescribed in larger amounts to speed recovery. When it comes to chronic disease, the passage of time contributes to the complete recovery of illness. If treated

---

44    Zhu Sha (*Cinnabaris*) contains significant amounts of mercury and is therefore considered highly toxic. Hence it is often replaced with Dan Zhu Ye (*Herba Lophatheri Gracilis*), which also has a similar effect on calming the spirit and clearing Heat. The standard dosage of Dan Zhu Ye is 7.5g, but in acute cases up to 26.25g can be used.

hastily, chronic illness has the tendency to return and is more difficult to treat the second time around. Some individuals will need to take the entire three-day dosage of Qing Fen (*Calomelas*), while others may need only one to two days. Occasionally, an individual may need to take the entire three-day course, take a break, and then start another three-day cycle.

I once successfully treated a So Yang Individual with numbness of her legs and illness of her throat, eyes, and nasal passages through three to four days of internal administration and inhalation of smoked Shui Yin (*Hydrargyrum*). After recovering from this illness, the individual must avoid sleeping in a cold room or being exposed to a draft, washing his or her hands and face regularly, changing into fresh clothes, or brushing his or her hair for a period of one month. Death cannot be avoided if these guidelines are not heeded. If a room is kept cold, for example, the Cold energy will enter the body and cause death. Yet the room should not be kept too warm, or vexation and discomfort of the chest will occur. Moreover, if a window is opened and a draft rushes in, death cannot be avoided. I have witnessed such occurrences with my own eyes. There was one individual who, after ten days of recovery, changed into a new set of clothes and suddenly died. Another individual who brushed their hair after 20 days of recovery also died suddenly. Yet another individual who inhaled the smoke of two herbal cigarettes of *Shuiyin Xunbi Fang* (Inhaled Mercury Formula) on the first day, and one herbal cigarette on the second day, felt stuffy and hot. He decided to open his window for a breath of fresh air and suddenly collapsed to his death.

I have heard that ingesting salt or soy sauce is contraindicated while taking Shui Yin (*Hydrargyrum*) because the fermentation process of soy [and the absorbency of salt] extracts its toxicity.[45] Since it is common to use toxic herbs to treat toxicity, this advice should be taken lightly.

## 17 Newly Discovered Formulae for the So Yang Individual (Formulated by Lee Je-ma)

### Hyungbang Peidok San
*Lee Je-ma's Schizonepeta and Ledebouriella Powder to Overcome Pathogenic Influences (Modified Jing Fang Bai Du San)*

| | | |
|---|---|---|
| Qiang Huo | *Rhizoma seu Radix Notopterygii* | 3.75g |
| Du Huo | *Radix Angelicae Pubescentis* | 3.75g |
| Chai Hu | *Radix Bupleuri* | 3.75g |
| Qian Hu | *Radix Peucedani* | 3.75g |
| Jing Jie | *Herba Schizonepetae* | 3.75g |
| Fang Feng | *Radix Saposhnikoviae* | 3.75g |
| Chi Fu Ling | *Poria Rubra* | 3.75g |
| Sheng Di Huang | *Radix Rehmanniae* | 3.75g |

---

45   Lee Je-ma is referring to the concept of "like treats like," in which the toxicity of Shui Yin (*Hydrargyrum*) contributes to its ability to treat toxic Heat accumulation within the body.

| Di Gu Pi | Cortex Lycii | 3.75g |
|---|---|---|
| Che Qian Zi | Semen Plantaginis | 3.75g |

This formula is for headaches and alternate chills and fever [during the initial stages of a Shang Han influence].

### Hyungbang Dojok San

*Lee Je-ma's Schizonepeta and Ledebouriella Guide the Red Powder (Modified Jing Fang Dao Chi San)*

| Sheng Di Huang | Radix Rehmanniae | 11.25g |
|---|---|---|
| Mu Tong | Caulis Akebiae | 7.5g |
| Xuan Shen | Radix Scrophulariae | 5.625g |
| Gua Lou Ren | Semen Trichosanthis | 5.625g |
| Qian Hu | Radix Peucedani | 3.75g |
| Qiang Huo | Rhizoma seu Radix Notopterygii | 3.75g |
| Du Huo | Radix Angelicae Pubescentis | 3.75g |
| Jing Jie | Herba Schizonepetae | 3.75g |
| Fang Feng | Radix Saposhnikoviae | 3.75g |

This formula is suitable for headaches and an unsettled sensation in the chest accompanied with vexation.

### Hyungbang Sabaek San

*Lee Je-ma's Schizonepeta and Ledebouriella, Clear the White Powder*

| Sheng Di Huang | Radix Rehmanniae | 11.25g |
|---|---|---|
| Fu Ling | Poria Alba | 7.5g |
| Ze Xie | Rhizoma Alismatis | 7.5g |
| Shi Gao | Gypsum Fibrosum | 3.75g |
| Zhi Mu | Rhizoma Anemarrhenae | 3.75g |
| Qiang Huo | Rhizoma seu Radix Notopterygii | 3.75g |
| Du Huo | Radix Angelicae Pubescentis | 3.75g |
| Jing Jie | Herba Schizonepetae | 3.75g |
| Fang Feng | Radix Saposhnikoviae | 3.75g |

This formula is suitable for headaches with extensive lower back and hip pain.

### Joryong Chajonja Tang
*Lee Je-ma's Polyporus and Plantago Seed Decoction*

| | | |
|---|---|---|
| Ze Xie | *Rhizoma Alismatis* | 7.5g |
| Fu Ling | *Poria Alba* | 7.5g |
| Zhu Ling | *Polyporus* | 5.625g |
| Che Qian Zi | *Semen Plantaginis* | 5.625g |
| Zhi Mu | *Rhizoma Anemarrhenae* | 3.75g |
| Shi Gao | *Gypsum Fibrosum* | 3.75g |
| Qiang Huo | *Rhizoma seu Radix Notopterygii* | 3.75g |
| Du Huo | *Radix Angelicae Pubescentis* | 3.75g |
| Jing Jie | *Herba Schizonepetae* | 3.75g |
| Fang Feng | *Radix Saposhnikoviae* | 3.75g |

This formula is recommended for headaches with abdominal pain and diarrhea.

### Hwalsok Gosam Tang
*Lee Je-ma's Talcum and Sophora Decoction*

| | | |
|---|---|---|
| Ze Xie | *Rhizoma Alismatis* | 7.5g |
| Fu Ling | *Poria Alba* | 7.5g |
| Hua Shi | *Talcum* | 7.5g |
| Ku Shen | *Radix Sophorae* | 7.5g |
| Chuan Huang Lian | *Rhizoma Coptidis* | 3.75g |
| Huang Bai | *Cortex Phellodendri* | 3.75g |
| Qiang Huo | *Rhizoma seu Radix Notopterygii* | 3.75g |
| Du Huo | *Radix Angelicae Pubescentis* | 3.75g |
| Jing Jie | *Herba Schizonepetae* | 3.75g |
| Fang Feng | *Radix Saposhnikoviae* | 3.75g |

This formula is suitable for abdominal pain without diarrhea.

### Dokhwal Jihwang Tang
*Lee Je-ma's Angelica Pubescens and Rehmannia Decoction*
*(Modified Liu Wei Di Huang Tang)*

| | | |
|---|---|---|
| Shu Di Huang | *Radix Rehmanniae Preparata* | 15g |
| Shan Zhu Yu | *Fructus Corni Officinalis* | 7.5g |
| Fu Ling | *Poria Alba* | 5.625g |

| Ze Xie | *Rhizoma Alismatis* | 5.625g |
| Mu Dan Pi | *Cortex Moutan* | 3.75g |
| Fang Feng | *Radix Saposhnikoviae* | 3.75g |
| Du Huo | *Radix Angelicae Pubescentis* | 3.75g |

This formula is suitable for fullness in the chest due to food stagnation.

### *Hyungbang Jihwang Tang*

*Lee Je-ma's Schizonepeta, Ledebouriella, and Rhemannia Decoction*

| Shu Di Huang | *Radix Rehmanniae Preparata* | 7.5g |
| Shan Zhu Yu | *Fructus Corni Officinalis* | 7.5g |
| Fu Ling | *Poria Alba* | 7.5g |
| Ze Xie | *Rhizoma Alismatis* | 7.5g |
| Che Qian Zi | *Semen Plantaginis* | 3.75g |
| Qiang Huo | *Rhizoma seu Radix Notopterygii* | 3.75g |
| Du Huo | *Radix Angelicae Pubescentis* | 3.75g |
| Jing Jie | *Herba Schizonepetae* | 3.75g |
| Fang Feng | *Radix Saposhnikoviae* | 3.75g |

The following herbs should be added to the above formula according to symptomatic presentation.

- Coughing: Add Qian Hu (*Radix Peucedani*).

- Bleeding disorders: Add Xuan Shen (*Radix Scrophulariae*), Mu Dan Pi (*Cortex Moutan*).

- Parietal headaches: Add Huang Lian (*Rhizoma Coptidis*), Niu Bang Zi (*Fructus Arctii*).

- Fullness and distension due to food stagnation: Add Mu Dan Pi (*Cortex Moutan*).

- For spleen Fire: Add Shi Gao (*Gypsum Fibrosum*) (Shan Zhu Yu (*Fructus Corni Officinalis*) should be removed in this case).[46]

- For headache with an unsettled feeling in the chest and anxiety: Add Sheng Di Huang (*Radix Rehmanniae*).

Jing Jie (*Herba Schizonepetae*), Fang Feng (*Radix Saposhnikoviae*), Qiang Huo (*Rhizoma seu Radix Notopterygii*), and Du Huo (*Radix Angelicae Pubescentis*) help preserve the Yin energy of the body. Jing Jie (*Herba Schizonepetae*) and Fang Feng (*Radix Saposhnikoviae*) are particularly effective in clearing the chest and epigastric area and extinguishing Wind. Qiang Huo (*Rhizoma seu Radix Notopterygii*) and Du Huo (*Radix Angelicae Pubescentis*) are

---

46  Shan Zhu Yu (*Fructus Corni Officinalis*) should be eliminated from the formula whenever treating Heat syndromes because its astringent nature can trap Heat accumulation within the body.

particularly effective at preserving the True Yin[47] of the urinary bladder and eliminating headaches, abdominal pain and fullness, and diarrhea. I have prescribed these herbs with several deficient patients, and after administering up to several hundred packs, there is no doubt of their effect.

### Shipimi Jihwang Tang
*Lee Je-ma's Twelve Ingredient Rehmennia Decoction
(Modified Liu Wei Di Huang Tang)*

| Shu Di Huang | Radix Rehmanniae Preparata | 15g |
|---|---|---|
| Shan Zhu Yu | Fructus Corni Officinalis | 7.5g |
| Fu Ling | Poria Alba | 5.625g |
| Ze Xie | Rhizoma Alismatis | 5.625g |
| Mu Dan Pi | Cortex Moutan | 3.75g |
| Di Gu Pi | Cortex Lycii | 3.75g |
| Xuan Shen | Radix Scrophulariae | 3.75g |
| Gou Qi Zi | Fructus Lycii | 3.75g |
| Fu Pen Zi | Fructus Rubi | 3.75g |
| Che Qian Zi | Semen Plantaginis | 3.75g |
| Jing Jie | Herba Schizonepetae | 3.75g |
| Fang Feng | Radix Saposhnikoviae | 3.75g |

This formula addresses the So Yang Individual's vomiting of blood.

### Jihwang Baekho Tang
*Lee Je-ma's White Tiger Decoction with Rehmennia (Modified Bai Hu Tang)*

| Shi Gao | Gypsum Fibrosum | 18.75–37.5g |
|---|---|---|
| Sheng Di Huang | Radix Rehmanniae | 15g |
| Zhi Mu | Rhizoma Anemarrhenae | 7.5g |
| Fang Feng | Radix Saposhnikoviae | 3.75g |
| Du Huo | Radix Angelicae Pubescentis | 3.75g |

For the So Yang Individual's fever, headache, dysuria, and more than 24 hours without a bowel movement.

---

47   True Yin, or *Zhen Yin* (眞陰), is the body's inherent Yin energy, which accumulates in the kidneys and spreads through the body via the urinary bladder. Its role is to distribute Yin and keep Yang from excess. Source Yang, or *Yuan Yang* (元陽), is the body's inherent Yang energy, which accumulates in the spleen, and spreads throughout the body via the thoracic cavity. It is responsible for distributing Yang and controlling excessive Yin.

### Yang Dok Baek Ho Tang
*Lee Je-ma's White Tiger Decoction to Eliminate Yang Toxin (Modified Bai Hu Tang)*

| Shi Gao | Gypsum Fibrosum | 18.75–37.5g |
|---|---|---|
| Sheng Di Huang | Radix Rehmanniae | 15g |
| Zhi Mu | Rhizoma Anemarrhenae | 7.5g |
| Jing Jie | Herba Schizonepetae | 3.75g |
| Fang Feng | Radix Saposhnikoviae | 3.75g |
| Niu Bang Zi | Fructus Arctii | 3.75g |

This formula is suitable for the treatment of scarlet fever with constipation.

### Yanggyuk Sanhwa Tang
*Lee Je-ma's Cool the Diaphragm and Disperse Heat Decoction (Modified Lian Ge San)*

| Sheng Di Huang | Radix Rehmanniae | 7.5g |
|---|---|---|
| Ren Dong Teng | Caulis Lonicerae | 7.5g |
| Lian Qiao | Fructus Forsythiae | 7.5g |
| Zhi Zi | Fructus Gardenia | 3.75g |
| Bo He | Herba Menthae | 3.75g |
| Zhi Mu | Rhizoma Anemarrhenae | 3.75g |
| Shi Gao | Gypsum Fibrosum | 3.75g |
| Fang Feng | Radix Saposhnikoviae | 3.75g |
| Jing Jie | Herba Schizonepetae | 3.75g |

This formula is prescribed for Upper *Jiao Xiao Ge* syndrome.

### Indongdeng Jigolpi Tang
*Lee Je-ma's Honeysuckle and Lycium Decoction*

| Ren Dong Teng | Caulis Lonicerae | 15g |
|---|---|---|
| Shan Zhu Yu | Fructus Corni Officinalis | 7.5g |
| Di Gu Pi | Cortex Lycii | 7.5g |
| Chuan Huang Lian | Rhizoma Coptidis | 3.75g |
| Huang Bai | Cortex Phellodendri | 3.75g |

| Xuan Shen | *Radix Scrophulariae* | 3.75g |
|---|---|---|
| Ku Shen | *Radix Sophorae* | 3.75g |
| Sheng Di Huang | *Radix Rehmanniae* | 3.75g |
| Zhi Mu | *Rhizoma Anemarrhenae* | 3.75g |
| Zhi Zi | *Fructus Gardenia* | 3.75g |
| Gou Qi Zi | *Fructus Lycii* | 3.75g |
| Fu Pen Zi | *Fructus Rubi* | 3.75g |
| Jing Jie | *Herba Schizonepetae* | 3.75g |
| Fang Feng | *Radix Saposhnikoviae* | 3.75g |
| Jin Yin Hua | *Flos Lonicerae* | 3.75g |

This formula is prescribed for Middle *Jiao Xiao Ge* syndrome.

### Sukjihwang Gosam Tang
*Lee Je-ma's Processed Rhemannia and Sophora Decoction*

| Shu Di Huang | *Radix Rehmanniae Preparata* | 15g |
|---|---|---|
| Shan Zhu Yu | *Fructus Corni Officinalis* | 7.5g |
| Fu Ling | *Poria Alba* | 5.625g |
| Ze Xie | *Rhizoma Alismatis* | 5.625g |
| Zhi Mu | *Rhizoma Anemarrhenae* | 3.75g |
| Huang Bai | *Cortex Phellodendri* | 3.75g |
| Ku Shen | *Radix Sophorae* | 3.75g |

This formula is prescribed for Lower *Jiao Xiao Ge* syndrome.

### Moktong Daean Tang
*Lee Je-ma's Akebia Great Relief Decoction*

| Mu Tong | *Caulis Akebiae* | 18.75g |
|---|---|---|
| Sheng Di Huang | *Radix Rehmanniae* | 18.75g |
| Chi Fu Ling | *Poria Rubra* | 7.5g |
| Ze Xie | *Rhizoma Alismatis* | 3.75g |
| Che Qian Zi | *Semen Plantaginis* | 3.75g |
| Chuan Huang Lian | *Rhizoma Coptidis* | 3.75g |
| Qiang Huo | *Rhizoma seu Radix Notopterygii* | 3.75g |
| Fang Feng | *Radix Saposhnikoviae* | 3.75g |
| Jing Jie | *Herba Schizonepetae* | 3.75g |

The formula is suitable for superficial edema. In severe cases, a total of 100 packs should be prescribed. Huang Lian (*Rhizoma Coptidis*) and Ze Xie (*Rhizoma Alismatis*) may be omitted from the above formula if they are difficult to obtain.

### Hwangyon Chongjang Tang
*Lee Je-ma's Coptis Clear the Intestine Decoction*

| | | |
|---|---|---|
| Sheng Di Huang | *Radix Rehmanniae* | 15g |
| Mu Tong | *Caulis Akebiae* | 7.5g |
| Fu Ling | *Poria Alba* | 7.5g |
| Ze Xie | *Rhizoma Alismatis* | 7.5g |
| Zhu Ling | *Polyporus* | 3.75g |
| Che Qian Zi | *Semen Plantaginis* | 3.75g |
| Chuan Huang Lian | *Rhizoma Coptidis* | 3.75g |
| Qiang Huo | *Rhizoma seu Radix Notopterygii* | 3.75g |
| Fang Feng | *Radix Saposhnikoviae* | 3.75g |

This formula is suitable for dysentery. For gonorrhea, remove Mu Tong (*Caulis Akebiae*) and add Jing Jie (*Herba Schizonepetae*).

### Jusa Ikwon San
*Lee Je-ma's Cinnabar Support the Source Powder*

| | | |
|---|---|---|
| Hua Shi | *Talcum* | 7.5g |
| Ze Xie | *Rhizoma Alismatis* | 3.75g |
| Gan Sui | *Radix Euphorbiae Kansui* | 1.875g |
| Zhu Sha[48] | *Cinnabaris* | .375g |

Grind the above ingredients into a fine powder and mix with warm water or water drawn from a well at daybreak. This formula is suitable for cooling the body and clearing Heat-induced syndromes.

### Kamsu Chonil Wan
*Lee Je-ma's Divine Gan Sui Pill*

| | | |
|---|---|---|
| Gan Sui | *Radix Euphorbiae Kansui* | 1.875g |
| Qing Fen | *Calomelas* | .375g |

48  Zhu Sha (*Cinnabaris*) contains significant amounts of mercury and is therefore considered highly toxic. Hence it is often replaced with Dan Zhu Ye (*Herba Lophatheri Gracilis*), which also has a similar effect on calming the spirit and clearing Heat. The standard dosage of Dan Zhu Ye is 7.5g, but in acute cases up to 26.25g can be used.

Grind the above into fine powder, form into a paste, coat with Zhu Sha (*Cinnabaris*)[49] and shape into ten pills. This formula is suitable for acute cases of *Jie Xiong* syndrome.

The pills may dry out and become difficult to break down after being stored for a long period of time. If so, they can be wrapped in two or three sheets of paper, pounded in a mortar, and then cut into three to five slices. Place each slice one at a time in the patient's mouth and have him/her drink water drawn from a well at daybreak to melt and wash it down. If diarrhea doesn't occur within six to eight hours, then insert two more slices in the mouth. Three bouts of diarrhea after the second ingestion indicates improvement, and six bouts will produce significant relief. Rice porridge should be prepared ahead of time and provided after two to three bouts of diarrhea to replenish fluids. If this precaution is not taken, the patient will get weaker and have difficulty recovering from his or her illness. This formula can also assist with *Jie Xiong* syndrome marked by vomiting after the ingestion of water.

If ten pills made from 3.75g of Gan Sui (*Radix Euphorbiae Kansui*) and 1.875g of Qing Fen (*Calomelas*) are used, the formula is called *Kyungbun Kamsu Yongho Dan* (Lee Je-ma's Calomel and Kan Sui Root Dragon Tiger Pill). If ten pills made from equal amounts of Gan Sui (*Radix Euphorbiae Kansui*) and Qing Fen are used, the formula is referred to as *Kyungbun Kamsu Jaung Dan* (Lee Je-ma's Euphorbia and Calomelas Opposing Forces Pill). If 30 pills made from 3.75g and 1.875g of Ru Xiang (*Resina Olibani*), Mo Yao (*Myrrhae*), and Gan Sui (*Radix Euphorbiae Kansui*) are used, the formula is then called *Yuhyang Moyak Kyungbun Wan* (Lee Je-ma's Myrrh, Frankincense, and Calomelas Pill).

Qing Fen (*Calomelas*) promotes sweating, while Gan Sui (*Radix Euphorbiae Kansui*) decreases water retention by promoting diarrhea. In most cases, only .375g of Qing Fen (*Calomelas*) is enough to elicit an effect. Even as little as .1875g can suffice in some cases. In most cases, only .5625g of Gan Sui (*Radix Euphorbiae Kansui*) will elicit an effect. Even as little as .2625–.3g can be enough for some. Since both of the above herbs are toxic, they should be administered carefully and never exceed more than .375g, their prescribed dosage. Once the extent of illness is carefully determined, prescribe Gan Sui (*Radix Euphorbiae Kansui*) and Qing Fen (*Calomelas*) appropriately. Qing Fen (*Calomelas*) should be prescribed as the king herb to clear Fire from the head and brain, whereas Gan Sui (*Radix Euphorbiae Kansui*) as the king herb eliminates water accumulation from the chest.

The herbs prescribed for the So Yang Individual should not be dry-fried (until black), dry-fried with honey, or roasted.

---

49    Zhu Sha (*Cinnabaris*) is no longer used for coating pills due to its toxicity.

Chapter 8 —————————————————————————

# The Tae Eum Individual's Illness

*Section 1*

## The Tae Eum Individual's Esophageal Cold Causing Exterior Cold Syndrome[1]
太陰人胃脘受寒表寒病

張仲景이 曰太陽傷寒에 頭痛 發熱하며 身疼 腰痛하며 骨節皆痛하며 惡寒하며 無汗而喘이어든 麻黃湯을 主之니라.

According to Zhang Zhongjing, *Ma Huang Tang* (Ephedra Decoction) is prescribed when symptoms such as headaches, fever, body aches, lower back pain, joint pain, aversion to Cold, a lack of sweating, and shortness of breath occur during Shang Han illness.

註에 曰傷寒에 頭痛 身疼 腰痛하야 以至牽連하며 百骨節俱痛者는 此는 太陽傷寒이니 榮血이 不利故也니라.

He also delineates how symptoms such as headaches, general body aches, lower back pain, and discomfort of practically every joint in the body during a Shang Han illness are due to an imbalance of *Rong* and *Xue*.[2]

———————————————————

1    The Tae Eum Individual has four Esophageal Cold causing External Cold syndromes: External pathogen affecting the cervical spine, *Han Jue*, Cold esophagus syndrome, and Exterior Cold-induced Warm Febrile disease. The *Fu* organs (esophagus, small intestine) are associated with the Tae Eum and Tae Yang Individual's Exterior disorders, and the *Zhang* organs (lungs and liver) are associated with Interior disorders. The Tae Eum Individual's Esophageal Cold causing External Cold syndrome is due to an imbalance of his/her *Song* nature of joy and the feeling that others aren't assisting them. In this situation, they wish only to look out for and help themselves.

2    *Rong* (榮) is the pure, vs. turbid, energy of blood, and *Xue* (血) is translated as blood itself. When translated together *Rong Xue* (榮血) correlates with "nutrition," which is absorbed by the lungs and distributed to the rest of the *Zhang Fu* organs via the bloodstream. It also nourishes and fortifies the *Yuan* (Source) *Qi*. An imbalance of *Rong* and *Xue* occurs as a result of an external pathogen causing imbalance and impurity within the blood.

論曰此는 卽太陰人傷寒 背傾頁表病 輕證也니 此證에 麻黃湯을 非不當
用而桂枝 甘草는 皆爲蠱材니 此證에 當用麻黃發表湯이니라

As I see it, these symptoms indicate the Tae Eum Individual's External pathogen affecting the cervical spine.[3] *Ma Huang Tang* (Ephedra Decoction) can be used for this, but *Mahwang Balpyo Tang* (Ma Huang Release the Exterior Decoction) is more appropriate because it doesn't include two herbs incompatible with the Tae Eum Individual—Gui Zhi (*Ramulus Cinnamomi Cassiae*) and Gan Cao (*Radix Glycyrrhizae*).

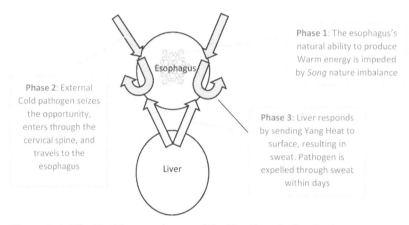

Phase 1: The esophagus's natural ability to produce Warm energy is impeded by *Song* nature imbalance

Phase 2: External Cold pathogen seizes the opportunity, enters through the cervical spine, and travels to the esophagus

Phase 3: Liver responds by sending Yang Heat to surface, resulting in sweat. Pathogen is expelled through sweat within days

*Figure 8.1: The Tai Yang syndrome of the Tae Eum Individual*

張仲景이 曰傷寒에 四五日而厥者는 必發熱이니 厥深者는 熱亦深하고
厥微者는 熱亦微하니라. 傷寒厥四日에 熱反三日하고 復厥五日은 厥多熱
少니 其病이 爲進이오 傷寒發熱四日에 厥反三日은 厥少熱多니 其病이
當自愈니라.

According to Zhang Zhongjing, if *Jue*[4] syndrome occurs after four to five days of Shang Han illness, then fever will inevitably follow. Acute fever will also come as severe cases of *Jue* syndrome advance. If *Jue* syndrome is minor, then the fever will be too. If after four days of *Jue* syndrome an additional three days of fever are followed by another five days of *Jue* in short spurts and then reduced fever, it means that the illness will continue onwards. If after four days of Shang Han illness pronounced fever is followed by three days of less pronounced *Jue*, a positive prognosis[5] can be expected.

---

3   The cervical spine and esophagus correlate with the *Pei Guk* (肺局), or lung system. Since the lungs are the weakest organ of the Tae Eum Individual, the cervical area, which is the external correlate of the lungs, is vulnerable to attack by external pathogens.

4   The term *Jue* (厥) is often used to describe the occurrence of extremely cold hands and feet as a result of a prolonged battle between *Zheng Qi* and pathogenic *Qi* within the body after the onset of a Shang Han illness. Lee Je-ma, however, interprets Zhang Zhongjing's inclusion of "*Jue*" in this sentence as indicating severe chills without fever rather than *Jue Ni*, extremely cold hands and feet.

5   Fever lasting longer than chills indicates the process of recovery. Shorter intervals of fever and longer intervals of chills indicate that the situation is getting worse.

論曰此謂之厥者는 但惡寒不發熱之謂也오 非手足厥逆之謂也라 太陰人 傷寒表證에 寒厥四五日後에 發熱者는 重證也니 此證에 發熱하고 其汗이 必自髮際而始通於額上하며 又數日後에 發熱而眉稜에 通汗하며 又數日後에 發熱而顴上에 通汗하며 又數日後에 發熱而脣⸢에 通汗하며 又數日後에 發熱而胸臆에 通汗也로되 而額上之汗이 數次而後에 達於眉稜하고 眉稜之汗이 數次而後에 達於顴上하고 顴上之汗이 數次而後에 達於脣⸢하고 脣⸢之汗은 不過一次而直達於胸臆矣라

From my perspective, this analysis of *Jue* involves an aversion to Cold with a lack of fever. It is not referring to *Jue Ni*[6] syndrome of the hands and feet. If fever occurs after four to five days of the Tae Eum Individual's *Han Jue*[7] due to the onset of a Shang Han illness, it can be viewed as a serious situation. When this illness occurs, fever will lead to sweating from the hairline (at both temples) to the forehead.

If after several days of fever there is sweating around the eyebrows, and after another few days of fever it spreads to the zygomatic arch, and after another few days of fever it spreads to the lips and chin, and after another few days of fever it spreads to the chest, and after a second bout of several days of forehead sweating it again travels upwards and spreads to the hairline and after another few days of sweating at the hairline it spreads to the zygomatic arch and after another few days of sweating at the zygomatic arch it spreads to the lips and after another few days of sweating at the lips it spreads to the chin, it will again follow the same course and then spread to the chest once again.

此證은 首尾幾近 二十日에 凡寒厥 六七次而後에 病解也니 此證을 俗謂之 長感病이라 凡太陰人病이 先額上眉稜에 有汗而一汗에 病不解하고 屢汗에 病解者를 名曰長感病이니라.

This illness, commonly referred to as *Zhang Gan Bing*,[8] usually takes about 20 days to recover from and six to seven bouts of *Han Jue*. It is marked by the onset of eyebrow-area sweating that doesn't result in immediate recovery. Only after the second bout of sweating will *Zhang Gan Bing* be resolved.

---

6 In this sentence, Lee Je-ma distinguishes between *Jue Ni* (厥逆) and Zhang Zhongjing's use of the single character *Jue* (厥). The former syndrome is due to the reversal of *Qi* movement, leading to a minute (or non-palpable) pulse, freezing-cold hands and feet, and loss of consciousness. The latter syndrome simply describes the occurrence of chills without fever after the onset of a Shang Han illness.

7 *Han Jue* (寒厥), or "Cold *Jue*," is another term for *Jue* (厥) syndrome. Lee Je-ma uses both of these terms interchangeably in this text. He states that, contrary to common belief, severe chills and a lack of sweating, rather than cold hands and feet, are the main symptoms of *Jue* or *Han Jue*.

8 *Zhang Gan Bing* (長感病), literally translated as "long-term Cold," is a severe form of *Han Jue* that is accompanied by repeated bouts of light sweating at the forehead and/or temples, but not enough sweating to recover once and for all. Hence, this illness lingers on for about 20 days.

太陰人病이 寒厥六七日而不發熱不汗出則死也라 寒厥二三日而發熱汗
出則輕證也오 寒厥四五日而發熱하고 得微汗於額上者를 此之謂長感
病이니 其病이 爲重證也라

If no sweating or fever appears after six to seven days of *Han Jue*, it is to be taken as a grave situation. If sweat and fever occur for two to three days after the onset of *Han Jue* occurrence, it is considered a minor situation. If there is fever but only limited sweating at the forehead after four to five days of *Han Jue* occurrence, it is a serious illness.

此證原委는 勞心焦思之餘에 胃脘이 衰弱而表局이 虛薄하여 不勝寒而
外被寒邪所圍하야 正邪相爭之形勢가 客勝主弱하니 譬如一團孤軍이 因
在垓心하야 幾於全軍覆沒之境하다가 先鋒一隊가 倖而跳出하야 決圍一
面하고 僅得開路나 後軍全隊가 尙在垓心하야 將又屢次力戰然後라야 方
爲出來則爻象이 正是凜凜之勢也라額上通汗者는 卽先鋒一隊가 決圍跳
出之象也오 眉稜通汗者는 卽前軍全隊가 決圍全面하고 氣勢勇敢之象
也오 顴上通汗者는 中軍半隊가 緩緩出圍之象也니

This illness is the result of excess worry and stress,[9] which weaken the esophagus,[10] making it difficult to battle off External pathogenic Cold. Furthermore, the pathogenic *Qi* surrounds the *Zheng Qi*, which tries to fight it off. Hence, the pathogenic "guest" proceeds to defeat the weakened *Zheng Qi* of the "host." This situation can be compared to a stranded platoon that is surrounded by its enemy and almost completely annihilated but, at the last minute, a front-line soldier pokes his way through the enemy line and paves the escape route for his platoon. Yet, still trapped, the rear guard fights onward alongside one another with all their might. Fighting onward, they too make their escape, yet still give the advantage to the opposing army. Sweating at the forehead can also be compared to the front-line soldier fighting his way through the enemy line.

此病에 汗出眉稜則快免危也오 汗出額上則必無危也니라. 太陰人汗은 無
論額上 眉稜 顴上하고 汗出이 如黍粒하여 發熱稍久而還入者는 正强邪
弱이니 快汗也오 汗出이 如微粒커나 或淋漓無粒타가 乍時而還入者는
正弱邪强이니 非快汗也니라.

Sweating from the eyebrows indicates an escape from the worst scenario, and sweating from the zygomatic arch indicates a complete escape from danger. Hence,

---

9   "Excess worry and stress" is a translation of *Noshim Josa* (勞心焦思), which literally means "labored heart and worrisome thoughts." These thoughts occur when the Tae Eum Individual cannot balance their *Song* nature of joy.

10  The esophagus is the Yang correlate of the lungs, which is the weakest organ of the Tae Eum Individual, vulnerable to External pathogenic influence.

recovery from this illness depends on whether or not there is sweating from the forehead, eyebrow, or zygomatic arch. Drops of sweat the size of a millet kernel with substantial, persistent fever indicate a weakening of the pathogen and strengthening of the *Zheng Qi*. Small kernel-sized or unshaped[11] and unsubstantial sweat indicates a weakening of the *Zheng Qi* and strengthening of the pathogen, signaling a poor prognosis.

太陰人이 背部後面 自腦以下에 有汗而面部髮際以下에 不汗者는 凶證也오 全面에 皆有汗而耳門左右에 不汗者는 死證也니라 大凡太陰人汗은 始自耳後高骨 面部髮際하야 大通於胸臆間하면 而病解也니 髮際之汗은 始免死也오 額上之汗은 僅免危也오 眉稜之汗은 快免危也오 顴上之汗은 生路寬闊也오 脣頥之汗은 病已解也오 胸臆之汗은 病大解也니라.

If the Tae Eum Individual sweats from the occiput to the thoracic spine but not from the anterior hairline or face, it is an unfavorable situation. Sweating throughout the face except for around the ears points to a grave situation. Ample sweating that starts from the ears and makes its way to the zygomatic arch, anterior hairline area, face, and then chest signifies imminent recovery. Sweating that only occurs at the hairline [and doesn't travel downwards] indicates a grave situation. If it descends to the forehead, then it is considered somewhat critical but not grave. Sweating at the temple indicates the escape from a critical stage. Sweating at the zygomatic arch is a clear sign of recovery. If it occurs around the lips and chin, then recovery has already begun. Chest sweating indicates full recovery.

嘗見此證에 額上汗이 欲作眉稜汗者는 寒厥之勢가 不甚猛也오 額上汗이 欲作脣頥之汗者는 寒厥之勢가 甚猛하야 至於寒戰叩齒하여 完若動風而其汗이 直達兩腋하나니 張仲景所云 厥深者는 熱亦深하고 厥微者는 熱亦微라함이 蓋謂此也니라此證에 寒厥之勢가 多日者는 病重之勢也오 寒厥之勢가 猛峻者는 非病重之勢也니라.

From past experience, I noticed that sweat starting from the forehead and moving to the temple(s) indicates a lighter, less detrimental form of *Han Jue*. If sweating starts from the zygomatic arch and spreads to the lips and chin, it indicates a stronger, more serious form of *Han Jue*, which will inevitably be accompanied by sweating from the armpits and severe shivering to the point of resembling *Dong Feng*[12] syndrome. Zhang Zhongjing referred to this situation when stating that fever

---

11  "Unshaped" refers to sweat that covers the skin without a bead-shaped appearance, and instead forms a thin film covering the skin. This type of sweat is an indication of weakening *Zheng Qi* and the escape of Yang through the skin pores. It is also the hallmark symptom of the So Eum Individual's *Mang Yang* syndrome.

12  *Dong Feng* (動風) syndrome, literally translated as "Moving Wind," is a result of External Wind pathogen making its way interiorly, and is marked by convulsions. Lee Je-ma illustrates how the shivering of *Han Jue* syndrome can be so severe that it appears as if the individual is convulsing.

will also be pronounced following severe cases of *Jue*, while in lighter cases, it is less pronounced. The latter situation indicates a serious illness, but the former, more pronounced *Han Jue* syndrome indicates a lighter, non-critical form of *Han Jue*.[13]

此證을 京畿道人이 謂之長感病이라하고 咸鏡道人이 謂之四十日痛 或謂之無汗乾病이라하니 時俗所用에 荊防敗毒散과 藿香正氣散과 補中益氣湯이 個個誤治로되 惟熊膽이 雖或盲人直門이나 然이나 又連用他藥하면 病勢更變하나니

In Kyoung-Gi Province, this illness is referred to as *Janggan Byung*,[14] whereas, in Ham Kyoung Province, it is called *Sashipil Byung*[15] or *Muhangon Byung*.[16] In the past, *Jing Fang Bai Du San* (Schizonepeta and Saposhnikoviae Powder to Overcome Pathogenic Influences), *Hou Xiang Zheng Qi San* (Agastache Powder to Rectify the Qi), or *Bu Zhong Yi Qi Tang* (Tonify the Middle and Augment the Qi Decoction) have been mistakenly prescribed. Actually, in my own experience, Xiong Dan (*Vessica Fellea Ursi*) is the most suitable medicine for this situation. If other medicines are given, then *Han Jue* can transform into other, yet more serious, illnesses.

古人所云 病不能殺人이오 藥能殺人者를 不亦信乎아 百病加減之勢를 以凡眼目으로 觀之컨대 固難推測而此證이 又有甚焉하니 此證之汗이 在眉稜 額上時에는 雖不服藥이라도 亦自愈矣而病人이 招醫하여 妄投誤藥則額上之汗이 還爲額上之汗而外證寒厥之勢則稍減矣니라 於是焉에 醫師가 自以爲信藥效하며 病人이 亦自以爲得藥效하야 又數日誤藥則額上之汗이 又不通而死矣니 此證은 當以汗之進退로 占病之輕重이오 不可以寒之寬猛으로 占病之輕重이니 張仲景이 曰其病이 當自愈云者는 豈非珍重無妄之論乎아 然이나 長感病에 無疫氣者는 待其自愈則好也而瘟病에疫氣重者는 若明知證藥하여 無疑則不可尋常置之니 待其勿藥自愈하면恐生奇證이니라.

In ancient times, there was a saying that medicine, rather than the illness itself, is often to blame when death occurs. I believe there is truth in this. With only moderate insight into the ebb and flow of disease, medical approaches are often devised by merely guessing, which inevitably makes matters worse. When it comes to *Han Jue*

---

13 In this sentence, Lee Je-ma argues that severe chills followed by high fever are not necessarily an indication of serious illness. On the contrary, it is considered moderate when compared to prolonged lighter cycles of chills followed by fever.

14 *Janggan Byung* is the Korean Romanization of the Chinese term *Zhang Gan Bing* (長感病), or "long-term Cold."

15 *Sashipil Byung* (四十日痛), literally "forty-day illness," is a form of *Han Jue*, which though similar to *Zhang Gan Bing* has a prolonged recovery time of approximately 40 days.

16 *Muhangon Byung* (無汗乾病), literally "lack of sweat and dryness-related illness," describes a critical form of *Han Jue* where sweating doesn't accompany fever. Note that significant sweating with relatively high fever is necessary to overcome *Han Jue*.

syndrome, if it is followed by significant sweating at the temple and zygomatic arch area, then even if medicine is not administered, recovery is imminent. If a doctor is sought at this point, it is possible that they would haphazardly prescribe medicine. If the temple area sweating stops and only the forehead sweating continues, indicating recovery from *Han Jue*, the doctor would mistakenly attribute it to the effects of intervention. Yet if after several more days of herbal treatment the sweating at the forehead disappears, death is inescapable. The extent of illness is determined by the existence or lack of sweating and the abruptness or delay of chills. Zhang Zhongjing stated that recovery from *Han Jue* occurs without intervention—surely an admonition against impulsive treatment, emphasizing the need to proceed with caution. While it is advisable to let *Zhang Gan Bing* take its course, if symptoms of epidemic or Warm Febrile disease are present, then this approach is not advisable. In such cases, the illness may advance if the doctor chooses not to interfere by prescribing medicine, with the hope that the patient will naturally recover. However, if the disease and its treatment are clearly planned out, even in severe situations, there is no need for worry.

論曰太陰人病이 寒厥四日而無汗者는 重證也오 寒厥五日而無汗者는 險證也니 當用熊膽散 或寒多熱少湯 加ㄷㄷ 五七九個하되 大便이 滑者는 必用乾栗 薏苡仁等屬하고 大便燥者는 必用葛根 大黃等屬하야 若額上 眉稜上에 有汗則待其自愈而病解後에 用藥調理니 否則恐生後病이니라.

From my perspective, if there is no sweating after four days of *Han Jue* onset, it is considered a serious illness. After five days of no sweating, it is considered a critical illness. In such cases, Xiong Dan (*Vessica Fellea Ursi*) or *Handa Yulso Tang* (Lee Je-ma's Greater Cold Lesser Heat Decoction) with four to nine pieces of Qi Cao (*Holotrichia*) should be prescribed without delay. If the stools are loose then Yi Yi Ren (*Semen Coicis*) and Gan Li (*Castania*) should be added. If the stools are dry then Ge Gen (*Radix Puerariae*) and Da Huang (*Radix et Rhizoma Rhei*) should be added. If there is significant sweating at the temple and zygomatic arch, then it is advisable to wait until the patient recovers naturally, and only afterwards should medicinal herbs be prescribed in order to prevent recurrence.

**Table 8.1: The different forms of the Tae Eum Individual's *Han Jue* syndrome**

| Syndrome | Common symptoms | Accompanying symptoms | Treatment approach |
|---|---|---|---|
| *Han Jue* (mild) | | Two to three days of *Han Jue* fever followed by ample sweating | No treatment necessary |
| *Han Jue* (severe)<br>1. *Zhang Gan Bing*<br>2. *Janggan Byung* | Extreme chills | Four to five days of *Han Jue* followed by fever and light sweating on the forehead and/or temples | Xiong Dan (*Vessica Fellea Ursi*) |
| *Han Jue* (critical)<br>1. *Muhangon Byung* | | Six to seven days of *Han Jue* followed by fever without sweating | 1. Xiong Dan (*Vessica Fellea Ursi*)<br>2. *Handa Yulso Tang* (Lee Je-ma's Greater Cold Lesser Heat Decoction) with four to nine pieces of Qi Cao (*Holotrichia*)<br>**If stools are loose:**<br>Add Yi Yi Ren (*Semen Coicis*) and Gan Li (*Castania*)<br>**If stools are dry:**<br>Add Ge Gen (*Radix Puerariae*) and Da Huang (*Radix et Rhizoma Rhei*) |

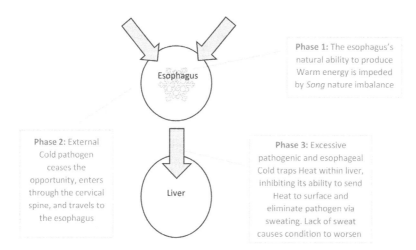

*Figure 8.2: The Han Jue syndrome of the Tae Eum Individual*

嘗治太陰人의 胃脘寒證瘟病할새 有一太陰人이 素有怔忡하고 無汗 氣
短 結咳矣더니 忽焉又添出一證하야 泄瀉가 數十日不止하니 卽表病之
重者也ㅣ라 用太陰調胃湯 加樗根皮 一錢하야 日再服十日하니 泄瀉方
止어늘 連用三十日하니 每日流汗滿面하고 素證도 亦減而忽其家五六
人이 一時瘟疫하니 此人이 緣於救病하야 數日不服藥矣라 此人이 又染
瘟病瘟證하야 粥食이 無味하여 全不入口어늘 仍以太陰調胃湯 加升麻
黃芩 各一錢하야 連用十日하니 汗流滿面하고 疫氣少減而有二日大便不
通之證이어늘 仍用葛根承氣湯 五日而五日內에 粥食이 大倍하고 疫氣가
大減而病解라 又用太陰調胃湯 加升麻 黃芩하여 四十日調理하니 疫氣가
旣減하고 素病도 亦完하니라.

I once treated a Tae Eum Individual suffering from a Warm Febrile disease, which began as Cold esophagus syndrome. He originally experienced palpitations, lack of sweat, shortness of breath, and a dry, hacking cough. In addition to these symptoms, he had consistent diarrhea lasting over 20 days, indicating a serious case of External Cold-induced illness. After two packs a day of *Tae Eum Jowi Tang* (Lee Je-ma's Regulate the stomach Decoction for the Tae Eum Individual) with 3.75g of Chun Gen Pi (*Cortex Ailanthi*), his diarrhea completely ceased. Throughout the entire 30 days of ingesting this decoction, he continued to sweat profusely from his face, and eventually overcame his other symptoms. Unexpectedly, however, all five members of his family were infected by the same Warm Febrile disease, and he was not provided the medicine I prescribed. Shortly afterwards, he contracted another Warm Febrile disease from a family member and couldn't eat even the slightest bit of food. As soon as I was informed of his condition, I prescribed *Tae Eum Jowi Tang* (Lee Je-ma's Regulate the stomach Decoction for the Tae Eum Individual) with 3.75g of Sheng Ma (*Rhizoma Cimicifugae*) and Huang Qin (*Radix Scutellariae*) for another ten days. He started to perspire profusely from his face, recovering slightly from his Warm Febrile disease. A bout of constipation followed for two days, so I prescribed *Kalgen Seunggi Tang* (Lee Je-Ma's Kudzu Support the Qi Decoction) for a further five days. Within this period of time his appetite returned and his symptoms gradually improved. I continued to prescribe another 40 days of *Tae Eum Jowi Tang* (Lee Je-ma's Regulate the stomach Decoction for the Tae Eum Individual) with 3.75g of Sheng Ma (*Rhizoma Cimicifugae*) and Huang Qin (*Radix Scutellariae*). Accordingly, he completely overcame the second bout of Warm Febrile disease and recovered from all underlying illness.

結咳者는 勉强發咳하야 痰欲出하나 不出而或出을 曰結咳니 少陰人結
咳를 謂之胸結咳오 太陰人結咳를 謂之頷結咳니라.

*Jie Ke*[17] is the term used to describe a distressing situation in which the desire to eliminate unproductive, or only slightly productive, phlegm leads to frequent coughing. The So Eum Individual's *Jie Ke* is referred to as Chest *Jie Ke*,[18] whereas the Tae Eum Individual's *Jie Ke* is referred to as Chin *Jie Ke*.[19]

大凡瘟疫은 先察其人素病如何則表裏虛實을 可知已니 素病寒者가 得瘟
病則亦寒證也오 素病熱者가 得瘟病則亦熱證也오 素病輕者가 得瘟病則
重證也오 素病重者가 得瘟病則險證也니라.

With Warm Febrile disease, the underlying illness must be clearly deciphered. Only then can the excesses and deficiencies of the Exterior and Interior be determined. If the underlying illness is due to Cold even when a Warm Febrile disease is present, it is still considered a Cold-related illness. If Heat underlies the occurrence of a Warm Febrile disease, it is considered a Heat-related illness. Even if the underlying disease is minor, then the influence of Warm Febrile disease will still be serious. If the underlying disease is serious, then the influence of Warm Febrile disease will be critical.

有一太陰人이 素病이 咽ㄱ乾燥而面色靑白하며 表寒或泄하니 蓋咽ㄱ乾燥
者는 肝熱也오 面色靑白하며 表寒或泄者는 胃脘寒也ㅣ니 此病은 表裏
俱病이니 素病之太重者也라 此人이 得瘟病하야 其證이 自始發日로 至
于病解히 二十日에 大便이 初滑或泄하며 中滑末乾하야 每日二三四次
無日不通이라 初用寒多熱少湯하고 病解後에 用調理肺元湯하야 四十日
調理하니 僅僅獲生하니라.

I once treated a Tae Eum Individual with a dry throat, pale complexion, and diarrhea. In most cases, a dry throat indicates Internal liver Heat syndrome, while a pale complexion and diarrhea indicate an External Esophageal Cold syndrome. Hence, this was a very serious condition in which both the Exterior and Interior were inflicted with illness. I concluded that this individual had contracted a Warm Febrile disease, which took 20 days for him to overcome. During the first six days of illness, his stools were occasionally loose with bouts of diarrhea. The second six days were marked by loose stools without diarrhea, while the remainder of the time he experienced dry stools with two to four bowel movements daily. At first, I prescribed

---

17   *Jie Ke* (結咳) translates literally as "binding cough."

18   Recall in Chapter 4 how, after ingestion, the *Go* fluids travel from the stomach to the chest. This process is impeded due to the So Eum Individual's weaker spleen and stomach. A lack of flow from the stomach to the chest may result in the stagnation of *Go* fluids, resulting in Chest *Jie Ke*.

19   Recall in Chapter 4 how, after ingestion, the *Jin* fluids travel from the esophagus to the chin or sublingual area. This process is impeded due to the Tae Eum Individual's weaker lung and esophagus. A lack of flow from the esophagus to the chest may result in the stagnation of *Jin* fluids, resulting in Chin *Jie Ke*.

*Handa Yulso Tang* (Lee Je-ma's Greater Cold Lesser Heat Decoction) to get him through the acute phase, followed by *Jori Peiwon Tang* (Lee Je-ma's Regulate the Interior and Replenish the lung Source Decoction) for 40 days in order to support his weakened constitution and save his life.

此病이 始發에 大便이 或滑或泄하며 而六七日內에 有額汗 眉稜汗 顴汗하고 飮食起居는 有時如常이어늘 六日後에 始用藥하니 七日에 全體面部 髮際以下로 至于脣┌히 汗流滿面하야 淋漓洽足而汗後에 面色帶青하며 有語訥證하더니 八日九日에 語訥耳聾而脣汗이 還爲額汗하고 額汗이 還爲眉稜汗하며 汗出微粒하야 乍出乍入而只有額汗하며 呼吸이 短喘矣호니 至于十日夜하야 額汗이 還入而語訥耳聾이 尤甚하며 痰涎이 壅喉하야 口不能咯하고 病人이 自以手指로 探口拭之而出하고 十一日에 呼吸短喘이 尤甚하니 至于十二日하야 忽然食粥을 二碗하니 斯時에 若論其藥則熊膽散이 或者可也而熊膽이 闕材하니 自念此人이 今夜에 必死矣호라 當日初昏에 呼吸이 暫時少定하고 十三日鷄鳴時에 髮際에 有汗하고 十四日 十五日 連三日을 食粥二三碗하며 額汗眉稜汗顴汗이 次次發出하며 面色이 脫靑하고 十六日에 臆汗이 始通하며 稍能咯痰하며 語訥이 亦癒하고 至于二十日하야 臆汗이 數次大通하고 遂能起立房中하야 諸證이 皆安而耳聾證則自如也호니 病解後에 用藥調理四十日하니 耳聾目迷가 自祛하더라.

As we have seen, from the onset of his illness, this individual experienced both loose stools and diarrhea. After six days of illness, sweat began to appear on his forehead, temple, and then his zygomatic arch. At this point, his appetite and daily activity level occasionally returned to normal. He began my herbal regime on the sixth day of illness. The next day he began to sweat profusely from the frontal hairline downward to the lips and chin. However, shortly afterwards, his lips turned a purplish color and his speech became unclear. On the eighth and ninth days, not only did his speech remain unclear, but he also experienced a loss of hearing. At this point, he stopped sweating around his lips but began to sweat at the zygomatic arch. Shortly afterwards, he stopped sweating at the zygomatic arch and began to sweat at the temple. This sweat, which was shaped like small rice grains, appeared and then disappeared, and then reappeared again at his forehead, followed by labored breathing. On the night of the tenth day of illness, his forehead sweat disappeared and his unclear speech and lack of hearing became significantly worse. His throat was so congested with stagnant phlegm that he tried to scoop it out with his finger. On the 11th day, his shortness of breath worsened, but on the 12th day, he was surprisingly capable of ingesting two bowls of rice porridge.

For the above situation, I felt that Xiong Dan (*Vessica Fellea Ursi*) would be the medicine of choice, but since it was not available, I thought that he would definitely not survive the evening. However, his breathing began to improve early that evening and, at dawn of the next day, he began to sweat from his temple. From the 14th to the 17th day, he was able to consume two to three bowls of rice porridge. During this time, he started to sweat little by little from the forehead, temple, and zygomatic arch, while his purplish complexion began to lighten. On the 16th day, he started to sweat from his chest and was gradually able to expectorate phlegm, which helped to improve the clarity of his speech. On the 20th day, he began to sweat profusely from his chest and he was finally able to walk around his room. At this point, despite his recovery from the second bout of Warm Febrile disease, his hearing didn't improve. However, his hearing and impeded eyesight finally improved after prescribing a total of 40 days of *Jori Peiwon Tang* (Lee Je-ma's Regulate the Interior and Replenish the lung Source Decoction).

**Table 8.2: The Tae Eum Individual's Warm Febrile disease beginning with the onset of External Cold syndrome**

| Syndrome | Common symptoms | Additional symptoms | Treatment approach |
|---|---|---|---|
| Warm Febrile disease (early stage) | Sudden onset of severe chills and high fever | Palpitations, lack of sweat, shortness of breath, and a dry, hacking cough | *Tae Eum Jowi Tang* (Lee Je-ma's Regulate the stomach Decoction for the Tae Eum Individual) **With diarrhea:** Add 3.75g of Chun Gen Pi (*Cortex Ailanthi*) |
| Warm Febrile disease (mid-stage) | | Palpitations, lack of sweat, shortness of breath, a dry, hacking cough, and a lack of appetite | *Tae Eum Jowi Tang* (Lee Je-ma's Regulate the stomach Decoction for the Tae Eum Individual) with 3.75g of Sheng Ma (*Rhizoma Cimicifugae*) and Huang Qin (*Radix Scutellariae*) **With constipation:** *Kalgen Seunggi Tang* (Lee Je-Ma's Kudzu Support the Qi Decoction) |
| Warm Febrile disease (severe stage) | | Dry throat, pale complexion, and diarrhea (combination of excess Cold and Heat symptoms) | *Handa Yulso Tang* (Lee Je-ma's Greater Cold Lesser Heat Decoction) |
| Warm Febrile disease (recovery stage) | | Absence of or mild lingering symptoms with fatigue and weakened *Zheng Qi* | *Jori Peiwon Tang* (Lee Je-ma's Regulate the Interior and Replenish the lung Source Decoction) |

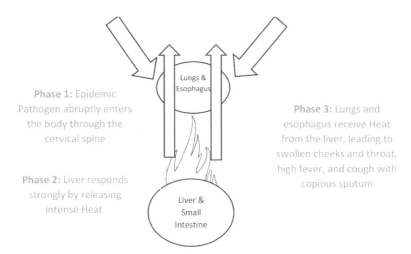

*Figure 8.3: The Warm Febrile syndrome of the Tae Eum Individual*

*Section 2*

# The Tae Eum Individual's Liver Heat Causing Interior Heat Syndrome[1]

太陰人肝受熱裏熱病

朱肱이 曰陽毒은 面赤 斑斑如 錦紋하며 咽喉痛하며 唾膿血이니 宜葛根
解肌湯 黑奴丸이니라 陽毒及壞傷寒은 醫所不治나 精魄이 已竭이라도
心下가 尙煖하거든 幹開其口하고 灌黑奴丸이면 藥下咽에 卽活이니라.

According to Zhu Gong, Yang toxin, which is characterized by a swollen, red-spotted face with a silky texture, sore throat, and expectoration of blood-streaked sputum, should be treated with *Ge Gen Jie Ji Tang* (Kudzu Clear the Flesh Decoction) or *Hei Nu Wan* (Black Servant Pill). Most doctors classify Yang toxin and *Huai Zheng*[2] as incurable diseases. However, Zhu Gong maintained that even if there is a loss of consciousness following these illnesses, if the area below the epigastrium is warm, then opening the mouth and administering *Hei Nu Wan* (Black Servant Pill) could save a life.

李 ┌이 曰微惡寒發熱에 宜葛根解肌湯이오 目疼鼻乾하며 潮汗 閉澁하며
滿渴狂譫에는 宜調胃承氣湯이니라 熱在表則目疼不眠이니 宜解肌
湯이오 熱入裏則狂譫이니 宜調胃承氣湯이니라.

According to Li Ting, minor chills with fever call for *Ge Gen Jie Ji Tang* (Kudzu Clear the Flesh Decoction). If the eyes are painful, the nasal passages are dry with accompanying Yin deficiency symptoms, there is spontaneous sweating with difficult defecation and urination, a swollen abdomen, and thirst, then *Tiao Wei Cheng Qi Tang* (Regulate the stomach Order the Qi Decoction) should be prescribed. If Heat is located at the Exterior, then painful eyes and insomnia will follow. In this case, *Ge Gen Jie Ji Tang* (Kudzu Clear the Flesh Decoction) is appropriate. If Heat is located in the Interior, there will be delirium with incoherent speech, for which *Tiao Wei Cheng Qi Tang* (Regulate the stomach Order the Qi Decoction) is appropriate.

---

1   The spleen and kidneys control absorption and excretion of food and fluid, and the lungs and liver control inhalation and exhalation respectively. Since inhalation and exhalation are at the core of the Tae Eum and Tae Yang Individual's health, imbalance of the liver and lungs will lead directly to Internal disorders. The Tae Eum Individual's liver Heat causing Internal Heat syndrome is due to an inability to regulate his/her *Jung* emotion of complacency, causing laziness and the desire to satisfy one's own, rather than others', needs and desires.

2   *Haui Zheng* (壞症), literally translated as "collapsing syndrome," is a Shang Han illness characterized by severe chills and eruption of red, rice grain-shaped hives throughout the body. It occurs after miscalculation of Shang Han treatment or relapse of illness before full recovery, and is characterized by a Warm Febrile disease following the invasion of an External Heat pathogen. It may also occur after contracting malaria from the invasion of an External Cold-induced pathogen or Internal Wind following the invasion of an External Wind pathogen.

龔信이 曰陽明病은 目疼 鼻乾 不得臥니 宜葛根解肌湯이니라. 三陽病이
深하면 變爲陽毒하야 面赤眼紅하며 身發斑黃하며 或下利黃赤하며 六
脈이 洪大하니 宜黑奴丸이니라.

According to Gong Xin, in the case of Yang Ming stage illness, *Ge Gen Jie Ji Tang*
(Kudzu Clear the Flesh Decoction) should be prescribed if the eyes are painful, the
nasal passages are dry, and insomnia is a problem. He continued by stating that if
the illness spreads to all three Yang stages[3] then Yang toxin will accumulate, resulting
in a red complexion, reddened sclera, and yellowish skin color throughout the body.
There may also be yellowish-red[4] diarrhea and fullness of the six[5] pulses. In this case,
*Hei Nu Wan* (Black Servant Pill) should be prescribed.

論曰右諸證에 當用葛根解肌湯 黑奴丸이니라.

From my perspective, all of the above syndromes should be treated with *Kalgen
Heigi Tang* (Lee Je-ma's Kudzu Clear the Flesh Decoction) and *Hei Nu Wan* (Black
Servant Pill).

**Table 8.3: The Internal Heat Yang Ming syndrome of the Tae Eum Individual**

| Syndrome | Common symptoms | Additional symptoms | Treatment approach |
| --- | --- | --- | --- |
| Yang Ming stage | Sudden onset of severe chills and high fever | Painful eyes, the nasal passages are dry, insomnia, red complexion, reddened sclera, and yellowish skin color throughout the body | *Kalgen Heigi Tang* (Lee Je-ma's Kudzu Clear the Flesh Decoction)<br><br>*Hei Nu Wan* (Black Servant Pill) |

3   "All three Yang stages" refers to the spread of illness to the Tai Yang, Yang Ming, and Shao Yang levels.
4   Yellow and/or red stool is a sign of Internal Heat accumulation.
5   The "six pulses" refers to the *cun, guan,* and *chi* pulse positions of both wrists.

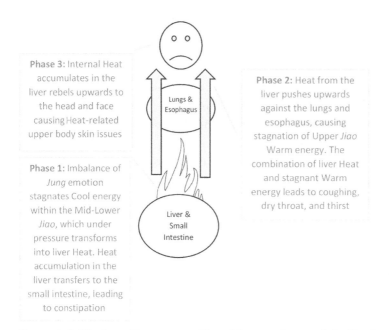

Phase 3: Internal Heat accumulates in the liver rebels upwards to the head and face causing Heat-related upper body skin issues

Phase 1: Imbalance of *Jung* emotion stagnates Cool energy within the Mid-Lower *Jiao*, which under pressure transforms into liver Heat. Heat accumulation in the liver transfers to the small intestine, leading to constipation

Lungs & Esophagus

Liver & Small Intestine

Phase 2: Heat from the liver pushes upwards against the lungs and esophagus, causing stagnation of Upper *Jiao* Warm energy. The combination of liver Heat and stagnant Warm energy leads to coughing, dry throat, and thirst

*Figure 8.4: The liver Heat causing Yang Ming syndrome of the Tae Eum Individual*

靈樞에 曰尺膚에 熱深하여 脈盛躁者는 病瘟也니라.

According to the *Ling Shu*, excessive Heat from the elbow to the wrist and full pulses are a sign of epidemic disease.

王叔和가 曰瘟病脈은 陰陽俱盛하니 病熱之極에는 浮之而滑하며 沈之散 澁하니라.

According to Wang Shu He, exuberant Yin and Yang aspects of the pulse[6] indicate the excessive Heat of an epidemic disease. If light pressure is applied, the pulse will feel slippery, and if heavier pressure is applied, it will be scattered and rough.

脈法에 曰瘟病이 二三日에 體熱 腹滿 頭痛하여 飮食如故하여도 脈直 而疾하면 八日에 死하고 瘟病이 四五日에 頭痛 腹滿而吐하며 脈來細 而强하면 十二日에 死하고 八九日에 頭身不痛하며 目不赤 色不變而 反利하고 脈來澁하야 按之不足하되 擧時大하며 心下堅하면 十七日에 死라.

According to the *Mai Jing* (*The Pulse Classic*), two to three days of fever, swelling of the abdomen, headaches, no loss of appetite, and strong and rapid pulses during an epidemic disease indicate a grave condition from which death occurs within eight days. If there are four to five days of headache, fullness sensation in the abdomen,

---

6    Exuberant Yin and Yang refers to the excessive nature of the pulse in both the superficial (Yang) and deep (Yin) positions.

vomiting, and a thin but strong pulse during an epidemic disease, death will occur within 12 days. If there are no headaches or body aches for eight to nine days, no redness of the sclera, no change in complexion, but diarrhea and a rough pulse that weakens under pressure but feels strong at the superficial layer when pressure is released, and hardness of the epigastric area during an epidemic disease, then death will occur within 17 days.

龔信이 日瘟病에 穰穰大熱하며 脈細小者는 死오 瘟病에 下利痛甚者도 死니라.

According to Gong Xin, excessive fever with a thin and minute pulse, diarrhea, and acute stomach pain during an epidemic disease signal imminent death.

萬曆丙戌에 余寓大梁한대 瘟疫이 大作하야 士民이 多斃라. 其證이 增寒壯熱하야 頭面項頰이 赤腫하며 咽喉腫痛하며 昏憒어늘 余가 發一秘方하고 名曰二聖救苦丸이니 大黃四兩 猪牙厂角二兩을 麵糊에 和丸綠豆大 五七十丸하야 一服卽汗하고 一汗卽愈니 稟壯者는 百發百中이니라. 皂角은 開關竅 發其表하고 大黃은 瀉諸火 通其裏하니라.

Gong Xin continued by stating that, in the year of the third stem and the 11th branch,[7] when he resided in Da Liang,[8] many farmers died after contracting an extremely prevalent form of epidemic illness, which was characterized by chills and severe fever with swelling and redness of the head, face, nape of the neck, and cheeks. These individuals also suffered from sore throats and swelling, and muddled consciousness. At this time he discovered a remedy called *Er Sheng Jiu Ku Wan* (Two Saints Rescue the Suffering Pill),[9] which consists of 225g of Da Huang (*Radix et Rhizoma Rhei*) and 75g of Zao Jiao (*Gleditsia Sinensis*). Gong Xin prepared this remedy by grinding it into a powder and shaping it into green pea-sized pills. After ingestion of 50 to 70 pills, sweating occurred without fail. Even after just one bout of sweat, there was a 100 percent chance of recovery among those who originally had a strong constitution. Zao Jiao (*Gleditsia Sinensis*) is capable of opening the orifices and expelling External pathogens, while Da Huang (*Radix et Rhizoma Rhei*) sedates Fire and promotes Interior flow.

---

7 The reference to "stems" and "branches" is a common method of recording time (year, month, day, and hour) according to the Chinese lunar calendar.

8 Da Liang (大梁), currently referred to as Kaifeng (開封), is a prefecture-level city in the east-central Henan Province of China, and formerly the capital of the Song Dynasty.

9 This formula first appeared in Gong Xin's *Wan Bing Hui Chun* (*Restoring Health from Tens of Thousands of Diseases*) and was later mentioned in the *Dongeui Bogam* (*The Mirror of Eastern Medicine*), written by Heo Jun.

感四時不正之氣하면 使人痰涎壅盛하고 煩熱하며 頭疼 身痛하며 增寒壯熱하야 項强睛疼하며 或飮食如常하며 起居依舊하되 甚至聲啞하며 或赤眼 口瘡하며 大小ᄀ腫하며 喉痺 咳嗽하고 稠粘噴嚏니라.

Unseasonal weather may lead to excess phlegm and saliva, headaches and body aches, chills, and fever with swelling of the throat and eye pain. In such cases the appetite is not affected and life carries on as usual; when severe, however, the throat will be so swollen that speech is impossible; the eyes will become red and swollen, mouth sores will form, as will boils on the cheeks, throat *Bi* syndrome will occur, with sneezing and coughing with copious sputum.

論曰右諸證에서 增寒壯熱 燥澁者는 當用ᄀ角大黃湯 葛根承氣湯이오 頭面項頰이 赤腫者도 當用皂角大黃湯 葛根承氣湯이오 體熱 腹滿自利者는 熱勝則裏證也니 當用葛根解肌湯이오 寒勝則表證而太重證也니 當用太陰調胃湯 加升麻 黃芩이니라.

From my perspective, if the above syndromes are accompanied by strong chills, excessive fever, and hard stool, then *Jogak Daehwang Tang* (Lee Je-ma's Honeylocust and Rhubarb Decoction) or *Kalgen Seunggi Tang* (Lee Je-ma's Kudzu Support the Qi Decoction) should be administered. These formulae should also be used if there is redness and swelling of the head, face, neck, and/or cheeks. With fever, fullness of the abdomen, and diarrhea with excessive Heat, it is classified as an Internal illness and should be treated with *Kalgen Heigi Tang* (Lee Je-ma's Kudzu Clear the Flesh Decoction). If these symptoms are accompanied with Exterior illness and excessive Cold symptoms, an extremely acute situation exists and should be treated with *Tae Eum Jowi Tang* (Lee Je-ma's Regulate the stomach Decoction for the Tae Eum Individual) with added Sheng Ma (*Rhizoma Cimicifugae*) and Huang Qin (*Radix Scutellariae*).

嘗治太陰人肝熱熱證 瘟病할새 有一太陰人의 素病이 數年來로 眼病이 時作時止矣호니 此人이 得瘟病이어늘 自始發日로 用熱多寒少湯하야 三四五日하니 大便이 或滑或泄하다가 至六日하야 有大便一日不通之 證이어늘 仍用葛根承氣湯하야 連三日하니 粥食大倍하고 又用三日하니 疫氣大減하니라 病解後에 復用熱多寒少湯하되 大便이 燥澁則加大黃 一錢하고 滑泄太多則去大黃하야 如此調理를 二十日하니 其人이 完健하니라.

I once treated a Tae Eum Individual suffering from Internal liver Heat syndrome due to the onset of a Warm Febrile disease. For several years prior, he also suffered from chronic insomnia, contributing to the onset of Internal liver Heat.[10] From the first

---

10    In this sentence, Lee Je-ma describes how epidemic (Warm Febrile) disease doesn't necessarily afflict everyone in its path. A lack of sleep contributed to the onset of liver Heat in the patient discussed, which in turn caused susceptibility to epidemic disease onset.

day of his Warm Febrile disease, I prescribed *Yulda Hanso Tang* (Lee Je-ma's Greater Heat and Lesser Cold Decoction), and after the third to fifth day of ingesting these herbs, he had reddish diarrhea. On the sixth day, he was not able to have a bowel movement, so I prescribed three days of *Kalgen Seunggi Tang* (Lee Je-ma's Kudzu Support the Qi Decoction). After he ingested this formula, his appetite increased significantly. Another three days of ingestion, and his Heat-related symptoms greatly improved. Following his recovery, I prescribed *Yulda Hanso Tang* (Lee Je-ma's Greater Heat and Lesser Cold Decoction), but his stools again became dry and hard to pass. I then either added or omitted 3.75g of Da Huang (*Radix et Rhizoma Rhei*) depending on whether [he was constipated] or his stools were too loose. I continued to attend his illness for another 20 days, leading to a full recovery.

此病이 始發에 嘔逆口吐하며 昏憒不省하야 重痛矣하더니 末境에 反爲 輕證하야 十二日而病解하니라.

During the early stages of his illness, this patient experienced an upset stomach, vomiting, muddled consciousness, and unbearable aches and pains. His condition improved as time went on, and by the 12th day he completely recovered.

一太陰人 十歲兒가 得裏熱瘟病하야 粥食을 全不入口하며 藥亦不入 口하고 壯熱穰穰하야 有時飮冷水호니 至于十一日則大便不通이 已四 日矣라. 怔忪 譫語曰有百蟲이 滿室이라하며 又有鼠入懷云하고 奔遑匍 匐하며 驚呼啼泣하다가 有時熱極生風하야 兩手厥冷하며 兩膝이 伸而不 屈이어늘 急用葛根承氣湯하야 不憚啼泣하고 强灌口中하니 卽日에 粥食 大倍하고 疫氣大解하야 倖而得生하니라.

I once treated a ten-year-old Tae Eum Individual who suffered from Internal liver Heat syndrome and contracted a Warm Febrile disease, causing a total loss of appetite and inability to ingest herbal medicine. His Heat syndrome was so acute that he continuously drank cold water. He first experienced 11 days of sporadic constipation, and then four days of absolutely no bowel movement whatsoever. In his anguish, he began to hallucinate, and complained of bugs piling up in his room and mice crawling within his chest. He would then lie on his stomach, screaming and crying. Occasionally his fever would decrease and he would contract *Feng* syndrome,[11] leading to extreme coldness of his hands and stiffness of his legs, making it impossible for him to bend his knees. I immediately prescribed *Kalgen Seunggi Tang* (Lee Je-ma's Kudzu Support the Qi Decoction) by forcing open his mouth to pour in the medicine despite his frantic crying. From that day onward, his

---

11   *Feng* (風) translates as "Wind." Hence, "*Feng* syndrome" refers to the stirring of Internal Wind, resulting in spasms, tremors, loss of consciousness, psychotic behavior, and/or stiffness of the extremities. In this chapter, Lee Je-ma discusses two types of *Feng* syndromes: *Man Jing Feng* (childhood convulsions/fright seizures) and *Zhong Feng* (Wind stroke).

appetite increased significantly, his epidemic illness greatly diminished, and his life was fortunately saved.

此病이 始發四五日에 飲食起居가 如常하야 無異平人矣하다가 末境에 反爲重證호니 十七日而病解하니라.

During the first four to five days of this illness, his appetite didn't change and he was able to carry out his daily affairs, appearing as if he were healthy. His symptoms became more serious towards the end of the illness, from which he recovered in 17 days.

**Table 8.4: The Internal Heat Warm Febrile disease syndrome of the Tae Eum Individual**

| Syndrome | Common symptoms | Additional symptoms | Treatment approach |
|---|---|---|---|
| Unseasonal weather leading to epidemic illness | **Early onset:** Phlegm and saliva, headaches and body aches, chills, and fever with swelling of the throat and eye pain<br><br>**Severe cases:** Strong chills and severe fever with swelling and redness of the head, face, nape of the neck, and cheeks, throat soreness and swelling, and muddled consciousness | Severe cases with hard stools, constipation | *Jogak Daehwang Tang* (Lee Je-ma's Honeylocust and Rhubarb Decoction)<br><br>or<br><br>*Kalgen Seunggi Tang* (Lee Je-Ma's Kudzu Support the Qi Decoction) |
| | | Severe cases with fullness of the abdomen, and diarrhea | *Kalgen Heigi Tang* (Lee Je-ma's Kudzu Clear the Flesh Decoction) |
| | | Extremely severe cases with excessive Cold signs and symptoms (combined Internal and External illness—extremely acute situation) | *Tae Eum Jowi Tang* (Lee Je-ma's Regulate the stomach Decoction for the Tae Eum Individual) with added Sheng Ma (*Rhizoma Cimicifugae*) and Huang Qin (*Radix Scutellariae*) |

內經에 曰諸澀에 枯 涸 皴揭는 皆屬於燥니라.

According to the *Nei Jing*, dryness of the skin throughout the body, malnutrition, azoospermia or amenorrhea, and dry cracking of the skin or peeling away of the finger—or toenails—are all associated with *Zao* syndrome.[12]

---

12  *Zao* (燥) translates as "dryness." Hence, *Zao* syndrome describes a lack of moisture and nourishment within the body. As Lee Je-ma said, this syndrome is due to long-term Internal liver Heat accumulation, which eventually scorches the bodily fluids. The character for *Zao* may also be translated as vexation, anxiousness, or worry. If left to their own devices, these emotions will eventually instigate Internal liver Heat and trigger *Zao* syndrome.

論曰太陰人이 面色靑白者는 多無燥證하고 面色黃赤黑者는 多有燥
證하니 蓋肝熱肺燥而然也니라

In my experience, if an individual has a bluish-pale complexion, then in most cases they will not have *Zao* syndrome. A yellowish-red or darkish complexion, in most cases, is a sign of *Zao* syndrome, which is due to Heat in the liver and dryness of the lungs.

嘗治太陰人 燥熱證 手指焦黑癍瘡病할새 自左手中指로 焦黑無力하야 二
年內에 一指黑血이 焦凝過掌心而掌背浮腫이어늘 以刀斷指矣하니 又一
年內에 癍瘡이 遍滿全體하야 大者는 如大錢하며 小者는 如小錢하니 得
病이 已爲三年而以壯年人으로 手力이 不能役勞一半刻하며 足力이 不
能日行步三十里라 以熱多寒少湯 用藁本 二錢 加大黃 一錢하야 二十八
貼用之호니 大便始滑하다가 不過一二日하야 又秘燥이어늘 又用二十
貼하니 人便不甚滑泄하며 而面部癍瘡이 少差하고 手力足力이 稍快有效
矣어늘 又用二十貼하니 其病이 快差하니라.

I once attended a Tae Eum Individual with *Zao* syndrome, whose fingers appeared charred with Heat-induced ulcerated sores. His illness began on the middle finger of his left hand, where his skin became dry and black, and lacked strength. Within two years, the dry and blackened skin spread from one finger to his entire palm, causing swelling of the palmar and dorsal aspect of his hand. I proceeded by slicing off the skin around the ulcer, but two years later, the ulcers reappeared and spread throughout his body. The larger ulcerative sores were the size of a quarter, while the smaller ones were the size of a nickel. After three years of illness, despite being at the prime of his life, his hands were so weak that he could not work for more than a half hour. With a loss of strength in his legs, he was unable to walk his regular seven miles per day.[13] His bowels became looser after I prescribed 28 packs of *Yulda Hanso Tang* (Lee Je-ma's Greater Heat and Lesser Cold Decoction) with 7.5g of Gao Ben (*Rhizoma Ligustici*) and 3.75g of Da Huang (*Radix et Rhizoma Rhei*), but within one to two days, they became hard and difficult to pass again. After 20 further packs, [his stools were much looser] with occasional light bouts of diarrhea, the ulcers on his face slowly began to heal, and his legs began to strengthen. After an additional 20 packs, he completely overcame his illness.

---

13  According to today's standards, seven miles a day may sound like a substantial walking distance. However, during Lee Je-ma's lifetime, walking was still the primary mode of transportation, likely making this an average daily walking distance for a healthy adult.

靈樞에 曰二陽結을 謂之消니 飮一溲二면 死不治니라. 註에 曰二陽結은 謂胃及大腸에 熱結也니라.

According to the *Ling Shu*, Xiao Ge syndrome is due to the binding together of the Two Yang Energies. In the terminal stage of this illness, after drinking one glass of water, there will be two or more times the output of urination. [According to the *Dongeui Bogam*,][14] the binding of the Two Yang refers to Heat stagnation of the stomach and the large intestine.

扁鵲難經에 曰消渴脈은 當得緊實而數이어늘 反得沈濇而微者는 死니라.

According to the *Bian Que Nan Jing*, Xiao Ge[15] is characterized by a tight, excessive, and rapid pulse. However, if it is accompanied by a deep, weak, rough, and minute pulse, then death is imminent.

張仲景이 曰消渴病에 小便反多하야 如飮水一斗에 小便亦一斗면 腎氣丸을 主之니라.

In the *Shang Han Lun*, Zhang Zhongjing states that *Xiao Ge* syndrome is characterized by excessive urine and that one sip of water, in this case, will yield the same amount of urine, for which *Jin Gui Shen Qi Wan* (kidney Qi Pill from the Golden Cabinet)[16] should be prescribed.

論曰此病은 非少陽人消渴也ㅣ오 卽太陰人燥熱也ㅣ니 此證에 不當用腎氣丸이오 當用熱多寒少湯 加藁本 大黃이니라.

From my perspective, this illness is not the *Xiao Ge* syndrome of the So Yang Individual, but instead the *Zao Re* syndrome of the Tae Eum Individual. *Yulda Hanso Tang* (Lee Je-ma's Greater Heat and Lesser Cold Decoction) with Gao Ben (*Rhizoma Ligustici*) and Da Huang (*Radix et Rhizoma Rhei*) should be prescribed instead of *Jin Gui Shen Qi Wan* (kidney Qi Pill from the Golden Cabinet).

---

14  In this sentence, Lee Je-ma refers to the *Difficult to Treat Illnesses* chapter of the *Dongeui Bogam*, which states: "According to the *Nei Jing*, the Two Yang is referred to as *Xiao* (消), which can be interpreted as the accumulation and blockage of Heat in the stomach and large intestine. The stomach and large intestine store Heat and disperse/eliminate *Su Gok* from the body." The Two Yang is another name for Yang Ming, which consists of two Yang organs: the stomach and large intestine. If excessive Heat accumulates in the Yang Ming, appetite and food intake will increase, but nourishment of the soft tissue will decrease, resulting in malnourishment and dryness, or *Xiao* (消).

15  *Xiao Ge* (消渴), as mentioned in the *stomach Heat Causing Internal Heat* section of Chapter 7, translates literally as "wasting and thirsting disorder." Lee Je-ma refers to this syndrome as *Xiao Re* (燥熱) of the Tae Eum Individual. The difference between both syndromes is that the former is due to stomach Heat eventually causing dryness and wasting of the So Yang Individual's weaker kidneys, while the latter comes from liver Heat eventually causing dryness and wasting of the Tae Eum Individual's weaker lungs.

16  Lee Je-ma doesn't refer to *Jin Gui Shen Qi Wan* elsewhere in this text and so its ingredients are listed here: Sheng Di Huang (*Radix Rehmanniae*) 24g, Shan Zhu Yu (*Fructus Corni Officinalis*) 12g, Shan Yao (*Radix Dioscoreae Oppositae*) 12g, Fu Zi (*Radix Aconiti*) 3g, Gui Zhi (*Ramulus Cinnomomi Cassiae*) 3g, Ze Xie (*Rhizoma Alismatis*) 9g, Fu Ling (*Poria Alba*) 9g, and Mu Dan Pi (*Cortex Moutan*) 9g. Source: *Jin Gui Yao Lue* (*Essentials from the Golden Cabinet*).

嘗治太陰人 年五十近衰者가 燥熱病에 引飲 小便多하며 大便秘者할새
用熱多寒少湯 用藁本 二錢 加大黃 一錢하야 二十貼하니 得效矣라 後一
月餘에 用他醫藥五貼하니 此人이 更病이어늘 復用熱多寒少湯 加藁本
大黃하야 五六十貼하니 用藥時間에는 其病이 僅僅支撑하다가 後에 終
不免死하고 又嘗治太陰人年少者가 燥熱病할새 用此方三百貼하야 得支
撑一周年하다가 此病이 亦不免死하니 此人이 得病一周年에 或間 用他
醫方인지 未知緣何故也로다. 蓋燥熱이 至於飲一溲二而病劇則難治니라.
凡太陰人이 大便秘燥하며 小便覺多而引飲者는 不可不早治豫防이니라.

I once treated a Tae Eum Individual, about 50 years old, who weakened with age, suffering from *Zao Re* syndrome. I successfully addressed his frequent urination and hardened stools by prescribing 20 packs of *Yulda Hanso Tang* (Lee Je-ma's Greater Heat and Lesser Cold Decoction) with 7.5g of Gao Ben (*Rhizoma Ligustici*) and 3.75g of Da Huang (*Radix et Rhizoma Rhei*). However, one month thereafter, he ingested about five packs of medicine from another doctor, whereupon his symptoms returned. I continued by prescribing 50 to 60 more packs of the above formula, and just when his symptoms started to resolve, he passed away.[17]

I later treated a Tae Eum adolescent with *Zao Re* syndrome with 300 packs of the same formula for about one year, but he too passed away. After one year of illness, he also occasionally ingested medicine prescribed from another doctor. Yet there is no way of knowing whether this had anything to do with his death.

In most cases, if an individual urinates twice the amount of his or her water intake, then treatment will be challenging. It is absolutely necessary to start treatment as early as possible if a Tae Eum Individual experiences hardened stools, excessive urination, and thirst.

此病은 非必不治之病也로되 此少年이 得病用藥一周年後에 方死하니 蓋
此病原委는 侈樂無厭하고 慾火外馳하야 肝熱大盛하며 肺燥太枯之故
也니라. 若此小年이 安心滌慾 一百日而用藥 則焉有不治之理乎아 蓋自始
病日로 至于終死日이 慾火가 無日不馳인 故也라. 諺에 曰先祖德澤은 雖
或不得一一個報而恭敬德澤은 必無一一不受報라하니 凡無論某病人하고
恭敬其心하며 蕩滌慾火하야 安靜善心하면 一百日則其病이 無不愈오 二
百日則其人이 無不完하리니 恭敬德澤之箇箇受報가 百事皆然而疾病이
尤甚하니라.

Despite the fact that the Tae Eum adolescent above eventually lost his life after a year of treatment, *Zao Re* syndrome itself is by no means incurable. As a general rule,

---

17    During the 1800s in Korea, one's lifespan was considerably shorter than now. Lee Je-ma himself passed away at age 63.

*Zao Re* is due to the inability to contain the fire of one's selfish desires,[18] leading to extreme liver Heat that in turn results in *Fei Zao* syndrome.[19] I would imagine that if this young man had calmed his mind and refrained from sexual intercourse for 100 days while taking medicine, how could his situation not have improved? I heard that from the start of his illness to the time of his death, there was not a single day in which his flame of desire was ever contained.

There is a saying that "no matter how much we try, there is no way to show enough patronage to our ancestors, yet they are rewarded day after day if we cultivate our heart and mind." It goes without question that anyone in the above situation would have improved their health if, for 100 days, they cultivated their mind, rid themselves of selfishness, and practiced kindness. And after 200 days, they would undoubtedly recover entirely from the illness. The Virtue of self-cultivation influences every action we take, day after day, especially when it comes to overcoming illness.

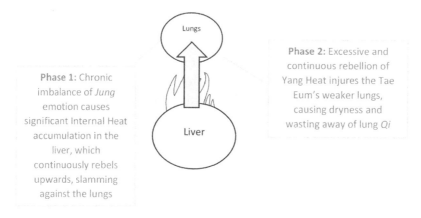

*Figure 8.5: The liver Heat causing Fei Zao syndrome of the Tae Eum Individual*

---

18  "Selfish desires" is a translation of the term *Chirak Muyom* (侈樂無厭), literally "Lacking Control of Indulgence and Complacency." As mentioned in Chapter 3, if the Tae Eum Individual doesn't control his or her *Song* nature of joy, then it can morph into the *Jung* emotion of complacency. The "fire of one's desire" is a translation of *Yok Hwa* (慾火), which is also interpreted as "sexual cravings." Lee Je-ma is likely referring to the fact that the above Tae Eum Individual engaged in excessive sexual activity.

19  *Fei Zao* (肺燥) translates literally as "lung dryness," a result of excessive liver Heat that burns away the moisture of the Tae Eum Individual's weakest organ, the lungs. Lee Je-ma also refers to this term simply as *Zao* (燥) elsewhere in this text.

危亦林이 曰陰血耗竭하야 耳聾 目暗하며 脚弱 腰痛이어든 宜用黑元
丹이니라. 凡男子가 方當壯年而眞氣猶怯은 此乃稟賦素弱이오 非虛而
然이라 滋益之方이 群品이 稍衆이로되 藥力이 細微하야 難見功效하니
但固天元一氣하야 使水升火降하면 則五臟이 自和하야 百病이 不
生하리니 宜用拱辰丹이니라.

According to Wei Yilin, exhaustion of Yin and blood is characterized by loss of hearing and vision, weakness of the legs, and pain of the lower back. He suggested that *He Yuan Dan* (Black Source Pill)[20] be prescribed for this. If a male experiences a loss of *Zhen Qi* in his middle age, it is due to a deficiency of pre-natal energy rather than age. Despite the availability of many different tonifying herbs, most of them are not strong enough to handle this. However, if herbs that focus on descending Fire and ascending Water are utilized in conjunction with supporting the *Yuan Qi*, then the Five *Zhang* will achieve balance, and no illness will go unchallenged. For this reason, he prescribed *Gong Chen Dan* (Embrace the King Pill).[21]

論曰此證에 當用黑元與拱辰丹이나 當歸 山茱萸는 皆爲蠹材라 藥力이
未全하니 欲收全力하거든 宜用拱辰黑元丹 鹿茸大補湯이니라.

From my perspective, *He Yuan Dan* (Black Source Pill) or *Gong Chen Dan* (Embrace the King Pill) are appropriate for use in the above situation, but since Dang Gui (*Radix Angelicae Sinensis*) and Shan Zhu Yu (*Fructus Corni Officinalis*) have no significant role to play here, they should be omitted. In order to achieve the most effective results, *Gongjin Hukwon Dan* (Lee Je-ma's Embrace the King Black Source Pill) or *Nogyung Daebo Tang* (Lee Je-ma's Deer Antler Great Tonification Decoction) should be prescribed.

20   Lee Je-ma doesn't mention *He Yuan Dan* elsewhere in this text, so here are its ingredients: Dang Gui (*Radix Angelicae Sinensis*) 80g, and Lu Rong (*Cornu Cervi Pantotrichum*) 40g. Preparation: Steep Dang Gui in alcohol and boil Lu Rong to remove milky residue and then roast until dry. Afterwards, grind these ingredients into powder and combine with plaster made from the flesh of Wu Mei (*Fructus Mume*). Form into oat-sized pills and then ingest 50 to 70 pills with warm rice wine. Source: *Dongeui Bogam* (*Mirror of Eastern Medicine*).

21   Lee Je-ma doesn't mention *Gong Chen Dan* elsewhere in this text, so its ingredients are listed here: Lu Rong (*Cornu Cervi Pantotrichum*) 160g, Dang Gui (*Radix Angelicae Sinensis*) 160g, Shan Zhu Yu (*Fructus Corni Officinalis*) 160g, and She Xiang (*Moschus*) 20g. Preparation: Boil Lu Rong to remove milky residue and then roast until dry. Grind these ingredients into powder and combine with flour paste. Form into oat-sized pills and then ingest 50 to 70 pills with a pinch of salt in warm rice wine. Source: *Dongeui Bogam* (*Mirror of Eastern Medicine*).

**Table 8.5: The Internal Heat *Zao Re* syndrome of the Tae Eum Individual**

| Syndrome | Common symptoms | Additional symptoms | Treatment approach |
|---|---|---|---|
| *Zao Re* syndrome | Frequent and/or excessive urination | With hardened stools and thirst | *Yulda Hanso Tang* (Lee Je-ma's Greater Heat and Lesser Cold Decoction) with 7.5g of Gao Ben (*Rhizoma Ligustici*) and 3.75g of Da Huang (*Radix et Rhizoma Rhei*) |
| | | Three to four bouts of nocturnal emissions within a month; it is considered a serious illness due to exhaustion and overwork | *Yulda Hanso Tang* (Lee Je-ma's Greater Heat and Lesser Cold Decoction)<br><br>**If constipated:**<br>Add 3.75g of Da Huang (*Radix et Rhizoma Rhei*) |
| | | Loss of hearing and vision, weakness of the legs, and pain of the lower back especially after meals (after onset of serious internal illness), coughing | *Gongjin Hukwon Dan* (Lee Je-ma's Embrace the King Black Source Pill) |
| | | Loss of *Yuan Qi* in middle age | *Nogyung Daebo Tang* (Lee Je-ma's Deer Antler Great Tonification Decoction) |

# A Synopsis of Tae Eum Illness

# 泛論

太陰人證에 有食後痞滿과 腿脚無力病하니 宜用拱辰黑元丹 鹿茸大補湯 太陰調胃湯 調胃升淸湯이니라.

If a Tae Eum Individual experiences fullness of the chest and abdomen and a loss of leg strength after meals, then *Gongjin Hukwon Dan* (Lee Je-ma's Embrace the King Black Source Pill), *Nogyung Daebo Tang* (Lee Je-ma's Deer Antler Great Tonification Decoction), *Tae Eum Jowi Tang* (Lee Je-ma's Regulate the stomach Decoction for the Tae Eum Individual), or *Jowi Seungchong Tang* (Lee Je-ma's Regulate the stomach Support and Clear Decoction) are advised.

太陰人證에 有泄瀉病하니 表寒證泄瀉는 當用太陰調胃湯이오 表熱證泄 瀉는 當用葛根蘿卜子湯이니라.

If a Tae Eum Individual experiences diarrhea in conjunction with an Exterior Cold-induced syndrome, then *Tae Eum Jowi Tang* (Lee Je-ma's Regulate the stomach Decoction for the Tae Eum Individual) should be prescribed. If they experience diarrhea in conjunction with Exterior Heat-induced syndrome, then *Kalgen Nabokja Tang* (Lee Je-ma's Kudzu Root and Radish Seed Decoction)[1] is pertinent.

太陰人證에 有咳嗽病하니 宜用太陰調胃湯 鹿茸大補湯 拱辰黑元 丹이니라.

For cough-related illness of the Tae Eum Individual, *Tae Eum Jowi Tang* (Lee Je-ma's Regulate the stomach Decoction for the Tae Eum Individual), *Nogyung Daebo Tang* (Lee Je-ma's Deer Antler Great Tonification Decoction), or *Gongjin Hukwon Dan* (Lee Je-ma's Embrace the King Black Source Pill) should be prescribed.

太陰人證에 有哮喘病하니 重證也라 當用麻黃定喘湯이니라.

Wheezing is considered a serious illness of the Tae Eum Individual and should be treated with *Mahwang Jongchun Tang* (Lee Je-ma's Ma Huang Ephedra Arrest Wheezing Decoction).

---

1    Lee Je-ma doesn't mention *Kalgen Nabokja Tang* elsewhere in this text, so its ingredients are listed here: Ge Gen (*Radix Puerariae*) 15g, Lai Fu Zi (*Semen Raphani*) 7.5g, Huang Qin (*Radix Scutellariae*) 3.75g, Jie Geng (*Radix Platycodi*) 3.75g, Gao Ben (*Rhizoma Ligustici*) 3.75g, Bai Zhi (*Radix Angelicae Dahuricae*) 3.75g, Sheng Ma (*Rhizoma Cimicifugae*) 3.75g, and Da Huang (*Radix et Rhizoma Rhei*) 3.75g. Source: *Dongeui Sasang Chobangjup* (*Collection of Sasang Medical Prescriptions*).

太陰人證에 有胸腹痛病하니 危險證也라 當用麻黃定痛湯이니라.

The combination of chest and abdomen pain constitutes a critical illness of the Tae Eum Individual and should be treated with *Mahwang Jongtong Tang* (Lee Je-ma's Ephedra Decoction for Pain).

太陰人小兒가 有泄瀉十餘次 無度者는 必發慢驚風하니 宜用補肺元 湯하야 豫備慢風이니라.

If a Tae Eum infant experiences ten or more bouts of diarrhea, then they will inevitably experience *Man Jing Feng* syndrome.[2] In order to prevent this illness *Bopei Won Tang* (Lee Je-ma's Tonify the Source Qi of the lungs Decoction) should be prescribed.

太陰人이 有腹脹浮腫病하니 當用乾栗蹄[　湯이니라. 此病은 極危險證而 十生九死之病也丨라 雖用藥病愈라도 三年內에 不再發然後에 方可論 生이니 戒侈樂 禁嗜然하며 三年內에 宜恭敬心身이니 調養愼攝이 必在 其人矣니라. 凡太陰人病에 若待浮腫已發而治之則十病九死也니 此病은 不可以病論之而以死論之可也라. 然則如之何其可也오

For abdominal swelling and edema of the Tae Eum Individual, *Konyul Jaejo Tang* (Lee Jae-ma's Chestnut and Grub Decoction) should be prescribed. This illness is extremely critical and only one out of ten people afflicted will survive. Even if an individual survives one bout of this syndrome, if it recurs within three years, the chances of survival are even slimmer. After its occurrence, one must refrain from sexual activity, cultivate one's mind, regulate one's diet, and avoid anything that could interfere with one's health for three years. No matter what illness the Tae Eum Individual struggles with, if it is accompanied by edema, then nine out of ten people will not survive. This is not an issue of curing illness, but instead one of avoiding death. So how can there be a perfect cure?

凡太陰人이 勞心焦思하야 屢謀不成者가 或有久泄久痢와 或淋病 小便不 利와 食後痞滿과 腿脚無力病하니 皆浮腫之漸이니 已爲重險病而此時에 以浮腫論而蕩滌慾火하며 恭敬其心하고 用藥治之可也니라.

In general, if a Tae Eum Individual labors his or her mind, feels excessively worried and stressed,[3] or gets continuously disappointed from unsuccessful ventures, he or she will eventually experience long-term diarrhea, dysentery, gonorrhea, difficult urination, fullness in the chest and abdomen after eating, and/or weakness of the

---

2   *Man Jing Feng* (慢驚風) syndrome, translated as "childhood convulsions" or "fright seizures," occurs primarily in childhood, and is the result of excessive bouts of diarrhea or vomiting due to Warm Febrile disease, or administration of excessively Cold-natured herbs. It is characterized by frightful hallucinations, convulsions, seizures, and general body weakness and/or stiffness without the occurrence of fever.

3   "Laboring the mind, excess worry and stress" is a translation of *Noshim Josa* (勞心焦思)—it emerges from the Tae Eum Individual's inability to regulate their *Song* nature of joy.

legs. All of these symptoms indicate the onset of edema, and are already considered components of a serious illness. The perfect cure for this illness is nothing other than being aware that edema is likely to occur, being cautious, ridding oneself of selfish tendencies, and taking herbal medicine.

**Table 8.6: The Esophageal Cold syndrome of the Tae Eum Individual**

| Syndrome | General information | Common symptoms | Additional symptoms | Treatment approach |
|---|---|---|---|---|
| Esophageal Cold | First stage of Exterior Cold attack with *Zheng Qi* still intact | Chills and fever | Headaches, body aches, (possible) joint pain, a lack of sweating, and shortness of breath | *Mahwang Balpyo Tang* (Ma Huang Release the Exterior Decoction) |
| | A. External Cold pathogenic attack with concurrent indigestion/diarrhea due to Yin and food stagnation<br>B. First stage of Warm Febrile disease | | Palpitations, lack of sweat, shortness of breath, and a dry, hacking cough | *Tae Eum Jowi Tang* (Lee Je-ma's Regulate the stomach Decoction for the Tae Eum Individual) |
| | Strong pathogen and weakening *Zheng Qi* after long battle | | Fullness of the chest and abdomen and loss of leg strength after meals | *Tae Eum Jowi Tang* (Lee Je-ma's Regulate the stomach Decoction for the Tae Eum Individual)<br>*Jowi Seungchong Tang* (Lee Je-ma's Regulate the stomach Support and Clear Decoction)<br>*Nogyung Daebo Tang* (Lee Je-ma's Deer Antler Great Tonification Decoction) |
| | External attack with Cold toxin accumulation in chest, which leads to sinking of Yin Qi | | Indigestion with diarrhea | **With more External Cold signs:**<br>*Tae Eum Jowi Tang* (Lee Je-ma's Regulate the stomach Decoction for the Tae Eum Individual) with 3.75g of Chun Gen Pi (*Cortex Ailanthi*)<br>**With more External Heat signs:**<br>*Kalgen Nabokja Tang* (Lee Je-ma's Kudzu Root and Radish Seed Decoction) |

| Syndrome | General information | Common symptoms | Additional symptoms | Treatment approach |
|---|---|---|---|---|
| Esophageal Cold | Pathogenic attack with history of *Zheng Qi* deficiency | Chills and fever | Lingering cough (after Exterior pathogenic attack), fatigue<br><br>**Other potential symptoms:**<br><br>Frequent bouts of nocturnal emission, exhaustion and overwork | *Nogyung Daebo Tang* (Lee Je-ma's Deer Antler Great Tonification Decoction) |
| | Severe pathogenic Yin stagnation in the chest | | Wheezing and asthma | *Mahwang Jongchun Tang* (Lee Je-ma's Ma Huang Ephedra Arrest Wheezing Decoction) |
| | Severe/critical pathogenic Yin stagnation in the chest that spreads to abdomen | | Acute chest and abdomen pain | *Mahwang Jongtong Tang* (Lee Je-ma's Ephedra Decoction for Pain) |
| | Congenital *Zheng Qi* deficiency with External Cold influence | | Ten or more bouts of diarrhea leading to *Man Jing Feng* syndrome | *Bopei Won Tang* (Lee Je-ma's Tonify the Source Qi of the lungs Decoction) |
| | Critical/mortal pathogenic Yin stagnation in the abdomen | | Acute edema and swelling of the abdomen | *Konyul Jaejo Tang* (Lee Jae-ma's Chestnut and Grub Decoction) |

太陰人證에 有夢泄病하니 一月內에 三四發者는 虛勞라 重證也ㅣ니 大
便秘一日則宜用熱多寒少湯 加大黃 一錢하고 大便每日不秘則加龍骨 減
大黃하거나 或用拱辰黑元丹 鹿茸大補湯하라 此病은 出於謀慮太多하며
思想無窮하니라.

If a Tae Eum Individual experiences three to four bouts of nocturnal emissions within a month, it is considered a serious illness due to exhaustion and overwork. If there is even one day of constipation, then *Yulda Hanso Tang* (Lee Je-ma's Greater Heat and Lesser Cold Decoction) with 3.75g of Da Huang (*Radix et Rhizoma Rhei*) should be prescribed. If the stools are soft and flow regularly, then *Yulda Hanso Tang* (Lee Je-ma's Greater Heat and Lesser Cold Decoction) with Long Gu (*Os Draconis*), *Gongjin Hukwon Dan* (Lee Je-ma's Embrace the King Black Source Pill), or *Nogyung Daebo Tang* (Lee Je-ma's Deer Antler Great Tonification Decoction) should be prescribed. I have thorough experience treating this illness, as it occurs much more often than one would imagine.

太陰人證에 有卒中風病하니 胸臆이 格格有窒塞聲而目瞪者는 必用瓜蒂
散이오 手足拘攣하고 眼合者는 當用牛黃淸心丸이니라 素面色이 黃赤黑
者는 多有目瞪者하고 素面色이 靑白者는 多有眼合者하나니 面色이 靑
白而眼合者는 手足拘攣則其病이 急危也니 不必待拘攣하고 但見眼合而
素面色이 靑者에 必急用淸心丸이니 古方淸心丸이 每每神效하니라. 目瞪
者는 亦急發而稍緩死하고 眼合者는 急發急死나 然이나 目瞪者도 亦不
可以緩論而急治之니라.

Among the various illnesses of the Tae Eum Individual, there is one referred to as *Zhong Feng*[4] that involves gasping for air with audible wheezing and staring into space without recognition of one's surroundings. This illness should be treated with *Gwajae San* (Muskmelon Pedicle Powder). If the hands and feet are stiff and contracted, and the eyes remain shut, then *Uhwang Chongshim Wan* (Lee Je-ma's Cattle Gall Stone Pill to Clear the heart) should be administered. Those with these symptoms who originally have a yellowish-red or dark complexion will have a tendency to stare into space without recognizing their surroundings, while those who originally have a whitish-blue complexion are prone to keeping their eyes closed. If an individual originally has a whitish-blue complexion and experiences contraction and inability to straighten the extremities, it is considered an emergency situation, calling for *Uhwang Chongshim Wan* (Lee Je-ma's Cattle Gall Stone Pill to Clear the heart). This formula is a modification of *Niu Huang Qing Xin Wan* (Cattle Gall Stone Pill to Clear the heart), prescribed by many doctors of the past, yielding incredible results. Those who stare into space and experience sudden convulsive episodes tend to die slowly, while those who do not open their eyes and experience sudden compulsive episodes die more quickly. Just because the former situation is slightly less acute, it doesn't mean that treatment can be delayed.

---

4    *Zhong Feng* (中風病), translated literally as "Wind stroke," is marked by gasping for air, wheezing sounds, staring into space, or sudden and complete loss of consciousness often followed by hemiplegia. Physiologically, this syndrome is commonly due to the occurrence of a cerebral infarction. The lungs are responsible for sending Yang energy to the head and upper body. Born with smaller (energetically weaker) lungs, the deficient Tae Eum is prone to circulatory issues from the neck upwards. Hence, stroke most frequently occurs with this constitution type.

**Table 8.7: The Internal Heat *Zhong Feng* (stroke) syndrome of the Tae Eum Individual**

| Syndrome | Original complexion before onset | Common symptoms | Treatment approach |
|---|---|---|---|
| Liver Heat *Zhong Feng* | Yellowish-red or dark | Gasping for air with audible wheezing and staring into space without recognizing one's surroundings | *Gwajae San* (Muskmelon Pedicle Powder) |
| Esophageal Cold *Zhong Feng* | Bluish-pale | | *Ungdam San* (Bear Gallbladder Powder) |
| | | | *Sokchangpo Wonji San* (Lee Je-ma's Sweetflag and Senega Powder) |
| | | | If the complexion is originally bluish-pale, hands and feet are stiff and contracted, and the eyes remain shut then administer: |
| | | | *Wuhwang Chongshim Tang* (Lee Je-ma's Cattle Gall Stone Pill to Clear the heart) |

**Table 8.8: Treatment according to everyday complexion before the onset of *Zhong Feng* (stroke) syndrome**

| Complexion color | Meaning |
|---|---|
| Yellowish-red or dark | Chronic Internal liver Heat syndrome |
| Bluish-pale | Chronic External Esophageal Cold syndrome |

牛黃淸心丸은 非家家必有之物이니 宜用遠志 石菖蒲末 各一錢을 灌口하고 因以ㄱ角末 三分을 吹鼻하라. 此證에 手足拘攣而項直則危也니 傍人이 以兩手로 執病人兩手腕하고 左右撓動兩肩하며 或執病人足腕하고 屈伸兩脚이니 太陰人中風에 撓動病人肩脚은 好也라 少陽人中風은 大忌 撓動病人手足이오 又不可抱人起坐오 少陰人中風에 傍人이 抱病人起坐 則可也而不可撓動兩肩이오 可以徐徐按摩手足이니라. 中風 吐瀉에 宜用 麝香이니라.

Because *Uhwang Chongshim Wan* (Lee Je-ma's Cattle Gall Stone Pill to Clear the heart) is not readily available in every household, I suggest preparing a powder with 3.75g of Yuan Zhi (*Radix Polygoni*) and Shi Chang Pu (*Rhizoma Acori Graminei*), which can be placed in the mouth, and 1.13g of Zao Jiao (*Gleditsia Sinensis*) powder, which can be blown into the nose. If *Zhong Feng* is accompanied by spasms of the hands and feet and stiffness of the neck, then it is an emergency. In this situation, one person should brace the individual's ankles, while another grasps and shakes his or her shoulders. Otherwise, one person can grasp the ankles and proceed to bend and straighten the legs over and over again. For the Tae Eum Individual suffering from stroke, both the shoulders and the legs should be shaken. The So Yang Individual, however, strongly abhors having their hands and feet shaken in this condition. Instead it is suitable to help them stand up, not allowing them to sit back down. For the So Eum Individual, I recommend having another person help them into a seated position and slowly massaging their hands and feet instead of having others shake their shoulders.

She Xiang (*Moschus*) is suitable for vomiting and diarrhea if food poisoning is suspected.

## The Tae Eum Individual's Four Formulae from Zhang Zhongjing's *Shang Han Lun*

### Ma Huang Tang
*Ephedrae Decoction*

| Ma Huang | Herba Ephedrae | 11.25g |
|---|---|---|
| Gui Zhi | Cortex Cinnamoni | 7.5g |
| Gan Cao | Radix Glycyrrhizae | 2.25g |
| Xing Ren | Semen Armeniacae Amarum | 10 Pieces |
| Sheng Jiang | Rhizoma Zingiberis Recens | 3 Slices |
| Da Zao | Fructus Jujubae | 2 Pieces |

### Gui Ma Ge Ban Tang
*Combined Cinnamon Twig and Ephedra Decoction*

| Ma Huang | Herba Ephedrae | 5.625g |
|---|---|---|
| Bai Shao Yao | Paeoniae Alba | 3.75g |
| Gui Zhi | Cortex Cinnamoni | 3.75g |
| Xing Ren | Semen Armeniacae Amarum | 3.75g |
| Gan Cao | Radix Glycyrrhizae | 2.625g |
| Sheng Jiang | Rhizoma Zingiberis Recens | 3 Slices |
| Da Zao | Fructus Jujubae | 2 Pieces |

### Tiao Wei Cheng Qi Tang
*Regulate the Stomach and Order the Qi Decoction*

| Da Huang | Radix et Rhizoma Rhei | 15g |
|---|---|---|
| Mang Xiao | Natrii Sulfas | 7.5g |
| Gan Cao | Radix Glycyrrhizae | 2.25g |

### Da Chai Hu Tang
*Major Bupleurum Decoction*

| Chai Hu | *Radix Bupleurum* | 15g |
|---|---|---|
| Huang Qin | *Radix Scutellariae* | 9.375g |
| Bai Shao Yao | *Paeoniae Alba* | 9.375g |
| Da Huang | *Radix et Rhizoma Rhei* | 7.5g |
| Zhi Shi | *Fructus Aurantii Immaturus* | 5.625g |

This formula is suitable for a Shao Yang stage illness, which transfers into a Yang Ming stage illness, marked by fever without chills, hardness of the stools, reddish urine, incoherent speech, distention of the abdomen, and hot flashes.

## The Tae Eum Individual's Nine Formulae Presented by Doctors of the Tang, Song, and Ming Dynasties

### Shi Chang Pu Yuan Zhi San
*Sweetflag and Senega Powder*

| Shi Chang Pu | *Rhizoma Acori Tatarinowii* |
|---|---|
| Yuan Zhi | *Radix Polygoni* |

Grind equal amounts of the above ingredients into powder and mix 3.75g with rice porridge or wine. If ingested three times a day, this formula can assist with vision and hearing.

This formula was extracted from Sun Simiao's book entitled *Qian Jin Fang* (*Thousand Golden Essential Prescriptions*).

### Tiao Zhong Tang
*Regulate the Middle Decoction*

| Da Huang | *Radix et Rhizoma Rhei* | 5.625g |
|---|---|---|
| Huang Qin | *Radix Scutellariae* | 3.75g |
| Jie Geng | *Radix Platycodi* | 3.75g |
| Ge Gen | *Radix Puerariae* | 3.75g |
| Bai Zhu | *Radix Atractylodis Macrocephalae* | 3.75g |
| Bai Shao Yao | *Radix Paeoniae Lactiflorae* | 3.75g |
| Chi Fu Ling | *Poria Rubra* | 3.75g |
| Gao Ben | *Rhizoma Ligustici* | 3.75g |
| Gan Cao | *Radix Glycyrrhizae* | 3.75g |

This formula, which can be found in Zhu Gong's text *Hourenshu* (*Revive the People*), is suitable for *Zao Yi* (燥疫) syndrome, a summertime Warm Febrile disease characterized by acute thirst and swelling of the throat.

From my experience, Bai Zhu (*Radix Atractylodis Macrocephalae*), Bai Shao Yao (*Radix Paeoniae Lactiflorae*), and Gan Cao (*Radix Glycyrrhizae*), which are prescribed for the So Eum Individual, and Chi Fu Ling (*Poria Rubra*), which is prescribed for the So Yang Individual, should be omitted.

### Hei Nu Wan
*Black Servant Pill*

| Ma Huang | *Herba Ephedrae* | 75g |
|---|---|---|
| Da Huang | *Radix et Rhizoma Rhei* | 75g |
| Huang Qin | *Radix Scutellariae* | 37.5g |
| Fu De Mei | *Cauldron Soot* | 37.5g |
| Mang Xiao | *Natrii Sulfas* | 37.5g |
| Zao Yao Mo | *Furnace Ash* | 37.5g |
| Liang Shang Chen[26] | *Dust (on a crossbeam)* | 37.5g |
| Xiao Mai Nu | *Smutted Ear of Barley* | 37.5g |

Grind the above ingredients into powder and mix with honey to make pills the size of an empress tree seed. Ingest one pill at a time with well water. If the body starts to quiver and sweat, then recovery is imminent. It may take several dosages before results are evident.

Doctors have often claimed that Yang toxin and *Haui Zheng* are untreatable. However, even when there is loss of consciousness and lack of movement, if the epigastric area is still warm, there is still hope. This pill should be divided into small pieces and inserted directly into the patient's mouth.

This formula originates from Zhu Gong's *Hourenshu* (*Revive the People*). In my thorough review, I have concluded that Mang Xiao (*Natrii Sulfas*), which is only useful for the So Yang Individual, should be omitted.

### Sheng Mai San
*Generate the Pulse Powder*

| Mai Men Dong | *Tuber Ophiopogonis* | 7.5g |
|---|---|---|
| Ren Shen | *Radix Ginseng* | 3.75g |
| Wu Wei Zi | *Fructus Shizandrae* | 3.75g |

This formula, within Li Chan's text entitled *Yuxuerumen* (*Introduction to Medicine*), is intended to cause a significant increase in energy if ingested in place of water during the summer.

After reviewing this formula I have concluded that Ren Shen (*Radix Ginseng*), which is useful for the So Eum Individual, should be omitted.

---

5   Liang Shang Chen (樑上塵), dust that accumulates upon a crossbeam, pillar, or girder, is blown into the nose with a straw to induce sneezing and strongly stimulate the nervous system. It is often utilized after stroke to avoid relapse and/or loss of consciousness.

### *Chun Gen Pi Wan*
*Ailanthus Bark Pill*

Chun Gen Pi    *Cortex Ailanthi*

Grind this herb into fine powder, mix with liquor to make a paste, then form into green pea-size pills. This formula, mentioned in Li Chan's text *Yuxuerumen* (*Introduction to Medicine*), is prescribed for nocturnal emissions and spermatorrhea. Since this formula has both a cool and dry nature, it should not be ingested long term.

### *Er Sheng Jiu Ku Wan*
*Two Saints Rescue the Suffering Pill*

| | | |
|---|---|---|
| Da Huang | *Radix et Rhizoma Rhei* | 150g |
| Zhu Ya Zao Jiao | *Fructus Gleditschiae Sinensis* | 75g |

Grind the above ingredients into fine powder, mix with flour and water to make a paste, then form into green pea-sized pills. Sweating will occur after just a single dose of 50 to 70 pills, indicating recovery. This formula, mentioned in Gong Xin's text entitled *Manbing Huichun* (*Ten Thousand Illnesses Return to Spring*), is indicated for the treatment of epidemic Warm Febrile disease.

### *Ge Gen Jie Ji Tang*
*Kudzu Clear the Flesh Decoction*

| | | |
|---|---|---|
| Ge Gen | *Radix Puerariae* | 3.75g |
| Sheng Ma | *Rhizoma Cimicifugae* | 3.75g |
| Huang Qin | *Radix Scutellariae* | 3.75g |
| Jie Geng | *Radix Platycodi* | 3.75g |
| Bai Zhi | *Radix Atractylodis Macrocephalae* | 3.75g |
| Chai Hu | *Radix Bupleurum* | 3.75g |
| Bai Shao Yao | *Radix Paeoniae Lactiflorae* | 3.75g |
| Qiang Huo | *Rhizoma seu Radix Notopterygii* | 3.75g |
| Shi Gao | *Gypsum Fibrosum* | 3.75g |
| Gan Cao | *Radix Glycyrrhizae* | 1.875g |

This formula, mentioned in Gong Xin's text *Yijianshu* (*Mirror of Eastern Medicine*), is indicated for painful eyes, dry nasal passages, and insomnia from Yang Ming stage illness.

After a thorough evaluation, I have concluded that Chai Hu (*Radix Bupleurum*), Qiang Huo (*Rhizoma seu Radix Notopterygii*), and Shi Gao (*Gypsum Fibrosum*), which is useful for the So Yang Individual, and Gan Cao (*Radix Glycyrrhizae*), which is useful for the So Eum Individual, should be omitted.

### Niu Huang Qing Xin Wan
*Cattle Gall Stone Pill to Clear the Heart*

| | | | |
|---|---|---|---|
| Shan Yao | *Rhizoma Dioscoreae* | 26.25g | |
| Zhi Gan Cao | *Radix Glycyrrhizae* | 18.75g | (Stir-fried with honey) |
| Ren Shen | *Radix Ginseng* | 9.375g | |
| Pu Huang | *Typhae Pollen* | 9.375g | |
| Shen Qu | *Massa Fermentata Medicinalis* | 9.375g | |
| Xi Jiao | *Cornu Rhinoceri* | 7.5g | |
| Zhi Da Dou Huang | *Soybean Sprouts (Dried)* | 6.375g | (Dry-fried) |
| Rou Gui | *Cortex Cinnamomi* | 6.375g | |
| E Jiao | *Colla Corni Asini* | 6.375g | |
| Bai Shao Yao | *Radix Paeoniae Lactiflorae* | 5.625g | |
| Mai Men Dong | *Tuber Ophiopogonis* | 5.625g | |
| Huang Qin | *Radix Scutellariae* | 5.625g | |
| Dang Gui | *Radix Angelicae Sinensis* | 5.625g | |
| Bai Zhu | *Radix Atractylodis Macrocephalae* | 5.625g | |
| Fang Feng | *Radix Saposhnikoviae* | 5.625g | |
| Zhu Sha Shui | *Cinnabaris* | 5.625g | (Highly refined powder) |
| Chai Hu | *Radix Bupleurum* | 4.875g | |
| Jie Geng | *Radix Platycodi* | 4.875g | |
| Xing Ren | *Semen Armeniacae Amarum* | 4.875g | |
| Fu Ling | *Poria Alba* | 4.875g | |
| Chuan Xiong | *Radix Ligustici Chuanxiong* | 4.875g | |
| Niu Huang | *Calculus Bovis* | 4.5g | |
| Ling Yang Jiao | *Cornu Saigae Tataricae* | 3.75g | |
| Long Nao | *Borneolum* | 3.75g | |
| She Xiang | *Moschus* | 3.75g | |
| Xiong Huang | *Realgar* | 3g | |
| Bai Lian | *Radix Ampelopsis* | 2.625g | |
| Pao Gan Jiang | *Rhizoma Zingiberis Preparata* | 2.625g | |
| Jin Bo | *Gold Sheets* | 140 Sheets | (Dry-fried until black) |
| Da Zao | *Fructus Jujubae* | 20 Pieces | |

To prepare this formula, grind the above ingredients, excluding Da Zao (*Fructus Jujubae*), with 40 sheets of Jin Bo (*Gold Sheets*) into a fine powder. Boil 20 pieces of Da Zao, with seeds removed, and then puree after removing the skin.[6] Mix Da Zao puree and honey with the above powdered ingredients to form a paste. Then shape into ten pills for each 37.5g of paste. Finally, wrap each pill with Jin Bo. A total of 40 out of 140 sheets of Jin Bo should be utilized, while the rest should be ground and mixed with this combination. Ingest a single pill dissolved in warm water per dose.

This formula, presented in Gong Xin's text entitled *Yijianshu* (*Mirror of Eastern Medicine*), is indicated for sudden occurrence of stroke leading to loss of consciousness, abundant phlegm, fading consciousness, speech impairment, and/or hemiplegia of the face, arms, and legs.

After a thorough review, I have concluded that Chai Hu (*Radix Bupleurum*), Bai Fu Ling (*Poria Alba*), Shen Qu (*Massa Fermentata Medicinalis*), Niu Huang (*Calculus Bovis*), E Jiao (*Colla Corni Asini*), and Zhu Sha (*Cinnabaris*), which are useful for the So Yang Individual, and Bai Zhu (*Radix Atractylodis Macrocephalae*), Ren Shen (*Radix Ginseng*), Gan Cao (*Radix Glycyrrhizae*), Bai Shao Yao (*Radix Paeoniae Lactiflorae*), Rou Gui (*Cortex Cinnamomi*), Dang Gui (*Radix Angelicae Sinensis*), Chuan Xiong (*Radix Ligustici Chuanxiong*), Gan Jiang (*Rhizoma Zingiberis*), honey, and Da Zao (*Fructus Jujubae*), which are useful for the So Eum Individual, should be omitted.

### Ma Huang Ding Chuan Tang
*Ephedra Arrest Wheezing Decoction*

| Ma Huang | *Herba Ephedrae* | 11.25g | |
|---|---|---|---|
| Xing Ren | *Semen Armeniacae Amarum* | 5.625g | |
| Huang Qin | *Radix Scutellariae* | 3.75g | |
| Ban Xia | *Rhizoma Pinelliae* | 3.75g | |
| Sang Bai Pi | *Cortex Mori* | 3.75g | |
| Su Zi | *Cortex Perillae* | 3.75g | |
| Kuan Dong Hua | *Flos Farfarae* | 3.75g | |
| Gan Cao | *Radix Glycyrrhizae* | 3.75g | |
| Bai Guo | *Semen Ginkgo* | 21 Pieces | (Stir-fried, cortex removed |

---

6   The soft flesh of the Da Zao (*Fructus Jujubae*) can be extracted by pressing or squeezing with cheesecloth after boiling.

There is a *Yellow Song,*[7] which exclaims: "Every disease has an appropriate herbal treatment." Yet, from my experience, it is especially difficult to address issues related to snoring and asthma.

This formula, mentioned in Gong Xin's text *Manbing Huichun* (*Ten Thousand Illnesses Return to Spring*), is surprisingly effective in treating asthma. Only after the ingestion of this pill could its miraculous effects be discovered.

After a thorough review, I have concluded that Ban Xia (*Rhizoma Pinelliae*), Su Zi (*Cortex Perillae*), and Gan Cao (*Radix Glycyrrhizae*), which are useful for the So Eum Individual, should be omitted.

## 24 Newly Discovered Formulae for the Tae Eum Individual (Formulated by Lee Je-ma)

### Tae Eum Jowi Tang
*Lee Je-ma's Regulate the Stomach Decoction for the Tae Eum Individual*

| Yi Yi Ren | Semen Coicis | 11.25g |
|---|---|---|
| Gan Li | Castania | 11.25g |
| Lai Fu Zi | Semen Raphani | 7.5g |
| Wu Wei Zi | Fructus Shizandrae | 3.75g |
| Mai Men Dong | Tuber Ophiopogonis | 3.75g |
| Shi Chang Pu | Rhizoma Acori Graminei | 3.75g |
| Jie Geng | Radix Platycodi | 3.75g |
| Ma Huang | Herba Ephedrae | 3.75g |

### Kalgen Heigi Tang
*Lee Jae-ma's Kudzu Clear the Flesh Decoction*

| Ge Gen | Radix Puerariae | 11.25g |
|---|---|---|
| Huang Qin | Radix Scutellariae | 5.625g |
| Gao Ben | Rhizoma Ligustici | 5.625g |
| Jie Geng | Radix Platycodi | 3.75g |
| Sheng Ma | Rhizoma Cimicifugae | 3.75g |
| Bai Zhi | Radix Atractylodis Macrocephalae | 3.75g |

---

7  The *Yellow Songs*, or *Huang Ge* (黃歌), are poems written in ancient China that emphasized significant medicinal concepts in a format that made it easier to remember, through the use of rhyming or similarly structured Chinese characters. These "songs," memorized by doctors and commoners alike, were deeply embedded in daily life as everyday decisions were often based on ancient medicinal advice.

## *Jowi Seungchong Tang*
### *Lee Jae-ma's Regulate the Stomach Support and Clear Decoction*

| Yi Yi Ren | Semen Coicis | 11.25g |
|---|---|---|
| Gan Li | Castania | 11.25g |
| Lai Fu Zi | Semen Raphani | 5.625g |
| Ma Huang | Herba Ephedrae | 3.75g |
| Jie Geng | Radix Platycodi | 3.75g |
| Mai Men Dong | Tuber Ophiopogonis | 3.75g |
| Wu Wei Zi | Fructus Shizandrae | 3.75g |
| Shi Chang Pu | Rhizoma Acori Graminei | 3.75g |
| Yuan Zhi | Radix Polygoni | 3.75g |
| Tian Men Dong | Radix Asparagi | 3.75g |
| Suan Zao Ren | Semen Ziziphi Spinosae | 3.75g |
| Long Yan Rou | Arillus Longan | 3.75g |

## **Chongshim Yonja Tang**
### *Lee Je-ma's Lotus Seed Purify the Heart Decoction*

| Lian Zhi Rou | Semen Nelumbinis | 7.5g |
|---|---|---|
| Shan Yao | Rhizoma Dioscoreae | 7.5g |
| Tian Men Dong | Radix Asparagi | 3.75g |
| Mai Men Dong | Tuber Ophiopogonis | 3.75g |
| Yuan Zhi | Radix Polygoni | 3.75g |
| Shi Chang Pu | Rhizoma Acori Graminei | 3.75g |
| Suan Zao Ren | Semen Ziziphi Spinosae | 3.75g |
| Long Yan Rou | Arillus Longan | 3.75g |
| Bai Zhi Ren | Semen Platycladi | 3.75g |
| Huang Qin | Radix Scutellariae | 3.75g |
| Lai Fu Zi | Semen Raphani | 3.75g |
| Ju Hua | Flos Chrysanthemi | 1.125g |

## *Mahwang Jongchun Tang*
### *Lee Je-ma's Ephedra Arrest Wheezing Decoction*

| Ma Huang | Herba Ephedrae | 11.25g |
|---|---|---|
| Xing Ren | Semen Armeniacae Amarum | 5.625g |

| Huang Qin | Radix Scutellariae | 3.75g |
| Lai Fu Zi | Semen Raphani | 3.75g |
| Sang Bai Pi | Cortex Mori | 3.75g |
| Jie Geng | Radix Platycodi | 3.75g |
| Mai Men Dong | Tuber Ophiopogonis | 3.75g |
| Kuan Dong Hua | Flos Farfarae | 3.75g |
| Bai Guo | Semen Ginkgo | 21 Pieces |

### Mahwang Jongtong Tang
*Lee Je-ma's Ephedra Decoction for Pain*

| Yi Yi Ren | Semen Coicis | 11.25g |
| Ma Huang | Herba Ephedrae | 7.5g |
| Lai Fu Zi | Semen Raphani | 7.5g |
| Xing Ren | Semen Armeniacae Amarum | 3.75g |
| Shi Chang Pu | Rhizoma Acori Graminei | 3.75g |
| Jie Geng | Radix Platycodi | 3.75g |
| Mai Men Dong | Tuber Ophiopogonis | 3.75g |
| Wu Wei Zi | Fructus Shizandrae | 3.75g |
| Shi Jun Zi | Fructus Quisqualis | 3.75g |
| Long Yan Rou | Arillus Longan | 3.75g |
| Bai Zhi Ren | Semen Platycodi | 3.75g |
| Gan Li | Castania | 7 Pieces |

### Yulda Hanso Tang
*Lee Je-ma's Greater Heat Lesser Cold Decoction*

| Ge Gen | Radix Puerariae | 15g |
| Huang Qin | Radix Scutellariae | 7.5g |
| Gao Ben | Rhizoma Ligustici | 7.5g |
| Lai Fu Zi | Semen Raphani | 3.75g |
| Jie Geng | Radix Platycodi | 3.75g |
| Sheng Ma | Rhizoma Cimicifugae | 3.75g |
| Bai Zhi | Radix Atractylodis Macrocephalae | 3.75g |

### Handa Yulso Tang
*Lee Je-ma's Greater Cold Lesser Heat Decoction*

| | | |
|---|---|---|
| Yi Yi Ren | *Semen Coicis* | 11.25g |
| Lai Fu Zi | *Semen Raphani* | 7.5g |
| Mai Men Dong | *Tuber Ophiopogonis* | 3.75g |
| Jie Geng | *Radix Platycodi* | 3.75g |
| Huang Qin | *Radix Scutellariae* | 3.75g |
| Xing Ren | *Semen Armeniacae Amarum* | 3.75g |
| Ma Huang | *Herba Ephedrae* | 3.75g |
| Gan Li | *Castania* | 7 Pieces |

### Kalgen Seunggi Tang
*Lee Je-Ma's Kudzu Support the Qi Decoction*

| | | |
|---|---|---|
| Ge Gen | *Radix Puerariae* | 15g |
| Huang Qin | *Radix Scutellariae* | 7.5g |
| Da Huang | *Radix et Rhizoma Rhei* | 7.5g |
| Sheng Ma | *Rhizoma Cimicifugae* | 3.75g |
| Jie Geng | *Radix Platycodi* | 3.75g |
| Bai Zhi | *Radix Atractylodis Macrocephalae* | 3.75g |

If 11.25g of Da Huang (*Radix et Rhizoma Rhei*) is used in this formula, it is referred to as *Kalgen Daeseunggi Tang* (Kudzu Greater Support the Qi Decoction). If 3.5g of Da Huang (*Radix et Rhizoma Rhei*) is used, it is referred to as *Kalgen Soseunggi Tang* (Kudzu Lesser Support the Qi Decoction).

### Jori Peiwon Tang
*Lee Je-ma's Regulate the Interior and Support the Lung Source Decoction*

| | | |
|---|---|---|
| Mai Men Dong | *Tuber Ophiopogonis* | 7.5g |
| Jie Geng | *Radix Platycodi* | 7.5g |
| Yi Yi Ren | *Semen Coicis* | 7.5g |
| Huang Qin | *Radix Scutellariae* | 3.75g |
| Ma Huang | *Herba Ephedrae* | 3.75g |
| Lai Fu Zi | *Semen Raphani* | 3.75g |

## Mahwang Balpyo Tang
*Lee Je-ma's Ephedra Release the Exterior Decoction*

| Jie Geng | *Radix Platycodi* | 11.25g |
|---|---|---|
| Ma Huang | *Herba Ephedrae* | 5.625g |
| Mai Men Dong | *Tuber Ophiopogonis* | 3.75g |
| Huang Qin | *Radix Scutellariae* | 3.75g |
| Xing Ren | *Semen Armeniacae Amarum* | 3.75g |

## Bopei Won Tang
*Lee Je-ma's Tonify the Lung Source Decoction*

| Mai Men Dong | *Tuber Ophiopogonis* | 11.25g |
|---|---|---|
| Jie Geng | *Radix Platycodi* | 7.5g |
| Wu Wei Zi | *Fructus Shizandrae* | 3.75g |

## Nogyung Daebo Tang
*Lee Je-ma's Deer Antler Great Tonification Decoction*

| Lu Rong | *Cornu Cervi Pantotrichum* | 7.5g, 11.25g, or 15g |
|---|---|---|
| Mai Men Dong | *Tuber Ophiopogonis* | 5.625g |
| Yi Yi Ren | *Semen Coicis* | 5.625g |
| Shan Yao | *Rhizoma Dioscoreae* | 3.75g |
| Tian Men Dong | *Radix Asparagi* | 3.75g |
| Wu Wei Zi | *Fructus Shizandrae* | 3.75g |
| Xing Ren | *Semen Armeniacae Amarum* | 3.75g |
| Ma Huang | *Herba Ephedrae* | 3.75g |

This formula is suitable for the acute Exterior Cold syndrome of a deficient Tae Eum Individual.

### Gongjin Hukwon Dan
*Lee Je-ma's Embrace the King Black Source Pill*

| Lu Rong | *Cornu Cervi Pantotrichum* | 150g, 187.5g, or 225g |
|---|---|---|
| Shan Yao | *Rhizoma Dioscoreae* | 150g |
| Tian Men Dong | *Radix Asparagi* | 150g |
| Ji Cao | *Holotrichia Diomphalia Bates* | 37.5–75g |
| She Xiang | *Moschus* | 18.75g |

To prepare this formula, boil several pieces of Wu Mei (*Fructus Mume*) flesh, with seed omitted, until soft and then puree. Grind together the above ingredients and then mix with pureed Wu Mei to form a paste. Shape into pills the size of an empress tree seed and ingest 50 to 70 pills per dose with warm water or ingested with rice wine. This formula is suitable for the deficient Tae Eum Individual with significant Internal[8] illness.

### Jogak Daehwang Tang
*Lee Je-ma's Honeylocust and Rhubarb Decoction*

| Sheng Ma | *Rhizoma Cimicifugae* | 11.25g |
|---|---|---|
| Ge Gen | *Radix Puerariae* | 11.25g |
| Da Huang | *Radix et Rhizoma Rhei* | 3.75g |
| Zao Jiao | *Gleditsia Sinensis* | 3.75g |

Do not exceed three to four doses of this formula because 11.25g of Sheng Ma (*Rhizoma Cimicifugae*) and 3.75g of Da Huang (*Radix et Rhizoma Rhei*) and Zao Jiao (*Gleditsia Sinensis*) have a very strong combined effect.

### Kalgen Bupyong Tang
*Lee Je-ma's Kudzu and Spirodela Decoction*

| Ge Gen | *Radix Puerariae* | 11.25g |
|---|---|---|
| Lai Fu Zi | *Semen Raphani* | 7.5g |
| Huang Qin | *Radix Scutellariae* | 7.5g |
| Zi Bei Fu Ping | *Herba Spirodelae* | 3.75g |
| Da Huang | *Radix et Rhizoma Rhei* | 3.75g |
| Ji Cao | *Holotrichia Diomphalia Bates* | 10 Pieces |

This formula addresses superficial edema caused by Internal illness.

---

8    Internal illness refers to the Tae Eum Individual's liver Heat causing Internal Heat syndrome.

## Konyul Jaejo Tang
*Lee Je-ma's Chestnut and Grub Decoction*

| Ji Cao | *Holotrichia Diomphalia Bates* | 10 Pieces |
| Gan Li | *Castania* | 7 Pieces |

The above ingredients can either be ingested as a tea, roasted and eaten directly, or made into a powder. In order to prepare the powder, grind ten pieces of Ji Cao (*Holotrichia Diomphalia Bates*) and drink with warm tea made from Gan Li (*Castania*). This formula addresses superficial edema caused by External[9] illness.

## Konyul Jogenpi Tang
*Lee Je-ma's Chestnut and Ailanthus Decoction*

| Chun Gen Bai Pi | *Cortex Ailanthi* | 11.25–18.75g |
| Gan Li | *Castania* | 7 Pieces |

This formula addresses dysentery of the Tae Eum Individual. These ingredients can be ingested as a tea or made into pills. To prepare pills, omit Gan Li (*Castania*) and simply prepare with 18.75g of Chu Gen Bai Pi (*Cortex Ailanthi*).

## Gwajae San
*Gua Di San (Chinese)—Muskmelon Pedicle Powder*

| Gua Di | *Melo Pedicellus* | (Stir-fried until yellow) |

Roast this ingredient until golden-brown, then grind into powder and ingest 1.125–1.875g mixed with warm water. For immediate use, boil 3.75g of dried muskmelon and drink as tea.

This formula is suitable for acute stroke, crackling and wheezing sounds in chest while gasping for air, and/or catatonia. It should not be used for other illnesses or symptoms, and should especially be avoided when there is chest and abdominal pain, coughing, or wheezing due to External Cold invasion or indigestion.

If a deficient individual with a pale complexion, who originally experienced an External Cold attack, suddenly suffers from the onset of a stroke, they should be prescribed *Ungdam San* (Bear Gallbladder Powder), *Wuhwang Chongshim Tang* (Lee Je-ma's Cattle Gall Stone Pill to Clear the heart), or *Sokchangpo Wonji San* (Lee Je-ma's Sweetflag and Senega Powder). *Gwajae San* (Muskmelon Pedicle Powder) should be avoided in such situations.

## Ungdam San
*Xiong Dan San (Chinese)—Bear Gallbladder Powder*

| Xiong Dan | *Fel Ursi* | 1.125–1.875g |

Prepare this ingredient as a herbal tea and ingest while still warm.

---

9    External illness refers to the Tae Eum Individual's Esophageal Cold causing External Cold syndrome.

### Sahyang San
*She Xiang San (Chinese)—Moschus Powder*

| She Xiang | *Moschus* | 1.125–1.875g |
|---|---|---|

She Xiang can be ingested with warm water or warm liquor.

### Sokchangpo Wonji San
*Lee Je-ma's Sweetflag and Senega Powder*

| Yuan Zhi | *Radix Polygoni* | 3.75g |
|---|---|---|
| Shi Chang Pu | *Rhizoma Acori Graminei* | 3.75g |
| Zhu Ya Zao Jiao | *Fructus Gleditschiae Sinensis* | 1.125g |

Grind the above ingredients into powder and mix with warm water, drink while still warm. Zhu Ya Zao Jiao (*Fructus Gleditschiae Sinensis*) can also be blown into the nose, while Yuan Zhi (*Radix Polygoni*) and Shi Chang Po (*Rhizoma Acori Graminei*) are ingested as a powder mixed with warm water.

### Maekmundong Wonji San
*Lee Je-ma's Ophiopogon and Senega Powder*

| Mai Men Dong | *Tuber Ophiopogonis* | 11.25g |
|---|---|---|
| Yuan Zhi | *Radix Polygoni* | 3.75g |
| Shi Chang Pu | *Rhizoma Acori Graminei* | 3.75g |
| Wu Wei Zi | *Fructus Shizandrae* | 1.875g |

### Uhwang Chongshim Wan
*Lee Je-ma's Cattle Gall Stone Pill to Clear the Heart*

| Shan Yao | *Rhizoma Dioscoreae* | 26.25g | |
|---|---|---|---|
| Zhi Pu Huang | *Pollen Typhae* | 9.375g | (Dry-fried) |
| Xi Jiao | *Cornu Rhinoceri* | 7.5g | |
| Zhi Da Dou Huang Juan | *Dried Soybean Sprouts* | 6.375g | (Dry-fried) |
| Mai Men Dong | *Tuber Ophiopogonis* | 5.625g | |
| Huang Qin | *Radix Scutellariae* | 5.625g | |
| Jie Geng | *Radix Platycodi* | 4.875g | |
| Xing Ren | *Semen Armeniacae Amarum* | 4.875g | |

| Niu Huang | *Calculus Bovis* | 4.5g |
| Ling Yang Jiao | *Cornu Saigae Tataricae* | 3.75g |
| Long Nao | *Borneolum* | 3.75g |
| She Xiang | *Moschus* | 3.75g |
| Bai Lian | *Radix Ampelopsis* | 2.625g |
| Jin Bo | *Gold Sheets* | 70 Sheets |

To prepare this formula, grind the above herbs into a fine powder and mix with a paste made from 20 pieces of steamed Wu Mei (*Fructus Mume*). Then shape into 20 pills for each 37.5g of paste. Finally, wrap each pill with Jin Bo (*Gold Sheets*). Ingest a single pill per dose dissolved in warm water.

As a general rule, the twinned seeds, husk, and both tips of Xing Ren (*Semen Armeniacae Amarum*) should always be discarded. The cores of Mai Men Dong (*Tuber Ophiopogonis*) and Yuan Zhi (*Radix Polygoni*) should also be removed. Bai Guo (*Semen Ginkgo*) and Gan Li (*Castania*) should be removed from their shells. Da Huang (*Radix et Rhizoma Rhei*) can be prepared in alcohol or used raw depending on the situation. Zao Jiao (*Gleditsia Sinensis*) should always be prepared by dry-frying with wine. Lastly, Suan Zao Ren (*Semen Ziziphi Spinosae*), Xing Ren (*Semen Armeniacae Amarum*), and Bai Guo (*Semen Ginkgo*) should always be prepared by dry-frying.

太
陽
人
論

# The Tae Yang Individual's Illness

*Section 1*

## The Tae Yang Individual's Externally Contracted Illness Affecting the Lumbar Spine[1]

## 太陽人外感腰脊病論

內經에 日尺脈이 緩澁을 謂之解㑊이니라.

According to the *Nei Jing*, if the *chi* position of the pulse feels sluggish and rough, it indicates *Xie Yi*[2] syndrome.

───────────────

1   Unlike the other three Sasang constitutions, Lee Je-ma refers to the spine, rather than the organs, when entitling the Tae Yang Individual's External illness. Actually, in earlier writings, Lee Je-ma also referred to the spine when describing the External illnesses of the other constitutions, but later modified them to emphasize the primary role of the *Song* nature and its correlating organ in the onset of illness. According to Lee Je-ma, the weakest area of the spine is indeed where pathogenic influences enter the body, whereas the Tae Eum Individual's External pathogen enters through the cervical spine (correlating with the lung group), the So Eum Individual's External pathogen enters through the thoracic spine (correlating with the spleen group), and the So Yang Individual's External pathogen enters through the sacral area (correlating with the kidney group). Yet these areas aren't vulnerable to pathogenic influence when the *Song* nature of each constitution is balanced. The Tae Yang Individual's Externally contracted illness affecting the lumbar spine, or *Yochuk Byung* (腰脊病), occurs as a result of an External pathogen entering the Tae Yang Individual's lumbar spine area. The lumbar spine, along with the small intestine, is a member of the liver group, the weakest area of the Tae Yang Individual's body, and is therefore vulnerable to attack from External pathogens. If the Tae Yang Individual balances his/her sorrowful *Song* nature, then the stronger lungs will send ample energy to the weaker lumbar spine, protecting it from External pathogens.

2   *Xie Yi* (解㑊) syndrome is marked by difficult-to-differentiate symptoms such as slight chills, slight fever, slight fatigue, slight energy, and weakness of the lower extremities without visual signs of emaciation or necrotic bone/muscle tissue. *Xie Yi*, literally translated as "inconclusive diagnosis," was given its name because the diagnosis and recognition of this obscure syndrome was historically an unrelenting challenge.

釋曰尺爲陰部니 肝腎이 主之니 緩爲熱中이오 澁爲亡血인 故로 謂之解㑊이라 解㑊者는 寒不寒하며 熱不熱하며 弱不弱하며 壯不壯하여 獰不可名이니 謂之解㑊也니라.

To further elaborate, the *chi* position correlates with the Yin, or liver and kidney, aspect of the body. A sluggish pulse signals Heat, while a rough pulse indicates Blood Collapse.[3] When combined, both pulse presentations indicate the occurrence of *Xie Yi* syndrome, which is marked by the simultaneous occurrence of unusual, difficult-to-differentiate symptoms, such as feeling chilly but not cold, warm but not hot, deficient but not weak, and energized but not energetic.

靈樞에 曰髓傷則消爍이니 胻痠體解「하여 然不去矣니 不去는 謂不能行去也니라

As written in the *Ling Shu*, exhaustion and withering of the bone marrow, such as in *Xie Yi* syndrome, leads to tingling and numbness of the calf muscles, making it difficult to walk. The inability to move here refers to the inability to travel a substantial distance by foot.

論曰此證은 卽太陽人腰脊病太重證也니라. 必戒深哀하고 遠嗔怒하고 修淸定然後에 其病이 可愈니 此證에 當用五加皮壯脊湯이니라.

From my perspective, this indicates an extremely serious condition, which I refer to as the Tae Yang Individual's [Externally contracted illness affecting the] lumbar spine. The only way to overcome this illness is to rid oneself of excessive sadness and anger, while cultivating one's mind and body. The administration of *Ohgapi Jangchok Tang* (Lee Je-ma's Acanthopanax Strengthen the Spine Decoction) is also suitable in this instance.

解㑊者는 上體完健而下體解㑊이나 然이나 脚力이 不能行去也而其脚이 自無痲痺腫痛之證이오 脚力이 亦不甚弱하나니 此가 所以弱不弱하며 壯不壯하며 寒不寒하며 熱不熱而其病이 爲腰脊病也라 有解㑊證者는 必無大惡寒發熱身體疼痛之證也니 太陽人이 若有大惡寒發熱身體疼痛之證則腰脊表氣가 充實也니 其病이 易治오 其人이 亦完健이니라.

The upper body remains strong and robust during *Xie Yi* syndrome, but the lower body becomes extremely deficient, making it difficult to walk. Yet there are no visible signs of paralysis, swelling, or even weakness aside from the legs. The patient may feel somewhat deficient, but not weak, somewhat energized, but not energetic, somewhat chilled, but not cold, and somewhat warm, but not hot. Such is the

3 Blood Collapse, or *Mang Xue* (亡血), refers to a significant loss of blood through urine, stools, or vomiting as a result of maltreatment of a Shang Han disease. According to the *Zhu Jie Shang Han Lun* (*The Annotated Shang Han Lun*), *Mang Xue* occurs as a result of excessive diaphoresis or laxative administration after the occurrence of a Shang Han disease.

obscurity of the Tae Yang Individual's lumbar spine illness, which, although it occurs in the Exterior, never produces excessive chills, fever, pain, or other discomfort. If a Tae Yang Individual does experience excessive chills, fever, or body pain, it is a sign of substantial External energy[4] of the lumbar spine, which is easy to treat, with full recovery expected.

**Table 9.1: The Tae Yang Individual's Externally contracted illness affecting the lumbar spine**

| Syndrome | Symptoms | Treatment approach |
|---|---|---|
| Externally contracted illness affecting the lumbar spine | Difficult-to-differentiate symptoms with extremely deficient lower body, leading to weakness of the lower legs and difficulty walking:<br><br>"The patient may feel somewhat deficient, but not weak, somewhat energized and but not energetic, somewhat chilled, but not cold, and somewhat warm, but not hot." | *Ohgapi Jangchok Tang* (Lee Je-ma's Wu Jia Pi Strengthen the Spine Decoction) |

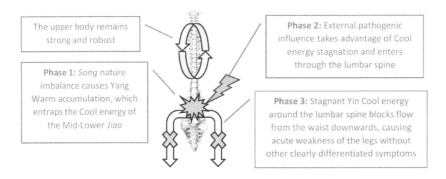

The upper body remains strong and robust

**Phase 1:** *Song* nature imbalance causes Yang Warm accumulation, which entraps the Cool energy of the Mid-Lower *Jiao*

**Phase 2:** External pathogenic influence takes advantage of Cool energy stagnation and enters through the lumbar spine

**Phase 3:** Stagnant Yin Cool energy around the lumbar spine blocks flow from the waist downwards, causing acute weakness of the legs without other clearly differentiated symptoms

*Figure 9.1: The Xie Yi syndrome of the Tae Yang Individual*

---

4    "Substantial External energy" refers to when the Tae Yang Individual has substantial *Zheng Qi*, giving him/her the ability to fight off Exterior pathogenic influences. Contrary to what one might expect, the occurrence of acute Internal or External symptoms is actually a sign of a lighter, easier-to-treat illness of the Tae Yang Individual, whose serious illness is often signified by the presence of obscure, difficult-to-differentiate symptoms.

*Section 2*

# The Tae Yang Individual's Internally Contracted Illness Affecting the Small Intestine[1]

## 太陽人內觸小腸病論

朱震亨이 曰噎膈反胃之病은 血液이 俱耗하여 胃脘이 乾枯니 其枯가 在
上近咽則水飮이 可行이나 食物이 難入하며 入亦不多니 名之曰噎이오
其枯가 在下近胃則食雖可入이나 難盡入胃하며 良久에 復出이니 名之曰
膈이며 亦曰反胃니라. 大便이 秘少하여 若羊屎然하니 名雖不同이나 病
出一體니라.

According to Zhu Zhenheng, *Ye Ge Fan Wei*[2] is characterized by the depletion of the blood and bodily fluids, and drying of the esophagus. Even if esophageal dryness extends from the stomach to the throat, ingesting fluids is not difficult. Solid foods, however, pose a challenge, and can be ingested only in small amounts. Difficulty ingesting solid foods is referred to as *Ye*.[3] If the entire esophagus has dried out (from the stomach to the throat), then after ingestion, solid food will accumulate and have difficulty entering the stomach, eventually leading to vomiting. This is referred to as *Ge*[4] or *Fan Wei*.[5] [As a result of reduced food intake and dryness,] there will be limited, dry bowel movement, whose shape resembles that of lamb feces. Even though there are several names for this syndrome, they all indicate the same illness.

上焦噎膈은 食下則胃脘當心而痛타가 須臾에 吐出하며 食出하면 痛乃
止하고 中焦噎膈은 食物이 可下나 難盡入胃하며 良久에 復出하고 下
焦噎膈은 朝食暮吐하며 暮食朝吐니 氣血俱虛者는 口中에 多出沫이라
但見沫多出者는 必死오 大便이 如羊屎者는 難治오 不淡飮食者도 難
治니라.

---

1   Small intestine illness, or *Sojang Byung* (小腸病), occurs as a result of small intestine stagnation of the Tae Yang Individual. The lumbar spine, along with the small intestine, is a member of the liver group, the weakest area of the Tae Yang Individual's body, which is vulnerable to stagnation. If the Tae Yang Individual balances his/her angry *Jung* nature, then the stronger lungs will send ample energy to the weaker small intestine, promoting Internal flow.

2   *Ye Ge Fan Wei* (噎膈反胃) syndrome is actually a combination of three syndromes: *Ye* (噎), or "choking," syndrome; *Ge* (膈), or "diaphragm," syndrome; and *Fan Wei* (反胃), or "vomit," syndrome.

3   *Ye* (噎) translates as "choking." *Ye* syndrome is due to dryness of the esophagus leading to difficult passage of solid foods through the esophagus, which often results in choking, gagging, or vomit.

4   *Ge* (膈) translates as "diaphragm." *Ge* syndrome is also due to dryness of the esophagus, leading to difficult passage of solid food through the esophagus, often resulting in diaphragmic spasms.

5   *Fan Wei* (反胃) translates as "vomit" or "dry heaves." *Fan Wei* syndrome comes from dryness of the esophagus, leading to solid foods passing with difficulty through the esophagus, which often results in vomiting or dry heaves.

Zhu Zhenheng also states that if *Ye Ge*[6] syndrome occurs in the Upper *Jiao*, then after ingestion, food will stagnate in the esophagus, causing pressure pushing upwards and leading to pain and subsequent vomiting. Vomiting will completely relieve the pain. If *Ye Ge* syndrome occurs in the Middle *Jiao*, food will have difficulty entering the stomach [but still pass through the esophagus], with delayed vomiting. If *Ye Ge* syndrome occurs in the Lower *Jiao*, breakfast will be vomited in the evening, and supper vomited in the morning. If the *Qi* and blood are depleted as a result of *Ye Ge* syndrome, then there will be a significant amount of foamy sputum, which indicates imminent death. This illness will be difficult [but not impossible] to address, with the presence of lamb-shaped stools or difficulty ingesting food.

張鷄峯이 曰噎은 當是神思間病이니 惟內觀自養이라야 可以治之니라.

According to Zhang Ji Feng, the mind is the source of *Ye* syndrome. Only if the mind is cultivated, especially through relaxation, can this illness be overcome.[7]

龔信醫鑑에 曰反胃也와 膈也와 噎也는 受病이 皆同하니 噎膈之證은 不屬虛하며 不屬實하며 不屬冷하며 不屬熱이오 乃神氣中一點病耳니라.

According to Gong Xin, *Ye*, *Ge*, and *Fan Wei* syndromes all have the same source and are not due to deficiency, Cold, or Heat, but rather, to the state of one's mind.[8]

論曰此證은 則太陽人小腸病太重證也라 必遠嗔怒하고 斷厚味然後에 其病이 可愈니 此證에 當用獼猴藤植腸湯이니라.

From my perspective, this syndrome is nothing other than the Tae Yang Individual's [Internally contracted illness affecting the] small intestine, and is extremely serious. Only after refraining from anger and discontinuing the ingestion of excessively fatty foods can this illness be overcome. The administration of *Mihudeng Shikjang Tang* (Lee Je-ma's Kiwifruit Vine Support the Intestines Decoction) is also suitable in this situation.

食物이 自外入而有所防碍曰噎이오 自內受而有所拒格曰膈이오 朝食暮吐하며 暮食朝吐曰反胃라 然이나 朝食而暮吐하며 暮食而朝吐者는 非全食皆吐也오 有所防碍而拒格於胃之上口者는 經宿而自吐也니 則反胃도 亦噎膈也니라.

---

6    In this sentence, Zhu Zhenheng refers to *Ye* (噎) and *Ge* (膈) together, since they occur simultaneously and are actually the same syndrome.

7    This assertion is written in the *Complicated Disorders* chapter of the *Dongeui Bogam* (*The Mirror of Eastern Medicine*). No additional information about Zhang Ji Feng himself has been discovered.

8    In this sentence, "one's mind" is a translation of *Shen Qi* (神氣), or "Spirit *Qi*," which, according to Chinese philosophy, resides in the heart. In Sasang medicine, the *Shen* (神) correlates with the lung group and the Upper *Jiao*.

*Ye* syndrome is characterized by difficulty with the initial phase of food ingestion, which begins as soon as food enters the mouth and ends when it enters the stomach. *Ge* syndrome is characterized by difficulty with the second stage of digestion, once the food has entered the stomach. *Fan Wei* syndrome is marked by vomiting breakfast in the evening, and vomiting supper the following morning. With *Fan Wei*, it isn't either the entire breakfast or supper that is vomited, but only the food remaining stuck in the fundus. *Fan Wei* in this regard encompasses both *Ye* and *Ge* syndromes [since it involves both the first and second stages of food ingestion].

蓋噎膈者는 胃脘之噎膈也오 反胃者는 胃口之噎膈也니 同是一證也라 有噎膈證者는 必無腹痛腸鳴泄瀉痢疾之證也니 太陽人이 若有腹痛腸鳴泄瀉痢疾之證則小腸裡氣가 充實也니 其病은 易治오 其人은 亦完健이니라.

Generally speaking, *Ye* and *Ge* syndromes occur in the esophagus and *Fan Wei* syndrome in the fundal region, yet they all signify the same illness. Despite the occurrence of *Ye* or *Ge* syndrome, symptoms such as abdominal pain, borborygmos, diarrhea, dysentery, or other digestive issues will not be apparent. If a Tae Yang Individual does experience these symptoms, he/she has substantial[9] Internal blockage of small intestine energy, which is easy to treat, with full recovery to be expected.

解㑊과 噎膈은 俱是重證而重證之中에 有輕重之等級焉하니 解㑊而無噎膈則解㑊之輕證也오 噎膈而無解㑊則噎膈之輕證也니라. 若解㑊에 兼噎膈하며 噎膈에 兼解㑊則其爲重險之證을 不可勝言而重險中에 又有輕重也니 太陽人의 解㑊과 噎膈이 不至死境之前에는 起居飮食如常하여 人必易之視以例病인 故로 入於危境而莫可挽回也라.

*Xie Yi*, *Ye*, and *Ge* syndromes are all considered serious, but rank differently from lighter to more critical. If *Xie Yi* syndrome occurs without *Ye* or *Ge* syndromes, it is considered a lighter form of *Xie Yi*. If *Ye* or *Ge* syndromes occur without *Xie Yi* syndrome, it is a lighter form of *Ye* and *Ge* syndrome. It goes without saying that if *Xie Yi* syndrome is followed by *Ye* or *Ge* syndromes, or if *Ye* or *Ge* syndromes are followed by *Xie Yi* syndrome, the condition is critical. Yet even though both situations are considered critical, they can still be broken down into lesser and greater levels of severity. *Xie Yi*, *Ye*, and *Ge* syndromes often do not manifest until 2am onwards, so during the day, the Tae Yang Individual may continue to eat and live life as if nothing has happened. Despite the absence of symptoms, if this situation reaches a critical stage, it will be very difficult to relieve.

---

9   Contrary to what one might expect, the occurrence of acute Internal or External symptoms is actually a sign of a lighter, easier-to-treat illness of the Tae Yang Individual. The Tae Yang Individual's serious illness is often signified by the presence of obscure, difficult-to-differentiate symptoms.

余가 稟臟太陽人으로 嘗得此病하여 六七年嘔吐涎沫하여 數十年攝
身하여 幸而免夭하고 錄此以爲太陽人有病者戒하노니 若論治法컨데 一
言蔽曰遠嗔怒而已矣니라.

As a Tae Yang Individual myself, I suffered from six to seven years of this illness, with thick frothy sputum, excessive saliva, and vomiting. Once I discovered its nature, I spent several decades preserving my health, and fortunately escaped the claws of death. I sincerely hope that by recording my own experience, I can encourage other Tae Yang Individuals who become ill to cultivate their mind and body. If there was just one method that could cover the entire treatment protocol for this syndrome, it would be quite simple to control the tendency towards rage.

太陽人은 意强而操弱하니 意强則胃脘之氣가 上達而呼散者가 太過而越
也오 操弱則小腸之氣가 中執而吸聚者가 不支而餧也니 所以其病이 爲噎
膈反胃也니라

The Tae Yang Individual has strong willpower but lacks principle.[10] If the willpower is too strong, the excess energy of the esophagus will push upwards and outwards through the mouth. A lack of principle results in stagnation of the small intestine, leading to malabsorption and atrophy. Hence an imbalance of willpower and principle leads to *Ye*, *Ge*, and *Fan Wei* syndromes.

問하노니 朱震亨論에 噎膈과 反胃曰血液이 俱耗하고 胃脘이 乾枯하여
食物難入이라 하니 其說이 如何오 曰水穀이 納於胃而脾가 衛之하며 出
於大腸而腎이 衛之하나니 脾腎者는 出納水穀之府庫而迭爲補瀉者也오
氣液이 呼於胃脘而肺가 衛之하며 吸於小腸而肝이 衛之하나니 肺肝者는
呼吸氣液之門戶而迭爲進退者也라

Zhu Zhenheng was once asked: "What exactly do you mean when you say there is difficulty ingesting food due to depletion of the blood and bodily fluids caused by *Ye*, *Ge*, and *Fan Wei* syndromes?"

    He responded that the spleen controls the process of food ingestion from the mouth to the stomach, while the kidney controls food elimination through the large intestine. He taught us that the spleen and kidneys are granaries, which either stimulate or suppress the process of excretion and ingestion[11] of food. The lungs

---

10   "Strong will and weak principle" is an interpretation of the four Chinese characters *Yi Jiang Cao Ruo* (意强 操弱), which translate as "strong will, weak conduct." The two Chinese characters for "will" and "principle" (*Yi*, 意, and *Jiang*, 操) are often used together to describe an individual who is upright, moral, and with strong principle and integrity. According to Lee Je-ma, willpower resides in the Tae Yang Individual's stronger esophagus and principle in his/her small intestine. Hence the excessive willpower needs to be tamed, and the weaker principle nourished.

11   Ingestion, or *Nap* (納), is controlled by the stomach and spleen, which are the strongest organs of the So Yang Individual. Excretion, or *Chul* (出), is regulated by the kidneys and large intestine, which are the strongest organs of the So Eum Individual. Hence *Chul Nap* is associated primarily with So Yang and So Eum Individuals.

control the process of *Qi* and bodily fluid distribution from the esophagus, while the liver controls the absorption of *Qi* and bodily fluid in the small intestine. Therefore, he describes the lungs and liver as gates that control inhalation, exhalation,[12] advancement, and retreat of *Qi* and bodily fluid.

**Table 9.2: The metabolic process and organ function**

| Organ | Function | Inward/outward movement | Substance controlled |
|---|---|---|---|
| Spleen | Controls food ingestion from mouth to stomach | Ingestion | Food and drink |
| Kidneys | Control elimination from large intestine through anus | Excretion | |
| Lungs | Control the process of *Qi* and bodily fluid distribution from the esophagus | Distribution | *Qi* and bodily fluids |
| Liver | Control the process of *Qi* and bodily fluid absorption in the small intestine | Absorption | |

是故로 少陽人의 大腸出水穀陰寒之氣가 不足則胃中納水穀陽熱之氣가 必盛也오 太陽人의 小腸吸氣液陰涼之氣가 不足則胃脘呼氣液陽溫之 氣가 必盛也니 胃脘陽溫之氣가 太盛則胃脘血液이 乾枯는 其勢固然也라 然이나 非但乾枯而然也오 上呼之氣가 太過而中吸之氣가 太不支인 故로 食物이 不吸入而還呼出也니라.

Since the So Yang Individual has a deficiency of Yin Cold[13] energy, which controls the excretion of food in their large intestine, an excess of Yang Heat energy will be absorbed within the stomach.[14] Since the Tae Yang Individual has a deficiency of Yin Cool[15] energy, which controls the absorption of *Qi* and bodily fluid in the small intestine, there will be an excess of Yang Warm energy within the esophagus,[16] which distributes *Qi* and bodily fluid throughout the body. Excess outward distribution of *Qi* and bodily fluid will inevitably lead to *Qi* and fluid vacancy and dryness within the esophagus. Not only will the esophagus dry out, but there will also be a surge of upward-bearing energy due to an extreme lack of absorption [within the small

---

12  Inhalation, or *Hup* (吸), is controlled by the lungs and esophagus, which are the strongest organs of the Tae Yang Individual. Exhalation, or *Ho* (呼), is regulated by the liver and small intestine, which are the strongest organs of the Tae Eum Individual. Hence *Ho Hup* is associated primarily with the Tae Yang and Tae Eum Individuals.

13  As mentioned in Chapter 4, Cold energy is associated with the So Yang Individual's weaker organs, the kidneys and large intestine.

14  According to Lee Je-ma, the stomach is the source of Hot energy within the body.

15  As mentioned in Chapter 4, Cool energy is associated with the Tae Yang Individual's weaker organs, the liver and small intestine.

16  According to Lee Je-ma, the esophagus is the source of Warm energy within the body.

intestine]. Thus, a lack of energy devoted to drawing in food causes it to be expelled right back outwards.

或曰朱震亨所論에 噎膈反胃者를 安知非少陰少陽太陰人病而吾子가 必
名目曰太陽人病이라하며 內經所論에 解㑊者를 安知非少陰少陽太陰
人病而吾子가 必名目曰太陽人病이라 하니 莫非牽强附會耶아 願聞其
說하노라

Someone once asked me: "Why do you suppose that Zhu Zhenheng's *Ge, Ye,* and *Fan Wei* syndromes do not apply to the So Eum, So Yang, and Tae Eum constitutions but only to the Tae Yang Individual? How can you conclude that the *Nei Jing* confirms this observation? What principle could ever support such remarks? I certainly think this needs an explanation."

曰少陽人이 有嘔吐則必有大熱也오 少陰人이 有嘔吐則必有大寒也오 太
陰人이 有嘔吐則必病愈也니 今此噎膈과 反胃는 不寒不熱非實非虛則此
非太陽人病而何也오 解㑊者는 上體完健而下體가 解㑊然하여 胻痠不能
行去之謂也니 少陰少陽太陰人이 有此證則他證이 疊出而亦必無寒不寒
熱不熱弱不弱하며 壯不壯之理矣리라.

I answered by stating that the So Yang Individual's vomiting is always due to excessive Heat in the upper part of the body, whereas the So Eum Individual's is always due to excessive Cold. The Tae Eum Individual's vomiting is always a sign of recovery from illness. When it comes to *Ge, Ye,* and *Fan Wei* syndromes, there are no signs of Heat or Cold, excess or deficiency. If this is not an illness of the Tae Yang Individual, then what could it be? With *Xie Yi* syndrome, the upper body is in perfect health, yet the thighs are numb, making it difficult to walk. If the So Eum, So Yang, or Tae Eum Individual suffers from this illness, accompanying identifiable symptoms will definitely be present. Only the Tae Yang Individual will feel somewhat chilled but not cold, somewhat warm but not hot, somewhat weak but not really weak, and somewhat strong but not robust.

或曰吾子가 論太陽人解㑊病治法曰戒深哀하며 遠嗔怒하며 修清
定하라하고 論噎膈病治法曰遠嗔怒하며 斷厚味라하니 意者가 太陽人解㑊
病이 重於噎膈病而哀心所傷者가 重於怒心所傷乎아

Another individual once said: "You mentioned that controlling excessive sorrow, refraining from anger, and cultivating one's mind are methods of treatment for the Tae Yang Individual's *Xie Yi* syndrome, and that refraining from anger and avoiding *Hu Mi*[17] are the methods of treatment for the Tae Yang Individual's *Ge* and *Ye*

---

17  *Hu Mi* (厚味), or "food with excessive flavor," refers to foods that are excessively sweet, sour, bitter, and/ or acrid. Lee Je-ma also utilizes *Hu Mi* here to describe foods with high fat or protein content, which are particularly difficult for the Tae Yang Individual to digest.

syndromes. If *Xie Yi* syndrome is more severe than *Ge* and *Ye* syndromes, does it mean that sorrow[18] is more detrimental than anger[19] for the Tae Yang Individual?"

曰否라 太陽人의 噎膈病이 太重於解㑊病而怒心所傷者가 太重於哀心所傷也니 太陽人哀心이 深着則傷表氣하고 怒心이 暴發則傷裡氣인 故로 解㑊表證에 以戒哀와 遠怒로 兼言之也니라.

I countered this by explaining that actually *Ge* and *Ye* syndromes are more severe than *Xie Yi* syndrome and that anger is more detrimental than sorrow for the Tae Yang Individual. Sorrow affects the health of the [nose and lumbar spine in the] Exterior, while the explosion[20] of anger affects the [liver and small intestine in the] Interior. That is why I stated that sorrow should be overcome and anger avoided in cases of Externally contracted illness.

曰然則少陽人의 怒性이 傷口膀胱氣하며 哀情이 傷腎大腸氣하고 少陰人의 樂性이 傷目膂氣하며 喜情이 傷脾胃氣하고 太陰人의 喜性이 傷耳腦傾頁氣하며 樂情이 傷肺胃脘氣乎아 曰然하다.

Then he continued: "Therefore, anger[21] will affect the mouth and urinary bladder[22] and sadness[23] will affect the kidneys and large intestine of the So Yang Individual. Complacency[24] will affect the eyes and the thoracic spine and excessive joy[25] will affect the spleen and stomach of the So Eum Individual. Joy[26] will affect the ears and the cervical spine and cheerfulness[27] will affect the lungs and esophagus of the Tae Eum Individual."

I replied: "That is right."

---

18  Sorrow is the *Song* nature of the Tae Yang Individual. Imbalanced *Song* nature leads to Exterior vulnerability and External [lumbar spine] illness.

19  Anger is the *Jung* emotion of the Tae Yang Individual. Imbalanced *Jung* emotion leads to Internal [small intestine] illness.

20  As mentioned in Chapter 2, significant or chronic imbalance of one's *Song* nature leads to explosion, or acute outburst, of the *Jung* emotion.

21  Anger is the *Song* nature of the So Yang Individual. Imbalanced *Song* nature leads to Exterior vulnerability and External [spleen Cold] illness.

22  In this sentence, Lee Je-ma correlates the urinary bladder with the Exterior syndrome of the So Yang Individual. In Chapter 2, Lee Je-ma also refers to this area as the "sacrum" when associating it with the other areas of the spine. It is likely that he is referring to both the urinary bladder and the sacrum here.

23  Sorrow is the *Jung* emotion of the So Yang Individual. Imbalanced *Jung* emotion leads to Internal [stomach Heat] illness.

24  Complacency is the *Song* nature of the So Eum Individual. Imbalanced *Song* nature leads to Exterior vulnerability and External [kidney Heat] illness.

25  Joy is the *Jung* emotion of the So Eum Individual. Imbalanced *Jung* emotion leads to Internal [spleen Cold] illness.

26  Joy is the *Song* nature of the Tae Eum Individual. Imbalanced *Song* nature leads to Exterior vulnerability and External [Esophageal Cold] illness.

27  Complacency is the *Jung* emotion of the Tae Eum Individual. Imbalanced *Jung* emotion leads to Internal [liver Heat] illness.

太陽人의 大便이 一則宜滑也오 二則宜體大而多也며 小便이 一則宜多
也오 二則宜數也며 面色이 宜白不宜黑하며 肌肉이 宜瘦 不宜肥하고 鳩
尾下에 不宜有塊니 塊小則病輕而其塊가 易消오 塊大則病重而其塊가 難
消니라.

For the Tae Yang Individual, thick and abundant stool is an indication of health, but not as much as soft and easy-to-pass stools. Frequent urination also indicates health, but less than larger volume and less frequent urination. A pallid complexion is comparably healthier than a darker complexion, and a thinner Tae Yang Individual is generally healthier than a heavyset one. Hardness of the Tae Yang Individual's epigastric area is an indication of poor health. A smaller area of hardness indicates a lighter, easy-to-overcome illness, while a larger hard area indicates a more serious condition that is difficult to treat effectively.

**Table 9.3: The Tae Yang Individual's Internally contracted illness affecting the small intestine**

| Syndrome | Symptoms | Treatment approach |
|---|---|---|
| Internally contracted illness affecting the small intestine | Dysphagia followed by choking, diaphragm spasms, vomiting (of breakfast in the evening and dinner in the morning) and/or dry heaves, thick frothy sputum, and excessive saliva, *without* abdominal pain, borborygmos, diarrhea, dysentery, or other digestive issues | *Mihudeng Shikjang Tang* (Lee Je-ma's Kiwifruit Vine Support the Intestines Decoction) |

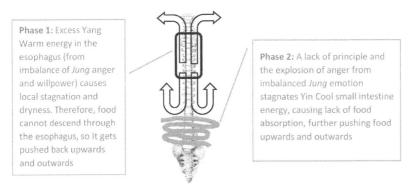

**Phase 1:** Excess Yang Warm energy in the esophagus (from imbalance of *Jung* anger and willpower) causes local stagnation and dryness. Therefore, food cannot descend through the esophagus, so it gets pushed back upwards and outwards

**Phase 2:** A lack of principle and the explosion of anger from imbalanced *Jung* emotion stagnates Yin Cool small intestine energy, causing lack of food absorption, further pushing food upwards and outwards

*Figure 9.2: The Ye Ge Fan Wei syndrome of the Tae Yang Individual*

## The Tae Yang Individual's Ten Herbs from the *Ben Cao Lun*, and Two Herbs Introduced by Li Chan and Gong Xin

本草日 五加皮는 治兩脚疼痺하며 骨節攣急痿厂하니라. 小兒三歲가 不能行에 服此하니 便行走하니라.

The *Ben Cao Lun* describes Wu Jia Pi (*Cortex Acanthopanacis*) as suitable for pain and numbness of the lower extremities, swelling of the knees and ankles, and difficulty walking. I once prescribed this herb for a Tae Yang adolescent unable to walk. After taking this herb as a tea, he was walking again.

松節은 療脚軟弱하니라.

Song Jie (*Lignum Pini Nodi*) is prescribed for weakness of the legs.

木瓜는 止嘔逆하니 煮汁飲之면 最佳니라.

Mu Gua (*Fructus Chaenomelis Lagenariae*) is prescribed for dry heaves, and is best prepared as a tea.

葡萄根은 止嘔厂하니 濃煎取汁하여 細細飲之면 佳니라.

Grape root (*Mahonia Aquifolium*) is also prescribed for dry heaves, and is best prepared as a strong tea ingested in small amounts.

獼猴桃는 治熱壅反胃하니 取汁服之니라. 藤汁은 至滑하여 主胃閉니 吐逆에는 煎取汁하여 服之면 甚佳니라.

Mi Hou Tao (*Fructus Actinidiae Sinensis*), also known as kiwifruit, clears excessive Heat causing vomiting and/or dry heaves, and is best prepared as a juice. The vine of Mi Hou Tao, also known as Mi Hou Teng (*Rhizoma Actinidiae Sinensis*), helps lubricate the stomach wall and prevent vomiting caused by stagnation of stomach energy. It is best to prepare the vine as a tea.

蘆根은 治乾嘔噎及五噎하며 煩悶하니라. 蘆根五兩을 水煎頓服一升하면 不過三升에 即差니라.

Lu Gen (*Rhizoma Phragmitisis*) is prescribed for dry heaves, *Wu Ye*[28] syndrome, and anxiety with fullness in the chest. Prepare 187.5g as a tea and drink with 64oz of water per dose. The patient will inevitably recover after drinking 192oz (three servings) of Lu Gen tea.

蚌蛤은 治反胃吐食하니라.

Bang Ha (*Solen Gouldii*) is prescribed for consistent vomiting following meals.

---

28    *Wu Ye* (五噎), translated as "five difficulties" syndrome, indicates illnesses stemming from one or more of the following five factors: worry, indigestion, overwork, *Qi* disharmony, and overthinking.

鮒魚는 治反胃하니라. 蓴和鮒魚를 作羹食之니라 主反胃 食不下하며 止嘔하니라.

Crucian Carp (*Carassius Carassius*) is for consistent vomiting after meals. Crucian Carp with Water Shield (*Bracenia Schreberi*) is also prescribed as a soup for consistent dry heaves and vomiting after meals.

蕎麥은 實腸胃하고 益氣力하니라.

Buckwheat (*Fagopyrum Esculentum*) strengthens the stomach and intestines while increasing stamina.

李ㅁ日杵頭糠은 主噎하며 食不下하며 咽喉塞하니라. 細糠一兩을 白粥淸에 調服하니라.

Li Chan once stated that Asian Rice Bran (*Furfur Oryza Sativa*) assists with dyspepsia and a feeling of blockage in the throat. Grind 37.5g of rice bran into fine powder and drink with rice water.

龔信曰蚌蛤은 治反胃하니라.

According to Gong Xin, Bang Ha (*Solen Gouldii*) assists with consistent vomiting or dry heaves after food intake.

## Two Newly Discovered Formulae for the Tae Yang Individual (Formulated by Lee Je-ma)

### Ohgapi Jangchuk Tang
*Lee Je-ma's Acanthopanax Strengthen the Spine Decoction*

| Wu Jia Pi | *Cortex Acanthopanacis* | 15g |
|---|---|---|
| Mu Gua | *Fructus Chaenomelis Lagenariae* | 7.5g |
| Song Jie | *Lignum Pini Nodi* | 7.5g |
| Grape Root | *Mahonia Aquifolium* | 3.75g |
| Lu Gen | *Rhizoma Phragmitisis* | 3.75g |
| Yu Li Ren | *Semen Pruni* | 3.75g |
| Buckwheat | *Fagopyrum Esculentum* | ½ Tablespoon |

Pine needles of good quality can be substituted if Song Jie (*Lignum Pini Nodi*) is not available. This formula is suitable for the Exterior syndrome of the Tae Yang Individual.

### *Mihudeng Shikjang Tang*
*Lee Je-ma's Kiwifruit Vine Support the Intestines Decoction*

| | | |
|---|---|---|
| Mu Gua | *Fructus Chaenomelis Lagenariae* | 18.75g |
| Grape Root | *Mahonia Aquifolium* | 18.75g |
| Mi Hou Tao | *Fructus Actinidiae Sinensis* | 15g |
| Lu Gen | *Rhizoma Phragmitisis* | 3.75g |
| Yu Li Ren | *Semen Pruni* | 3.75g |
| Wu Jia Pi | *Cortex Acanthopanacis* | 3.75g |
| Song Hua | *Pine Tree Flowers* | 3.75g |
| Asian Rice Bran | *Furfur Oryza Sativa* | ½ Tablespoon |

If fresh Mi Hou Tao (*Fructus Actinidiae Sinensis*) is not available, then Mi Hou Teng (*Rhizoma Actinidiae Sinensis*) can be substituted. This formula is suitable for the Tae Yang Individual's Interior syndrome.

Generally speaking, vegetables and fruit have a clear and neutral energy, making them beneficial for the liver. Most shells also have the ability to support the liver.

This section is limited in scope due to my lack of experience in treating the Tae Yang Individual, who since ancient times comprised only a small fraction of the total population. Hence there is very little written about the Tae Yang Individual's illness or appropriate treatment plan. Even though it may seem that *Ohgapi Jangchuk Tang* (Lee Je-ma's Acanthopanax Strengthen the Spine Decoction) and *Mihudeng Shikjang Tang* (Lee Je-ma's Kiwifruit Vine Support the Intestines Decoction) are unsophisticated and insufficient in scope, if they are carefully considered and adjusted after scrupulously evaluating the patient, then why worry about a lack of resources?

Part III

# ADDITIONAL TOPICS

## Chapter 10

廣
濟
說

# The Virtuous Path—Advice
# for Everyday Life

初一歲로 至十六歲를 曰幼오 十七歲로 至三十二歲를 曰少오 三十三
歲로 至四十八歲를 曰壯이오 四十九歲로 至六十四歲를 曰老니라.

Ages 1 through 16 can be considered childhood, 17 through 32 can be considered youth, 33 through 48 are the prime years, and 49 through 64, advanced age.

凡人이 幼年에 好聞見而能愛敬하니 如春生之芽하고 少年에 好勇猛而能
騰捷하니 如夏長之苗하고 壯年에 好交結而能修飭하니 如秋斂之實하고
老年에 好計策而能秘密하니 如冬藏之根하니라.

All people take pleasure in listening and looking, loving their parents, and looking up to their elders in childhood, which resembles a newly formed sprout emerging from the ground. In youth, courage and bravery take precedence. It makes sense for these youth to leap forward, like a seedling in the summer. During the prime years, teaching and self-cultivation become a priority, like ripened fruit in the fall. In advanced age, planning and keeping to oneself are a priority, which can be compared to a dormant root in the winter.

幼年에 好文字者는 幼年之豪傑也오 少年에 敬長老者는 少年之豪傑也오
壯年에 能汎愛者는 長年之豪傑也오 老年에 保可人者는 老年之豪傑也니
有好才能而又有十分快足於好心術者는 眞豪傑也오 有好才能而終不十分
快足於好心術者는 才能而已라.

Those who enjoy reading in their childhood often become extraordinary people, as do those who respect their parents and elders in their youth. Those who practice benevolence in their prime often become magnificent people. Those who have advanced skills and carry them out with a pure heart[1] will become extraordinary people. Those who have advanced skills but do not carry them out with a pure heart can only become skillful [but not magnificent].

幼年 七八歲前에 聞見이 未及而喜怒哀樂이 膠着則成病也니 慈母가 宜保護之也오 少年 二十四五歲前에 勇猛이 未及而喜怒哀樂이 膠着則成病也니 智父能兄이 宜保護之也오 壯年 三十八九歲前則賢弟良朋이 可以助之也오 老年 五十六七歲前則孝子孝孫이 可以扶之也니라.

If a child between seven and eight years of age doesn't engage in listening or observing enough and is easily overjoyed, angered, saddened, or cheerful, they will naturally be prone to illness and need their mother's protection. During one's youth, up to ages 24 or 25, if one lacks boldness, and is easily overjoyed, angered, saddened, or cheerful, one will be prone to illness, and will need their father's wisdom and their older brother's cleverness. During one's prime years, before ages 38 or 39, one must develop a close friendship with one's younger siblings in order to offer support and guidance. During one's senior years, up through ages 56 or 57, one will need the support of one's children and grandchildren.

善人之家에 善人이 必聚하고 惡人之家에 惡人이 必聚하나니 善人多聚則善人之臟氣가 活動하고 惡人多聚則惡人之心氣가 强旺하니라 酒色財權之家에 惡人이 多聚인 故로 其家孝男孝婦가 受病하니라.

Virtuous people will gather within the house of a virtuous person, while immoral people will gather in the house of an immoral person. If many virtuous people gather together, it will enhance the purification of their minds and bodies.[2] If many immoral people gather together, it will encourage negative thoughts and behavior.[3] Immoral people will often gather in households that indulge themselves in excessive alcohol, sex, riches, and authority. Even the virtuous man living in such a home will fall victim to illness.

好權之家는 朋黨이 比周하니 敗其家者는 朋黨也오 好貨之家는 子孫이 驕愚하니 敗其家者는 子孫也니라.

Immoral people will form groups, embrace, and flatter one another in a house that clings to authority, eventually suffering defeat from one of its own factions. Arrogance and stupidity prevail among the descendants of a home with accumulated riches. This home too will suffer defeat from one of its own descendants.

---

1   "Pure heart" is a translation of the term *Xin Shu* (心術), or "heart-centered skills." It denotes the ability to center one's mind and engage one's heartfelt sincerity.

2   "Purify the mind and body" is an interpretation of the phrase "臟氣가 活動하다," literally translated as "ample flow of organ energy."

3   "Negative thoughts and behavior" is an interpretation of the phrase "心氣가 强旺하니라," literally translated as "stiffening of the heart energy."

人家에 凡事不成하야 疾病이 連綿하며 善惡이 相持하야 其家將敗之
地에 惟明哲之慈父孝子라야 處之有術也니라.

Only a wise and affectionate father and the filial devotion of his child(ren) can save
a home that has failed in all of its endeavors, is incapable of shaking off illness, and
has lost sight of right and wrong.

驕奢가 減壽하고 懶怠가 減壽하고 偏急이 減壽하고 貪慾이 減壽하니라.
爲人驕奢하면 必耽侈色하고 爲人懶怠하면 必嗜酒色하고 爲人偏急하면
必爭權勢하고 爲人貪慾하면 必殉貨財하니라.

Arrogance, extravagance, laziness, hastiness, and selfishness will all shorten one's
lifespan.

An individual who is arrogant and extravagant will definitely chase after
beauty. An individual with a lazy nature will eventually abuse alcohol and indulge
in unhealthy eating habits. If a person is narrow-minded, they will always find
themselves at odds with those who wield power and influence. A greedy individual
will eventually destroy his/her health through an addiction to money and riches.

簡約이 得壽하고 勤幹이 得壽하고 警戒가 得壽하고 聞見이 得壽니라. 爲
人簡約이면 必遠奢色하고 爲人勤幹이면 必潔酒食하고 爲人警戒면 必避
權勢하고 爲人聞見이면 必淸貨財하니라

Simplification, diligence, self-reflection, and wisdom will lengthen one's lifespan.

A person who lives simply will distance him/herself from sexual attraction.
A diligent person will avoid alcohol and unhealthy eating habits. A self-reflective
person will abstain from bearing authority. A wise person will not stain his or her
purity with money or riches.

居處荒涼은 色之故也오 行身闊茸은 酒之故也오 用心煩亂은 權之故也오
事務錯亂은 貨之故也니라.

Excessive lust results in a lonely and desolate home. Excessive alcohol consumption
results in behavioral neglect. Excessive authority results in a mind lacking persistency
and always in a state of confusion and disarray. Excessive accumulation of wealth
results in difficulty with public affairs.

若敬淑女면 色得中道하고 若愛良朋이면 酒得明德하고 若尙賢人이면 權得正術하고 若保窮民이면 貨得全功하니라.

If a man accompanies[4] a virtuous wife, sexual intercourse between them is an act of virtue, while drinking alcohol with virtuous friends can also be seen in the same light. The yearning to be upright leads to fairness and honest leadership. If such an individual makes an effort to protect those who are widowed, orphaned, or without descendants, he or she will accumulate merit and wealth.

酒色財權을 自古所戒라 謂之四堵墙而比之牢獄하니 非但一身壽夭와 一家禍福之所係也라 天下治亂도 亦在於此하니 若使一天下酒色財權으로 乖戾之氣則庶幾近於堯舜周召南之世矣리라.

Since ancient times, our forefathers compared alcohol, sex, wealth, and authority to four "property markers" that may imprison an individual and determine the extent of his or her fortune or misfortune. Harmony, not just within a single family, but throughout the entire world, depends on the four "property markers." If everyone refrained from abuse and corruption of the four markers, then the entire world would achieve the extent of virtue accomplished by emperors Yao and Shun, and the rulers of Southern Zhou and Shao.[5]

凡人이 簡約而勤幹하며 警戒而聞見하야 四材圓全者는 自然上壽하고 簡約勤幹而警戒커나 或聞見警戒而勤幹하야 三材全者는 次壽하고 驕奢而勤幹하며 警戒而貪慾하거나 或簡約而懶怠하며 偏急而聞見하야 二材全者는 恭敬則壽하고 怠慢則夭하니라. 凡人이 恭敬則必壽하고 怠慢則必夭하며 勤幹則必壽하고 虛貪則必夭하니

If an individual remains pure, diligent, self-observant, and wise, he or she will naturally live a long and prosperous life. If an individual carries out three out of four of these qualities, such as purity, diligence, and self-observance [but not wisdom], or wisdom, self-observance, and diligence [but not purity], then he or she will live a fairly prosperous and long life. If an individual is cunning and extravagant, but diligent, self-observant, or pure and wise, but lazy and hasty, only if he or she is cautious about his/her behavior will prosperity and longevity await. But if he or she is overcome with laziness, then life will be short and unprosperous. An individual who shows respect to others will live a long time; if he becomes lazy, then life will

---

4   The word "accompany" is a translation of *Gyung* (敬), which also means "to respect" or "to honor." Hence although he lived in a time when wives were expected to be subordinate to their husbands, Lee Je-ma nevertheless acknowledges the importance of respecting and honoring one's virtuous wife.

5   In the *Confucian Analects*, Confucius asked his son: "Have you studied the Southern Zhou and Shao in the *Book of Poetry*? A lack of familiarity with the ways of the Southern Zhou and Shao is like standing in front of a wall blocking you from entering your own home." The Southern Zhou and Shao Dynasties were initiated by benevolent emperors whom Confucius often refers to when exemplifying virtue and propriety.

be short. If he is diligent, life will be expanded, but if he becomes indulgent, then he will not live a long life.

飢者之腸이 急於得食則腸氣가 蕩矣오 貪者之骨이 急於得財則骨力이 竭矣니라 飢而安飢則腸氣有守하고 貧而安貧則骨力有立하나니 是故로 飮食은 以能忍飢而不貪飽로 爲恭敬이오 衣服은 以能耐寒而不貪溫으로 爲恭敬이오 筋力은 以能勤勞而不貪安逸로 爲恭敬이오 財物은 以能謹實而不貪苟得으로 爲恭敬이니라.

Hunger that is hastily subdued leads to disharmony of the stomach and intestines. Poverty that leads to a hasty desire for wealth eventually causes weakness of the spirit. The ability to control hunger will lead to the strengthening of the stomach and intestines. The ability to cope with poverty will help solidify the spirit. The ability to control hunger and refrain from eating until full is worthy of respect. The ability to withstand colder temperatures and not overdress is worthy of respect. The desire to work hard and control a longing for relaxation is worthy of respect. The ability to avoid being excessively concerned about finances and a lack of desire for wealth is worthy of respect.

山谷之人이 沒聞見而禍夭하고 市井之人이 沒簡約而禍夭하고 農畝之人이 沒勤幹而禍夭하고 讀書之人이 沒警戒而禍夭하니라.

A mountain dweller who doesn't develop his/her desire to listen and observe will live a shortened life. A city dweller too, who doesn't remain pure, will live a shortened life. A farmer who is not diligent will live a shorter life. A scholar who is not self-observant will also live a shortened life.

山谷之人이 宜有聞見이니 有聞見則福壽하고 市井之人이 宜有簡約이니 有簡約則福壽하고 鄉野之人이 宜有勤幹이니 有勤幹則福壽하고 士林之人이 宜有警戒니 有警戒則福壽하니라.

A mountain dweller who develops a keen sense of hearing and sight will live a prosperous and long life. If a city dweller preserves the purity of their spirit, he or she will live a prosperous and long life. A diligent farmer will live a prosperous and long life. A scholar who focuses on polishing and cultivating their mind and body will live a prosperous and long life.

山谷之人이 若有聞見하면 非但福壽也라 此人은 卽山谷之傑也오 市井之人이 若有簡約하면 非但福壽也라 此人은 卽市井之傑也오 鄉野之人이 若有勤幹하면 非但福壽也라 此人은 卽鄉野之傑也오 林之人이 若有警戒하면 非但福壽也라 此人은 卽士林之傑也니라.

Not only will a mountain dweller with a keen sense of hearing and sight live a prosperous and long life, but they will also become an extraordinary mountaineer.

Not only will a city dweller with a pure heart live a prosperous and long life, but they will also become an extraordinary urbanite. Not only will a farmer who is diligent by nature live a prosperous and long life, but they will also become an extraordinary farmer. Not only will a scholar who focuses on polishing and cultivating their mind and body live a prosperous and long life, but they will also become an extraordinary scholar.

或이 曰農夫가 元來力作하니 最是勤幹者也而何謂沒勤幹하며 士人은 元來讀書하니 最是警戒者也인데 而何謂沒警戒耶아 曰以百畝之不治로 爲己憂者는 農夫之任也니 農夫而比之士人則眞是懶怠者也오 士人이 頗讀書인 故로 心恒妄矜하고 農夫는 目不識字인 故로 心恒佩銘하니 士人而擬之農夫則眞不警戒者也라. 若農夫가 勤於識字하며 士人이 習於力作則才性이 調密하고 臟氣가 堅固하니라.

Someone once asked me: "How can you say that a farmer who is diligent by trade is capable of being lazy, or a scholar who is self-observant by trade risks being ignorant?" I answered that a farmer who owns 100 rice fields will eventually be filled with worry. Field cultivation is the responsibility of a farmer, but such a farmer will become lazier than a scholar. A scholar who indulges himself in reading [without applying himself socially] will eventually become foolish and conceited. The farmer will always bear in mind his lack of literary skills, while the scholar doesn't keep watch over himself as much as the farmer. Thus, a farmer who makes an effort to become literate and a scholar who exerts himself like a farmer will not only increase their skills but also solidify his or her organ health.

嬌奢者之心은 藐視閭閻生活하며 輕易天下室家하야 眼界驕豪하야 全昧産業之艱難하고 甚劣財力之方略하나니 每爲女色所陷하야 終身不悔하니라

The well-off but arrogant and extravagant person will harbor resentment against the middle class, while carelessly engaging in his own family affairs. He will cling steadfastly to his opinions and ignore work-related and financial issues. He will have difficulty realizing that all of his affairs, which are based in lust [and greed], will eventually ruin his family and reputation.

懶怠者之心은 極其矗猛하야 不欲積工之寸累하고 每有虛大之甕算하니 蓋其心이 甚憚勤幹인 故로 欲逃其身於酒國하야 以姑避勤幹之計也라 凡懶怠者는 無不縱酒하니 但見縱酒者則必知其爲懶怠人心이 矗猛也니라.

The heart of a lazy-natured individual is always worn out and unstable. Instead of placing one foot forward, he or she sets impractical and absurd goals while abhorring hard work and drinking alcohol to escape from worry. This individual often devises schemes to avoid difficult tasks.

酒色之殺人者를 人皆曰酒毒이 枯腸하고 色勞가 竭精云하나 此는 知其
一이오 未知其二也니라. 縱酒者는 厭勤其身하니 憂患이 如山하고 惑色
者는 深愛其女하니 憂患이 如刀하야 萬端心曲이 與酒毒色勞로 幷力攻
之而殺人也니라.

Not all lazy-natured people indulge themselves in drinking. But those who do are
assuredly lazy, worn-out, and unstable. The phrase "alcohol and sex are murderous"
refers to the damaging effects of alcohol on the stomach and intestines, and to
the withering away of essence caused by excessive sexual intercourse. This phrase
doesn't, however, paint the full picture. Trouble will pile up as high as a mountain if
one abuses alcohol. Anxiety and worry will cut like a knife if an individual cannot
control his or her lust and overindulges in sexual activity.

狂童은 必愛淫女하고 淫女는 亦愛狂童하며 愚夫는 必愛妬婦하고 妬
婦는 必愛愚夫하나니 以物理觀之則淫女는 斷合狂童之配也오 愚夫는 亦
宜妬婦之匹也라. 蓋淫女妬婦는 可以爲惡人賤人之配匹也오 不可爲君
子貴人之配匹也니 七去惡中에 淫去 妬去 爲首惡而世俗이 不知妬字之
義리라. 但以憎疾衆妾으로 爲言하니 貴人之繼嗣가 最重則婦人이 必不
可憎疾貴人之有妾而亂家之本이 未嘗不在於衆妾則婦人之憎疾衆妾之邪
媚者는 猶爲婦人之賢德也니 何所當於妬字之義乎아 詩云桃之夭夭에 其
葉이 蓁蓁이로다 之子于歸에 宜其家人이라하니 宜其家人者는 好賢樂善
而宜於家人之謂也오 不宜其家人者는 妬賢嫉能而不宜於家人之謂也니라.

An uncultivated man will naturally fall in love with a lewd woman, while a lewd
woman will naturally fall in love with an uncultivated man. A foolish man will
inevitably fall in love with a jealous-natured woman, while a jealous-natured
woman will definitely fall in love with a foolish man. It goes without saying that
an uncultivated man and a lewd woman, or a foolish man and a jealous-natured
woman, make suitable couples. For the most part, lewd and jealous-natured wives
eventually marry malevolent and lowly, rather than learned or noble, men. Among
the *seven types of wives to avoid*,[6] those who are lewd or jealous are most certainly to
be avoided. Most people have trouble understanding the true meaning of jealousy
and equate it with a wife's hatred of a cheating husband. A wife [who cannot bear
a son] doesn't harbor hatred towards her husband's mistress, knowing that she may
assist in carrying on the family lineage.[7] Numerous mistresses, however, will likely

---

6    The *seven types of wives to avoid* (七去之惡) is the title of a section in the *Path of Marriage* chapter of the
    ancient text entitled *The Sayings of Confucius*. It advises against marriage and encourages divorce of a bride
    who is (1) not loyal to her parents, (2) infertile, (3) lavish, (4) jealous-natured, (5) plagued with chronic
    illness, (6) always gossiping, and (7) a kleptomaniac.

7    Lee Je-ma lived during the Joseon Dynasty (1392–1897) in Korea, which embraced the custom of entrusting
    the oldest son with carrying out his family heritage. He inherits most, if not all, of his family's property, and in
    return is expected to support his parents when they age. This custom, although fading quickly, is still practiced
    to an extent in present-day Korea.

cause a disturbance within the home. Hence it is an act of wisdom for a wife to single out those who are flattering and conniving. So what is meant by the Chinese character for "jealousy"? The *Book of Poetry* utilizes the peach as a metaphor for balance and harmony, because the blending of its flesh and leaves brings about exuberant beauty. It compares harmony to a bride who, after leaving her parents' home, brings balance and harmony to the groom's family who appreciate and enjoy a virtuous and kind-hearted bride. A family that is jealous of a virtuous bride and dislikes her talents cannot bring about unity and attain such stature.

凡人家에 疾病이 連綿하며 死亡이 相隨하며 子孫이 遇蚩하며 資産이 零落者가 莫非愚夫妬婦의 妬賢嫉能之所做出也니라.

The descendants of a family plagued with chronic disease and frequent death will often become irrational and destroy the family's remaining assets—a result of the combined efforts of foolish men and lavish women who envy the virtuous and loathe those who are capable. Their lives are all about devising schemes.

天下之惡이 莫多於妬賢嫉能이오 天下之善이 莫大於好賢樂善이니 不妬賢嫉能而爲惡則惡必不多也오 不好賢樂善而爲善則善必不大也니라.

The jealousy and hatred of benevolent people is the worst of all evils. The love of virtuous people and the joy of benefitting others is the greatest of all merits. If someone harbors jealousy towards virtuous people but doesn't hate those who are benevolent, their actions will not be ruthless. If someone dislikes virtuous people but enjoys benefitting others, their actions will not attain substantial merit.

歷稽往牒컨대 天下之受病이 都出於妬賢嫉能이오 天下之救病이 都出於好賢樂善이니 故로 曰妬賢嫉能은 天下之多病也오 好賢樂善은 天下之大藥也라하노라.

If one carefully heeds the ancient teachings, he or she will discover that all illness stems from the jealousy of virtuous people and the hatred of those who are benevolent. Moreover, these teachings emphasize how all illness can be overcome by admiring the virtuous and enjoying the act of benefitting others.

# Chapter 11 ───────

# Four Constitutional Classification and Diagnosis

四象人辨證論

太少陰陽人을 以今時目見하면 一縣萬人數로 大略論之則
太陰人이 五千人也오
少陽人이 三千人也오
少陰人이 二千人也오
太陽人數는 絶少하야 一縣中에 或三四人十餘人而已니라.

Years of observation led to my discovery that within a given population of 10,000 people, there are about 5000 Tae Eum Individuals, 3000 So Yang Individuals, and 2000 So Eum Individuals. Since there are so few Tae Yang Individuals, the total number will average about three to four, but no more than ten, out of 10,000 people.

太陽人 體形氣像은 腦佳頁之起勢가 盛壯而腰圍之立勢孤弱하고
少陽人 體形氣像은 胸襟之包勢가 盛壯而膀胱之坐勢孤弱하고
太陰人 體形氣像은 腰圍之立勢가 盛壯而腦佳頁之起勢孤弱하고
少陰人 體形氣像은 膀胱之坐勢가 盛壯而胸襟之包勢孤弱이니라.

The Tae Yang Individual has a well-developed head and cervical spine but a delicate and narrow waist. The So Yang Individual has a well-developed, wide chest and broad shoulders, but a loss of urinary bladder area muscle tone. The Tae Eum Individual has a well-developed waist but lacks a developed head and cervical spine. The So Eum Individual has superior muscle tone around their bladder but narrower shoulders and chest.

**Table 11.1: Developed and underdeveloped anatomy of each constitution**

| Constitution | Developed area of the body | Underdeveloped area of the body |
|---|---|---|
| Tae Yang | Head and cervical spine | Waist |
| So Yang | Chest and shoulders | Urinary bladder |
| Tae Eum | Waist | Head and cervical spine |
| So Eum | Urinary bladder | Shoulders and chest |

太陽人 性質은 長於疏通而材幹이 能於交遇하고
少陽人 性質은 長於剛武而材幹이 能於事務하고
太陰人 性質은 長於成就而材幹이 能於居處하고
少陰人 性質은 長於端重而材幹이 能於黨與하니라.

Generosity is a strong characteristic of the Tae Yang Individual, and is a skill born from *Kyo Uh*. Courage is a strong characteristic of the So Yang Individual, and is a skill born from *Sa Mu*. The sense of accomplishment is a strong characteristic of the Tae Eum Individual, and is a skill born from *Ko Cho*. Propriety is a strong characteristic of the So Eum Individual, and is a skill born from *Dang Yo*.[1]

太陽人 體形은 元不難辨而人數稀罕인 故로 最爲難辨也니 其體形이 腦
佳頁之起勢가 强旺하며 性質이 疏通하며 又有果斷하고 其病은 噎膈 反
胃 解㑊證이니 亦自易辨而病未至重險之前에는 別無大證하야 完若無病
壯健人也니라 少陰人老人이 亦有噎證하니 不可誤作太陽人治니라

Even though it is easy to decipher the body shape of a Tae Yang Individual, distinguishing them from other body types is still difficult since they are so few in number. This process is made easier by the fact that they have a well-developed head and neck, always seem energetic and resolute, and succumb to *Ye Ge Fan Wei* and *Xie Yi* syndromes. Moreover, they rarely manifest acute symptoms, always seeming healthy without illness. If an elder So Eum Individual contracts *Ye Ge Fan Wei* syndrome, the practitioner must practice extreme caution, and avoid mistreatment.

太陽女 體形이 壯實而肝小脇窄하야 子宮不足한 故로 不能生産이니 以
六畜으로 玩理컨대 而太陽牝牛馬 體形이 壯實而亦不能生産者하니 其
理를 可推니라.

Even though the Tae Yang female has a healthy and robust appearance, her waist will be narrow and her uterus undeveloped; hence she will have difficulty getting pregnant and/or giving birth. The Tae Yang female can be compared to a cow or horse that despite its robust and healthy appearance cannot reproduce easily.

---

1   Even though *Kyo Uh* is a strong characteristic of the Tae Yang, *Sa Mu* of the So Yang, *Ko Cho* of the Tae Eum, and *Dang Yo* of the So Eum Individual, they do not manifest of their own accord. These characteristics correlate with the *Jung* emotion of each constitution. Only when the *Jung* emotion is controlled and balanced do these strong characteristics manifest themselves.

少陽人 體形은 上盛下虛하며 胸實足輕하야 剽銳好勇而人數亦多하니 四象人中에 最爲易辨이니라.

The So Yang Individual has a developed upper body but deficient lower body. Hence the chest is well developed, but the legs are thin and narrow. The So Yang Individual is the easiest of the four constitutions to distinguish because of their hasty, harsh, straightforward, and masculine nature and high population density.

少陽人이 或有短小靜雅하야 外形이 恰似少陰人者하니 觀其病勢寒熱하야 仔細執證이오 不可誤作少陰人治니라.

The So Yang Individual may sometimes be confused with the So Eum Individual if they have a smaller body, a quiet nature, and a graceful disposition. Therefore, it is necessary to clearly decipher between Cold- and Hot-related syndromes and avoid prescribing So Eum herbs for the So Yang Individual and vice versa.

太陰少陰人 體形이 或略相彷彿하야 難辨疑似로대 而觀其病證則必無不辨이니
太陰人이 虛汗則完實也오 少陰人이 虛汗則大病也며
太陰人이 陽剛堅密則大病也오 少陰人이 陽剛堅密則完實也니라.
太陰人은 有胸膈怔忡證也오 少陰人은 有手足悗亂證也며
太陰人은 有目眥上引證하고 又有目睛內疼證也로대 少陰人則無此證也오
少陰人은 平時呼吸이 平均而間有一太息呼吸也나 太陰人則無此太息呼吸也오 太陰人은 瘧疾惡寒中에 能飮冷水로대 少陰人은 瘧疾惡寒中에 不飮冷水하고 太陰人脈은 長而緊이나 少陰人脈은 緩而弱하고 太陰人肌肉은 堅實이나 少陰人肌肉은 浮軟하고
太陰人 容貌詞氣는 起居有儀而修整正大하나
少陰人 容貌詞氣는 體任自然而簡易小巧하니라.
少陰人의 體形은 矮短而亦多有長大者하야 或有八九尺長大者며 太陰人의 體形은 長大而亦或有六尺矮短者니라.

The Tae Eum may also be confused with the So Eum, but symptomatic differences are not difficult to detect. A Tae Eum Individual with sweat due to deficiency may still be considered healthy, but a So Eum Individual would be considered seriously ill. Hard and thick skin is a sign of serious illness for the Tae Eum Individual, but a sign of health for the So Eum Individual. While the Tae Eum Individual has a tendency to experience palpitations, the So Eum Individual has a tendency to experience sudden shaking of the hands and feet [when overall health is compromised]. Unlike the So Eum Individual, some Tae Eum Individuals have eyes that arch upwards at the outer canthus or have sharp pain in their pupils. Unlike the Tae Eum Individual, some So Eum Individuals will occasionally gasp for air or let out a deep sigh. Unlike the So Eum Individual, the Tae Eum Individual can drink cold fluids even if they contract severe chills from malaria. The pulse of a Tae Eum Individual is long and firm, while the pulse of a So Eum Individual is slow and weak. The muscles and skin of the Tae Eum Individual have a solid texture, while the So Eum Individual has soft muscles and skin. The Tae Eum Individual often has a dignified appearance, strong voice, and upright lifestyle. They are often quick to correct their mistakes and don't have much of a private life. The So Eum Individual often has a natural and calm countenance, gentle speech, and has a casual gait as he or she walks, carrying a somewhat shrewd and clever air. The So Eum Individual is often short and occasionally dwarf-like in appearance, but may also be exceptionally tall, to the point of being eight to nine feet in height. The Tae Eum Individual is often tall and can grow up to six feet tall.

**Table 11.2: A comparison between the Tae Eum and So Eum Individual**

| Characteristic | Tae Eum Individual | So Eum Individual |
| --- | --- | --- |
| Sweating | Healthy even with deficient sweat | Deficient sweat indicates a lack of health |
| Skin | Hard and thick skin indicates serious illness | Hard and thick skin indicates health |
| Symptoms of deteriorating health | Palpitations | Shaking of the hands and feet |
| Eyes | Arch upwards at the outer canthus or pupil pain | These characteristics rarely exist |
| Sighing | Uncommon symptom | Common symptom |
| Cold fluids | Can drink cold fluids when experiencing chills | Cannot drink cold fluids when experiencing chills |
| Pulse | Long and firm | Slow and weak |
| Muscles and skin | Solid texture | Soft texture |
| Appearance | Dignified | Natural and calm |
| Voice | Strong | Soft |
| Height | Often taller | Often shorter |

太陰人은 恒有怯心하니 怯心이 寧靜則居之安하며 資之深而造於道也오 怯心이 益多則放心桎梏而物化之也라. 若怯心이 至於怕心則大病作而怔忡也니 怔忡者는 太陰人病之重證也니라.

The Tae Eum Individual is often fearful and must calm their fears and find tranquility of heart in order to enjoy a peaceful home. Only after the establishment of a firm inner foundation can the Tae Eum Individual embark on the journey of virtue. But depending on the situation, uncontrolled fear may lead to carelessness and a feeling of entrapment, restlessness, and/or vexation. Significant illness, accompanied by palpitations, will result if fear and cowardice lead to fright. The occurrence of palpitations [in all cases] indicate that the Tae Eum Individual is afflicted with a significant illness.

少陽人은 恒有懼心하니 懼心寧靜則居之安하며 資之深而造於道也오 懼心이 益多則放心桎梏而物化之也라. 若懼心이 至於恐心則大病作而健忘也니 健忘者는 少陽人病之險證也ㅣ니라.

The So Yang Individual always harbors fright. A peaceful home depends on the ability to calm fright and find tranquility of the heart. Only after the establishment of a firm inner foundation can the So Yang Individual embark on the journey of virtue. Uncontrolled fright will lead to a feeling of entrapment, restlessness, and/or vexation. Significant illness, accompanied by the sudden loss of memory, will result if fright leads to phobia or morbid thoughts. The sudden loss of memory [in all cases] indicates that the So Yang Individual is afflicted with a significant illness.

少陰人은 恒有不安定之心하니 不安定之心이 寧靜則脾氣가 卽活也오 太陽人은 恒有急迫之心하니 急迫之心이 寧靜則肝血이 卽和也니라.

The So Eum Individual always harbors unsettled feelings. Replacing these feelings with peace and tranquility will enliven the *Qi* of their weaker spleen.

The Tae Yang Individual always feels a sense of urgency. If these feelings are replaced with peace and tranquility, the Tae Yang Individual can balance his/her liver blood.

少陰人이 有咽喉證하니 其病은 太重而爲緩病也나 不可等閒任置니 當用 蔘桂八物湯 或用獐肝 金蛇酒니라.

Throat-related illness of the So Eum Individual indicates a critical situation that will take time and effort to overcome. Hence, [even when the throat is mildly sore] it is crucial not to overlook its severity. For this situation *Samgye Palmul Tang* (Lee Je-ma's Ginseng and Cinnamon Twig Eight Ingredient Decoction),[2] roe deer liver, or silver snake[3] should be prescribed.

太陽人이 有八九日 大便不通證하니 其病은 非殆證也라 不必疑惑而亦不可無藥이니 當用 獼猴藤五加皮湯이니라.

Even if the Tae Yang Individual goes without a bowel movement for eight to nine days, it is still not considered a dangerous situation, and there is no doubt of recovery. Yet if there is medicine at hand, *Mihudeng Ohgapi Tang* (Lee Je-ma's Kiwifruit and Acanthopanax Decoction)[4] may be prescribed.

---

2   Lee Je-ma doesn't give reference to *Samgye Palmul Tang* elsewhere in this text. It is likely that this formula is a combination of *Palmul Gunja Tang* (Lee Je-ma's Eight Ingredient Gentlemen Decoction) with added Gui Zhi (*Ramulus Cinnamomi Cassiae*), but the exact dosage of Gui Zhi could not be located. Please refer to the section on So Eum illness for the ingredients of *Palmul Gunja Tang*.

3   Silver snake isn't currently utilized in Sasang medicine, and further information about it could not be found.

4   Lee Je-ma doesn't refer to *Mihudeng Ohgapi Tang* elsewhere in this text. It is likely that it is an alternative name for *Mihudeng Shikjang Tang* (Lee Je-ma's Kiwifruit Vine Support the Intestines Decoction), which is included in the list of Tae Yang formulae (please see Chapter 9).

太陽人은 小便이 旺多則完實而無病이오
太陰人은 汗液이 通暢則完實而無病이오
少陽人은 大便이 善通則完實而無病이오
少陰人은 飮食이 善化則完實而無病이니라.

Regulated urination is a sign of the Tae Yang Individual's overall health and lack of illness. Uninhibited sweating is a sign of overall health and lack of illness for the Tae Eum Individual. Regular bowel movement is a sign of overall health and lack of illness for the So Yang Individual. The ability to digest food without complication is a sign of overall health and lack of illness for the So Eum Individual.

**Table 11.3: Health indications for each constitution**

| Constitution | Sign of health |
|---|---|
| Tae Yang | Smooth flow and regulated frequency of urine |
| Tae Eum | Sufficient sweating capability |
| So Yang | Smooth flow and regulated frequency of bowel movement |
| So Eum | Ability to digest food without complication |

太陽人이 噎膈則胃脘之上焦가 散豁如風하고
太陰人이 痢病則小腸之中焦가 窒塞如霧하고
少陽人이 大便不通則胸膈이 必如烈火하고
少陰人이 泄瀉不止則臍下가 必如氷冷하나니
明知其人而又明知其證則應用之藥이 必無可疑니라.

*Ye Ge Fan Wei* syndrome will cause the Tae Yang Individual's esophagus in the Upper *Jiao* to feel cool, like a [fall] breeze. The Tae Eum Individual's dysentery will cause the small intestine in the Mid-Lower *Jiao* to stagnate, like a thick fog. The So Yang Individual's lack of bowel movement will cause the chest and rib cage in the Mid-Upper *Jiao* area to feel hot like fire. The So Eum's consistent diarrhea will cause the area below the umbilicus in the Lower *Jiao* to feel as cold as ice. If one takes the time to clearly differentiate each constitution and accompanying symptoms, there is no reason to doubt which herbs are suitable for each condition.

人物形容을 仔細商量하야 再三推移하되 如有迷惑則參互病證하야 明見
無疑然後에 可以用藥이오 最不可輕忽而一貼藥을 誤投重病險證이면 一
貼藥이 必殺人이니라.

The careful observation of an individual's body shape should be repeated several times before a treatment protocol is established. If doubt lingers, then a thorough symptomatic investigation is warranted. Only after one takes precautions and no doubt remains should herbs be prescribed. Not even a single pack of herbs should be prescribed carelessly, since this can kill a patient who is seriously ill.

華佗曰養生之術이 每欲小勞니 但莫大疲니라.

According to the renowned physician Hua Tuo,[5] the secret to longevity is making suitable effort in one's affairs. Exhaustive effort made in vain [will shorten one's lifespan].

有一老人曰人可日再食而不四五食也며 又不可既食後添食이니 如此則必無不壽니라.

An elder once stated that two meals a day are adequate, while eating three or four meals per day should be avoided. He also advised against snacking between meals, adding that if such rules are followed, longevity will inevitably be achieved.

余足之曰太陰人은 察於外而恒寧靜怯心하고
少陽人은 察於內而恒寧靜懼心하고
太陽人은 退一步而恒寧靜急迫之心하고
少陰人은 進一步而恒寧靜不安定之心이니 如此則必無不壽니라.

In addition to these guidelines, I would like to add that if the Tae Eum Individual focuses more on external (societal) affairs while calming and quieting his/her timid mind, the So Yang Individual focuses more on internal (household) affairs while calming and quieting his/her frightful mind, the Tae Yang Individual retreats one step back while calming and quieting his/her hasty mind, and the So Eum Individual advances one step forward while calming and quieting his/her unsettled mind, then longevity will inevitably follow.

又曰太陽人은 恒戒怒心哀心하고 少陽人은 恒戒哀心怒心하고 太陰人은 恒戒樂心喜心하고 少陰人은 恒戒喜心樂心이니 如此則必無不壽니라.

Moreover, if the Tae Yang Individual controls his or her *Jung* emotion of anger and *Song* nature of sadness, the So Yang Individual controls his or her *Jung* emotion of sadness and *Song* nature of anger, the Tae Eum Individual controls his or her *Jung* emotion of complacency and *Song* nature of joyfulness, and the So Eum Individual controls his or her *Jung* emotion of joyfulness and *Song* nature of calmness, then longevity will be achieved.

---

5    Hua Tuo (華佗; 140–208 AD), a Chinese physician of the Eastern Han Dynasty, became well known for his superior surgical methods and ability as a skilled acupuncturist and herbologist. He was the first to use anesthesia during surgery with wine and a herbal decoction he referred to as *Ma Fei San* (麻沸散, Cannabis Boiling Powder). Hua Tuo also developed the *Exercise of the Five Animals*, or *Wu Qin Xi* (五禽戲), a martial arts technique to cultivate one's mind and body through imitating the movements of a tiger, deer, bear, ape, and crane.

大舜이 自耕稼陶漁로 無非取諸人以爲善하시고 夫子曰三人行에 必有
我師라하니 以此觀之則天下衆人之才能을 聖人이 必博學審問而兼之인
故로 大而化也니라.

The Great Emperor Shun learned how to till a rice field, use a kiln, hunt, and all other things from the common people for the sake of promoting benevolence. Confucius once said that if he travels with three people, surely one of them will be his guide. Further examination reveals how a sage, like the emperor who learns from the common people, always makes an earnest attempt to learn and inquire about everything, and compiles this wisdom [for the sake of future generations].

太少陰陽人 識見才局이 各有所長하야 文筆射御 歌舞揖讓으로 以至於博
奕小技 細鎖動作이 凡百做造가 面面不同하야 皆異其妙하니 儘乎衆人才
能之浩多於造化中也로라.

Each of the four constitutions has its own innate insights and skills [depending on the relative strength of the Four Major Organs]; everything from how sentences are structured, handwriting is written, a wagon is maneuvered, an arrow is shot, a dance is performed, modesty is expressed or yielding to others, and how Korean chess or *Paduk* strategy is implemented. Each individual has minute skills and actions that are all subtly different from one another. Yet the various skills of each person represent only a fraction of the countless variations in our infinite universe.

靈樞書中에 有太少陰陽五行人論而略得外形하고 未得臟理하니 蓋太少
陰陽人이 早有古昔之見而未盡精究也니라.

Even though the *Ling Shu* mentions Tae Yang, So Yang, Tae Eum, So Eum, and the Five Elemental Constitutions,[6] it refers to outward appearance rather than *Zhang* organ theory. Hence even though the Tae Yang, So Yang, Tae Eum, and So Eum Individuals had already been discovered in the distant past, precise examination was never undertaken.

---

6    In this sentence, Lee Je-ma refers to the 64th (*Yin and Yang and the Twenty-five Types of Men*) and 72nd (*Penetrating Heaven*) chapters of the *Ling Shu*. The former chapter states: "First establish the five appearances of Metal, Wood, Water, Fire, and Earth. Separate them into five colors. Differentiate them into five body types of man, and then the twenty-five types of mankind as a whole." The latter chapter states: "There is a Major Yin (Tai Yin) man, Minor Yin (Shao Yin) man, Major Yang (Tai Yang) man, Minor Yang (Shao Yang) man, and the balanced and harmonious Yin and Yang man. The total comprises five different types of men of different aspect. Their muscles, bones, *Qi*, and blood are all dissimilar" (Wu Jing-Nuan (1993) *Ling Shu or Spiritual Pivot*. University of Hawaii Press).

此書는 自癸巳七月十三日에 始作하야 晝思夜度하야 無頃刻休息하야 至于翌年 甲午四月十三日하니 少陰少陽人論則略得詳備하되 太陰太陽人論則僅成簡約하니 蓋經驗이 未遍而精力이 已憊故也ㅣ니라. 記에 曰開而不達則思라하니 若太陰太陽人을 思而得之則亦何損乎簡約哉리오.

I started to write this treatise on July 13, 1893. Without a moment of rest from my research, I completed it in the following year on April 13, 1894. However, as a result of limited clinical data and my failing health, I could only summarize the So Eum and So Yang sections and briefly touch on the Tae Eum and Tae Yang sections.

In ancient times it was written that if what is seen is not understood, then it requires further thought. If my concise analysis provided in the Tae Eum and Tae Yang sections is given ample thought, then what is there to be left misunderstood?

萬室之邑에 一人이 陶則器不足也오 百家之村에 一人이 醫則活人이 不足也니 必廣明醫學하야 家家知醫하며 人人知病然後에 可以壽世保元이라.

There would never be enough dishware if a county with 10,000 homes had only one potter, just as a single doctor is not sufficient to take care of a village with 100 homes. Longevity and the preservation of health throughout the world can only be accomplished through advancing medicine, and making it accessible in every household and comprehensible by all people.

光緒甲午四月十三日에 咸興에서 李濟馬가 畢書于漢南山中하니라.

Completed on April 13, 1894 by Lee Je-ma in Mt. Han Nam.

嗚呼라 公이 甲午에 畢書後하고 乙未에 下鄉하야 至于庚子까지 因本改草하기를 自性明論에서 至太陰人諸論까지는 各有增删이나 而太陽人以下三論은 未有增删인 故로 今以甲午舊本으로 開刊하니라.

I returned to my hometown a year after completing this manuscript in 1894. In the year 1900, I decided to add the *Tae Eum* and *Basic Principles of Medicine* sections without the chance to modify any remaining sections, and instead submitted this manuscript with the above additions for publication.

# Useful Resources

Despite its firm establishment and popularity in Korea, Sasang medicine is still in its infancy in the West, with limited material in English. Increasing interest will eventually lead to further availability of valuable Sasang-related information. With growing popularity will come well-meaning but misguided interpretations that depart from Lee Je-ma's original intentions. My annotated translation of his treatise aims to preserve fundamental Sasang principles, leaving them less open to misinterpretation and distortion.

For the student interested in continuing his or her study of Sasang medicine, I recommend choosing one or more of the following options:

1. The American Institute of Korean Traditional Medicine is currently offering an online *Introduction to Sasang Medicine* course accessible by clicking "Continuing Education Classes in Korean Medicine" on www.koreanmedicine.us. This course offers a detailed review of basic Sasang concepts and walks through the *Dongeui Susei Bowon*, highlighting key points along the way.

2. Sasang research articles in English are available and can be viewed by typing "Sasang medical research" in a Google, Yahoo, or other internet search engine.

3. Information about Sasang medicine that is currently scattered throughout the internet can be located by typing phrases such as "Sasang medicine," "Four Constitutional medicine," or "Korean constitutional medicine."

4. Readers interested in learning more about Sasang medicine and applying it to their daily lives may try going to www.sasangmedicine.com. This website provides general information, extensive research articles, videos, and food recipes for each Sasang constitution.

5. My book *Your Yin Yang Body Type* is also available to those who wish to develop a general understanding of Sasang medicine and enhance their health through constitutionally specific herbs, foods, and exercises.

6. I regularly update my YouTube channel with videos about Sasang medicine and Eastern philosophy. There is no fee to subscribe to this channel. Simply search for the word "sasangdoc" in the YouTube search engine and then click "subscribe."

7. To receive further information about Sasang medicine, please do not hesitate to contact me through www.harmonyclinics.com or the address and phone number below:

> Harmony Acupuncture and Herbs
> 21730 Willamette Dr.
> West Linn, OR 97068, USA
> (503) 722-5224

From the bottom of my heart, I thank the reader for his/her interest in Sasang medicine. May he/she find and promote inner peace and self-understanding through the study of Lee Je-ma's profound teachings.

# Index

Page numbers in *italics* refer to figures and tables.

abdomen
location 83
stature of 44–7
Abdominal Malaria syndrome 173, 174
acrid flavor 14
acupuncture 10, 20
Fire Acupuncture technique 172
Iron Water technique 172
points
CV 12 140
DU 26 147*n*21
GV 26 139, 141, 160, 165, 249
LI 4 174
ages of man 332–3
air, vata and 16
alcohol consumption 242, 334–5, 338
An Zi 43
anesthetics, herbal 94*n*10
anger
and the *Che/Yong* relationship 18
effects of 60, 61
flow of 57, 58, 59
and the Jung emotion of the Tae
Yang Individual 55, 61, 63, 65,
67, 72, 74, 76, 319*n*1, 324–5
and *Kyo Uh* 88
as one of the four constitutional
temperaments 12, 17, 20, 28
as one of the Seven Emotional
Disorders 12
and the So Eum Individual 72–3
and the Song nature of the So
Yang Individual 56, 61, 63,
68, 75*n*52, 75*n*56, 77*n*70
anterior body *41*
anus 84, 180
arsenic 173, 174
Asian Rice Bran (*Furfur
Oryza Sativa*) 328
astringent flavor 14
*The Attainment of Wisdom through
Examining the True Nature of All
Phenomena (Gyeukchigo)* 27
Ayurvedic medicine 10, 16

Ba Dou (*Semen Crotinis*) 115, 119,
121, 122, 135, 149, 151, 157,
166, 173, 180, 190, 198, 199
back, stature of 44–7
*Baek* 90
*Baek Hasuoh Buja Yijung Tang* (Lee
Je-ma's Fleeceflower and Aconite
Regulate the Middle Decoction)
134–5, 151, 201, 201–2
*Baek Hasuoh Yijung Tang* (Lee Je-
ma's Fleeceflower Regulate the
Middle Decoction) 134, 151
Baekje Dynasty 9
Bai He Shou Wu (*Radix Polygoni
Multiflori Alba*) 132

*Bai Hu Tang* (White Tiger Decoction)
212, 225, 226, 228, 232,
233, 234, 236, 237–8, 252
Bai Shao Yao (*Radix Paeoniae
Lactiflorae*) 121, 174
Bai Zhu (*Radix Atractylodis
Macrocephalae*) 118
*Ban Xia Tang* (Prepared Pinellia
Decoction) 176
*Ban Xia Xie Xin Tang* (Pinellia
Decoction to Drain the
Epigastrium) 135, 177–8
Bang Ha (*Solen Gouldii*) 327, 328
*Bang Ryak* (strategy) 37, 38*n*42, 39,
75*n*56, 75*n*58, 82, 152*n*27
Basic Characteristics, Four *see Sa Dan*
bears 9
*Bei* 98*n*23
Bell's palsy 216, 251
*Ben Cao Bu Yi* 96
*Ben Cao Lun* 93, 327–8
*Bencao Yanyi Buyi* 94*n*9, 97
benevolence 36*n*27, 41*n*60,
42–4, 46, 47, 49, 63
*Benshifang (Prescriptions of
Universal Benefit)* 183
beriberi 9
*Bi Fang Hwa Zhi Wan* (Secret
Transform Stagnation Pill) 189
*Bi* syndrome 135, 158–9, 250, 286
*Bi Yao* syndrome 116, 117,
120, 123–5, 126, 128
*Bi Ying* syndrome 108, 135
*Bian Que Nan Jing* 94, 290
bile 15
bites, dog and insect 250
bitter flavor 14
black bile 15
blood, as one of the four humors 15
Blood Collapse 317
blowfish eggs 250
*Bochung Ikgi Tang* (Lee Je-ma's Tonify
the Middle and Augments the
Qi Decoction) 105, 168, 193
bodily fluids 16, *16*, 57, *89*, *90*,
288*n*10, 319, 322–4, *323*
*see also Ek; Go; Jin; Jin Ye; Yu*
boils 9, 172, 286
*Bok* (anterior) 98*n*23
*Bol Shim* (self-praise) 40–1, 46, 81
*Bon Jo* 153–4, 155–6
bone, kaffa and 16
bones
bone marrow 317
formation *16*
fracture treatments 94*n*10
*Jung Hei* in 86, 89
*Book of Poetry* 335*n*5, 339
*Bopei Won Tang* (Lee Je-ma's Tonify
the Source Qi of the Lungs
Decoction) 296, 311

brain, the 71, 85, 87, 91
breasts 85, 92, 171
*Bu Zhong Yi Qi Tang* (Tonify the
Middle and Augment the Qi
Decoction) 94*n*7, 181, 274
Buckwheat (*Fagopyrum Esculentum*) 328
Buddha 54
bull horn 249
buttocks 37, 38, 41, 44–7, 75*n*56, 82

Cai Shu 44
calmness
effects of 60, *61*
flow of 57, *58*, 59
and the *Jung* emotion of the
Tae Eum Individual 76
and *Ko Cho* 88
as one of the four constitutional
temperaments 12, 13, 17, 28
and the So Yang Individual 73
and the Song nature of the
So Eum Individual 56,
61, 63, 69, 75*n*54, 78
and the Tae Eum Individual 73
*Cang Liao Ben Cao* 96
cannabis 346*n*5
Cao Cao, General 48
cervical spinal area 60, 71, 83, 270
Chai Hu (*Radix Bupleuri*) 113
*Chai Hu Tang* (Bupleurum
Decoction) 118
*Chai Ling Tang* (Bupleurum and
Poria Decoction) 213
*Chan Hou Feng* 248–9, 249*n*39
*Che*, and *Song* 36*n*26
*Che/Yong* relationship 17–18, *17*,
32*n*2, 32*n*3, 34*n*16, 38*n*43,
*38*, 45*n*74, 47*n*81,
54*n*12, 78*n*71, 91*n*27
Chen Pi (*Pericarpium Citri
Reticulatae*) 118, 132, 141, 163
Chen Zhang Qi 96
*Cheng Qi Tang* (Order the
Qi Decoction) 112,
119, 124, 128, 129
Cheng Wuji 118, 153–4
*Cheongung Gyeji Tang* (Lee Je-ma's
Lovage Root and Cinnamon Twig
Decoction) 105, 108, 173, 194
chest
location 83
stature of 44–7
*chi* pulse position 316–17
*Chi Shi Zhi Yu Yu Liang Tang*
(Halloysite and Limonite
Decoction) 136, 176
*Chi Shim* (extravagence) 41–2, 46, 82
children, dosage for 22
chin 36, 38, 40, 44–7, 80, 83
China
influence on Korea 9

use of local herbs in 10
Chinese characters, and their
    meanings 27–9
Chinese medicine
    compared with Sasang medicine
        11–14, *13*, *14*, *15*
    influence on Korean medicine 9, 10
    organ system 13
    translations of medical texts 9
    use of herbs 14, 207*n*5
    Yin and Yang theory 10
*Cho* 13
    *see also Jiao*
choleric temperament 15
*Chon Ki* (Heavenly Affairs)
    32–3, 34, *34*, 38, *38*
*Chon Shi* (divine meaning) 33, 34,
    36*n*22, 38, 49–50, 67, 69, 71, 87
*Chon Shim* (do as one pleases)
    41–2, 46, 81*nn*97–8
*Chon Song* (seed of heaven) 17, 18,
    *18* 38*n*43, 27, 38*n*43, 50*n*89
*Chong Mi Tang* (Lee Je-ma's Garlic
    and Honey Decoction) 198
*Chongshim Yonja Tang* (Lee Je-
    ma's Lotus Seed Purify the
    Heart Decoction) 308
Chuan Xiong (*Radix Ligustici
    Chuanxiong*) 14
Chun Gen Pi (*Cortex Ailanthi*) 277
*Chun Gen Pi Wan* (Ailanthus
    Bark Pill) 304
*Chun Zhong* 249
*The Classic of Herbal Medicine*
    *see Shennong Bencaojing*
*Clear Yang* 234, 238–40, 241, 247
*Clear Yin* 234
Climatic Factors, Six 12
Cold
    as a cause of illness 99
    conditions 15, 16, *16*
    and the large intestine 108–9
    nature of large intestine 84
    as one of the five temperatures 14
    as one of the Six Climatic Factors 12
    So Eum Individual and 112, 324
    So Yang Individual and 98*n*24, 323
    Tae Eum Individual and 98*n*24
Cold *Bi* syndrome 120
Cold esophagus syndrome 277
Cold-induced toxins, herbal
    prescriptions for 96*n*18
colds, common 21
*A Collection of Formulas from the Korean
    Elders of the Goguryeo Dynasty* 9
colors, pleasant and unpleasant 40
commoner, the 52–5, 62
compassion 17, 28, 36*n*25,
    53*n*7, 55*n*16, 76*n*59
complacency 63, 65, 68, 74, 325
complexion 137–42, 147, 154,
    161–3, 231, 278, 280, 283,
    285, 289, 299, *300*, 313, 326
*A Comprehensive Inventory of
    Local Korean Herbs* 10
conduct *see Jo*; *Myung*
*Confucian Analects* 10, 55*n*13, 335*n*5
Confucianism 10, 17, 26, 29,
    50*n*91, 78*n*71, 95*n*11, 242

Confucius 33*n*8, 33*n*10, 43, 55,
    244*n*32, 335*n*5, 338*n*6, 347
    The Great Learning 10, 27
    Ten Wings 32*n*3
constipation 113, 214, 225,
    233, 235, 251, 298
    remedies for 115, 116
constitutions, four 11, 51–66, *51*, *61*
    classification and diagnosis 340–8
        comparison between the Tae Eum
            and So Eum Individual *343*
        developed and underdeveloped
            anatomy of each
            constitution *341*
        health indications for each
            constitution *345*
    *see also* So Eum; So Yang;
        Tae Eum; Tae Yang
contemplation 12
Cool
    nature of small intestine 84
    as one of the five temperatures 14
    Tae Yang Individual and 323
coughs 122, 263, 278, 286, 295
cow meat 96*n*17
cows 50
Crucian Carp (*Carassius Carassius*) 328
Crucian Carp with Water Shield
    (*Bracenia Schreberi*) 328
cruelty 27
cysts 172, 249, 250

*Da Chai Hu Tang* (Major
    Bupleurum Decoction) 302
*Da Cheng Qi Tang* (Major Order the
    Qi Decoction) 115–16, 119, 120,
    130, 131, 134–5, 148, 180, 212
Da Huang (*Radix et Rizoma Rhei*)
    14, 115, 116*n*23, 117, 136, 275,
    285, 287, 289, 290, 291, 298
*Da Jie Xiong* syndrome 209
Da Liang (Kaifeng) 285
*Da Qing Long Tang* (Major Blue Green
    Dragon Decoction) 203–4, 253
*Da Xian Xiong Tang* (Major
    Sinking into the Chest
    Decoction) 208, 209, 253
*Dae In* ("magnificent one") 81–2
*Daejang Pahan* syndrome
    108*n*13, *109*, *110*
Dampness 12, 99, 161, 162, 188
Dang Gui (*Radix Angelicae
    Sinensis*) 10, 118, 293
*Dang Gui Si Ni Tang* (Tangkuei
    Decoction for Frigid
    Extremities) 128, 131, 177
*Dang Yo* (group responsibilities) 33,
    34, 37*n*33, 38, 69, 70, 72–3,
    74, 75*n*51, 78–9, 88, 341
*Danggui Baek Hasuoh Gwanjung
    Tang* (Lee Je-ma's Angelica
    and Fleeceflower Smooth the
    Middle Decoction) 198
*Danxi Xinfa* (*The Teachings of
    Danxi*) 119, 189, 259
*Dao* 244
*Dao Chi San* (Guide the Red
    Powder) 256–7
Daoism 10, 95*n*11
*De Xiao Fang* (*Shi Yi De Xiao Fang*) 105

death
    causes of 100–1, 131, 209, 217,
        219, 248–9, 260, 296
    indications of imminent
        115, 117, 285
deer
    antler decoction 293, 295, 298, 311
    liver 170, 344
Descartes, René 18–19
*Dexiaofang* (*Collection of Effective
    Prescriptions*) 183, 185, 188, 255
*Di Dang Tang* (Rhubarb and Leech
    Decoction) 107, 112, 179
diabetes 236–43, 247
diaphragm 83, 218, 233*n*11, 239,
    241, 249, 254–5, 265, 319*n*4
diarrhea 98, 108–9, 112, 120–1, 124,
    129, 134, 135–6, 139, 141, 146,
    *149*, 151, 156, 164, 165, 208,
    212, 219, 228–9, 234, 235, 262,
    277, 278–9, 295, 296, 345
    *see also* Mang Yin syndrome
diuretics 135–6
divine intervention *see Chon Shi*
dizziness 93, 98, 117*n*26,
    182, 183, 241, 255
*Do Ryang* (toleration) 36, 38*n*41, 39
*Doctrine of the Mean* 10
*Dokhwal Jihwang Tang* (Lee Je-
    ma's Angelica Pubescens and
    Rehmannia Decoction) 216,
    242, 245, 248, 262–3
*Doksam Buja Yijung Tang* (LeeJe-ma's
    Added Ginseng Regulate the
    Middle Decoction with Fu Zi) 168
*Doksam Gwangye Yijung Tang* (Lee
    Je-ma's Cinnamon Regulate
    the Middle Decoction with
    Added Ginseng) 169–70
*Doksam Palmul Tang* (Lee Je-ma's
    Added Ginseng Eight Ingredient
    Gentlemen Decoction) 119,
    131, 164, 168, 169
*Doksam Tang* (Lee Je-ma's
    Ginseng Decoction) 141
*Dong Feng* syndrome 274
*Dong Yuan Shu* (*The Writings of Li
    Dongyuan*) 149, 181, 188
*Dongeui Bogam* (*Mirror of Eastern
    Medicine*) 10, 95, 139*n*13, 285*n*7,
    290, 293*nn*18–19, 320*n*7
*Dongeui Susei Bowon* (*Eastern
    Medical Perspectives on
    Longevity and Wellbeing*)
    completion of 27
    translation of the title 11
*Dongmu Yugo* 14
*Dongyi Gangleiju* (Classified
    Prescriptions) 240, 241
dosage, and frequency 20–1, *21*
dreaming 91*n*27
Dryness 12
Du Huo (*Radix Angelicae
    Pubescentis*) 163
Du Ren 208
dualism 18
dyscratia 15
dysentery 171, 198, 248, 267, 296, 345

ears
  and Chon Shi 34, 49–50, 69, 71, 87
  and Heavenly Affairs 38
  *Jin Hei* and 91
  as a sensory organ 39–40, 90
  *Shin* in 85
  stature of 44
Eastern medicine 9, 10, 11, 21, 94
ecstasy 13
edema 123, 140–1, 163, 170–1,
  197, 208, 244, 246, 248,
  267, 296, 312, 313
*Ei see* sorrow
Eight Trigram Theory 44n67
*Ek* (essence) 16, *16*, 86, 89
*Ek Hei* 86, 88, 89, 91
The Elder at Mt. Panlong 214, 221
Emotional Disorders, Seven 12
emotions
  balancing 62
  directional flow of *58*, 67
emperors 54–5
  *see also* individual emperors
epidemics 10, 20, 26, 105, *144*,
  157, 185, 188, 284–5, 288
  *see also* Warm Febrile disease
epigastrium 135, 177–8
*Er Sheng Jiu Ku Wan* (Two Saints
  Rescue the Suffering Pill) 285, 304
Esophagal Cold causing Exterior
  Cold Syndrome *297–8*
esophagus 319, 321, 323–4
  connections 84
  *Jin* in 85, 89
  location 83
  and skin formation *16*
  Warm nature of 84
existence *see Ji Bang*
Existence, Four Phases of 57n19
Exterior Cold syndrome
  227–8, 295, 311
Exterior disorders
  definition 29
  etiology of 12
  release of pathogen from 14
  *Song* and 55n14
Exterior Heat-induced syndrome 295
External Cold syndrome 212, 278, *280*
external illness 98n24
eyes
  *Gi* in 85
  *Go Hei* and 91
  and Heavenly Affairs 38
  and Human Affairs 72
  and *Sei Wei* 34, 49–50, 70, 71, 87
  as a sensory organ 39–40, 90
  stature of 44
  visual problems 225, 282, 304

*Fan Wei* syndrome *see* Ye Ge
  Fan Wei syndrome
Fang Feng (*Radix Saposhnikoviae*)
  163, 227, 247
Fang Ji (*Radix Aristolochia*) 96n17
fear 12
*Fei Zao* syndrome 292, *292*
Fire Acupuncture technique 172
Fire Knife technique 172
Flavors, Five 14
  four, groups of 32n3
Fu Ling (*Poria Alba*) 163, 210

*Fu* organs *see* Organs, Four Major *Fu*
Fu Zi (*Radix Aconiti*) 121, 122–3,
  137n7, 138, 141, 156
*Fu Zi Tang* (Prepared Aconite
  Decoction) 142, 177

Galen 15
Gall Bladder 83n1, 97n22, 100
Gan Cao (*Radix Glycyrrhizae*)
  118, 173, 270
*Gan Cao Xie Xin Tang* (Licorice
  Decoction to Drain the
  Epigastrium) 135, 178
*Gan Huo Luan* syndrome 139–41
Gan Jiang (*Rhizoma Zingiberis
  Officinalis*) 156, 163
Gan Li (*Castania*) 275
Gan Sui (*Radix Euphorbiae
  Kansui*) 209–10, 212, 249
*Gangchul Gwanjung Tang* (Lee Je-ma's
  Ginger and Atractylodes Harmonize
  the Middle Decoction) 136, 149
Gao Ben (*Rhizoma Ligustici*)
  289, 290, 291
Gao Yao 62
garlic 9, 171, 198
*Ge Gen Jie Ji Tang* (Kudzu Clear the
  Flesh Decoction) 282, 283, 304–5
Ge Gen (*Radix Puerariae*) 96n17, 275
*Ge* syndrome *see* Ye Ge Fan
  *Wei* syndrome
*Gi see Qi*
ginger 135, 136, 149, 158,
  175, 178, 196, 228
ginseng 105, 108, 112, 118, 119,
  122, 130, 131, 138, 141, 152,
  153, 164, 168, 170, 171, 172,
  174, 176, 186, 191, 192,
  198–9, 199, 200, 202, 344
*Go Hei* 85, 87, 88, 91
*Go* (sticky fluids) 16, *16*, 85, 88, 89, 90
*Go* (sticky fluids) 90
Goguryeo Dynasty 9
golden-snake wine 171
*Gon Gong* 62n45
*Gong Chen Dan* (Embrace
  the King Pill) 293
Gong Tingxian 95n12
Gong Xin 95, 105, 132, 157, 182,
  184, 187, 206–7, 209, 241, 257–8,
  283, 285, 304, 304–7, 328
*Gongjin Hukwon Dan* (Lee Je-ma's
  Embrace the King Black Source
  Pill) 293, 295, 298, 312
gonorrhea 267, 296
Grape root (*Mahonia Aquifolium*) 327
The Great Learning 10, 27
Greater Cold and Lesser Heat
  syndrome 224, 226–7, 231n2
Greater Heat and Lesser Cold
  syndrome 231n2
Greater Yang *see* Tae Yang
Greater Yin *see* Tae Eum
Greece, ancient 15
greed 27
Gua Di (*Pedicellus Cucumeris
  Melonis*) 174
Gua Lou (*Semen Trichosantis*)
  215, 227, 247
*Guan Ge* syndrome 139–41, 151
Guan Shu 44

*Gui Bi Ge Ban Tang* (Combined
  Cinnamon Twig and
  Gypsum Decoction) 253
*Gui Ma Ge Ban Tang* (Combined
  Cinnamon Twig and Ephedra
  Decoction) 129, 131, 231, 301
*Gui Zhi Fu Zi Tang* (Cinnamon Twig
  and Aconite Decoction) 120
*Gui Zhi Fu Zi Tang* (Cinnamon
  Twig and Poria Pill) 185
Gui Zhi (*Ramulus Cinnamomi Cassiae*)
  113, 121, 148, 174, 270
*Gui Zhi Ren Shen Tang* (Cinnamon
  Twig Ginseng Decoction) 176
*Gui Zhi Tang* (Cinnamon
  Twig Decoction) 104,
  105, 116, 142, 175
*Gujin Yijian* (*Newly Amended
  Mirror of Ancient and Modern
  Medicine*) 95n12, 105, 158
gum bleeding 251
*Gung Shim* (self-conceit) 40–1, 80
*Gunggui Chongso Yijung Tang* (Lee
  Je-ma's Regulate the Middle
  Decoction with Lovage, Angelica,
  Scallion, and Perilla Leaf) 170
*Gunggwi Hyangsu San* (Lee Je-
  ma's Cyperus and Perilla Leaf
  Powder with Lovage and
  Angelica Root) 105, 194
*Gwa Shim* (boastfulness) 40–1, 46, 81
*Gwajae San* (Muskmelon Pedicle
  Powder) 299, 313
*Gwakhyang Jeonggi San* (Lee Je-ma's
  Agastach Powder to Rectify the
  Qi) 105, 109, 113, 136, 164, 195
*Gwangye Buja Yijung Tang* (Lee Je-ma's
  Cinnamon and Aconite Regulate
  the Middle Decoction) 136, 142,
  147, 149, 153, 154, 164, 200
*Gye Sam Go* (Lee Je-ma's Chicken
  Ginseng Paste) 198–9
*Gyebu Gwakjin Yijung Tang* (Lee
  Je-ma's Cinnamon Bark, Aconite,
  Agastache, and Tangerine
  Peel Decoction to Regulate
  the Middle) 140, 168
*Gyegung Yukgul* 152n27
*Gyeji Banha Senggang Tang* (Lee
  Je-ma's Cinnamon Pinellia and
  Ginger Decoction) 158, 196
*Gyeji Buja Tang* (Lee Je'ma's
  Cinnamon Twig and Prepared
  Aconite Decoction) 105
*Gyeukchigo* (*The Attainment of Wisdom
  through Examining the True
  Nature of All Phenomena*) 27

Hai Zang (Wang Hao Gu)
  94, 96, 118n29
hair
  brushing 251, 260
  in the lung group 85
  *Ni Hei* and 89
*Haizang Shu* (Hai Zang's
  Collection of Work) 118
Han Dynasty 94, 95, 115, 124
*Han Jue* syndrome 270–5, *276*
*Handa Yulso Tang* (Lee Je-ma's
  Greater Cold Lesser Heat
  Decoction) 275, 279, 310

haughtiness
    prevention of 36
    *see also* Kyo Shim
*Haui Zheng* 303
hawks 50
hawthorn 109, 113, 136, 164, 197
*He Dan* 161
*He Ren Yin* (Polygonum Multiflorum
    Root and Ginseng Decoction) 202
*He Yuan Dan* (Black Source Pill) 293
head
    *Chon Shim* in 41, 81*n*98
    *Ni Hei* and 89
    *Shik Kyun* in 37, 81*n*99
    stature of 44–7
    *Tal Shim* in 81
headaches 235–6, 260–2, 263, 264
Heart, So Eum Individual and 97*n*22
heart
    and the *Che/Yong* relationship 17
    in Chinese medicine 13
    Confucius on 33*n*8
    darkness and brightness of 50
    function 92
    and Human Affairs 35*n*21, 38*n*43
    influences on 46*n*76, 46*n*77
    location 92
    polishing 45
    and *Tai Chi* 11
    turbidity of 53
    and *Zhang* organs 52
Heart *Bi* syndrome 120
Heat
    as a cause of illness 99
    conditions 15, 16, *16*
    as one of the Six Climatic Factors 12
    So Eum Individual and 98*n*24
    So Yang Individual and 323, 324
    Tae Yang Individual and 98*n*24
Heat Clearing Method 113
heaven
    and the natural law of change 53
    relationship between man
        and 17, 27, *35*
    and the senses 90*n*26
    *see also* Chon Ki; Chon Song
*Hei Nu Wan* (Black Servant
    Pill) 282, 283, 303
hemiplegia 172, 244, 250,
    259, 299*n*23, 306
hemp seed 120
*Heng Gom* (reflection on actions)
    36, 38*n*41, 39, 81
Heo Jun 10, 95, 285*n*7
herbs, preparation of 21–2
Hippocrates 15
hips 60, 140, 261
hollow organs *see* Organs,
    Four Major, *Fu*
honey 120, 171, 179–80, 198
horses 50
Hot, as one of the five
    temperatures 14, 85
Hou Jun 95
*Hou Po Ban Xia Tang* (Prepared
    Pinellia and Magnolia Bark
    Decoction) 135, 176
Hou Po (*Magnolia Officinalis*) 117
*Hou Xiang Zheng Qi San* (Agastache
    Powder to Rectify the Qi) 274

*Hourenshu* (*Revive the People*)
    185–6, 302–3
*Hoyon Ji Gi* 19, 54
*Hoyon Ji Ri* 19, 54
*Hu Mi* 324–5
Hua Shi (*Talcum*) 226
Hua Tuo 346
*Huai Zheng* 282
Huan Dou 62
Huang Bai (*Cortex Phellodendri*) 225
Huang Di, Emperor 93, 95, 101
*Huang Di Neijing* (*Yellow Emperor's
    Inner Canon*) 93, 95, 101, 101–2
*Huang Ge* (*Yellow Songs*) 307
*Huang Lian Jie Du Tang* (Coptis
    Decoction to Relieve
    Toxicity) 238, 255
Huang Lian (*Rhizoma
    Coptidis*) 215, 227
Huang Qi (*Radix Astragali
    Membranacei*) 9, 121
Huang Qin (*Radix Scutellariae*)
    277, 286
*Huanggi Gyeji (Buja) Tang* (Lee Je-ma's
    Cinnamon Twig Astralagus and
    Aconite Decoction) 105, 108,
    121–2, 123, 131, 191, 194
*Hui see* joy
Human Affairs, Four 19, 32*n*2,
    33, 34, *34*, 38, *89*
human nature *see* Song
humanism 17
humility, virtue of 17, 33*n*6,
    33*n*11, 36*n*23, 37*n*36, 52,
    67*nn*4–5, 72*n*36, 72*n*41,
    75*n*52, 77*n*70, 78*n*71
humors, four 15, 16, *16*
*Hun* (ethereal aspect of the mind) 90
*Huo Luan* syndrome 141, 151
Huo Xiang (*Herba Pogostemonis*) 137*n*7
*Huo Xiang Zheng Qi San* (Agastache
    Powder to Rectify the Qi) 105, 136
*Huoren Shu* 94, 129–30
*Hwalsok Gosam Tang* (Lee Je-
    ma's Talcum and Sophora
    Decoction) 214, 216, 262
*Hwangyon Chongjang Tang* (Lee
    Je-ma's Coptis Clear the
    Intestine Decoction) 248, 267
*Hyang Buja Palmul Tang* (Lee Je-ma's
    Eight Ingredient Deciction
    with Cyperus Tuber) 196
*Hyangsa Yangwi Tang* (Lee Je-
    ma's Cyperus and Hawthorn
    Enliven the stomach Decoction)
    109, 113, 136, 164, 197
*Hyul* 88, 90
*Hyul Hei* (place where the blood
    resides) 86, 88, 89, 90, 91
*Hyungbang Dojok San* (Lee Je-ma's
    Schizonepeta and Ledebouriella
    Guide the Red Powder)
    205, 207–8, 210, 261
*Hyungbang Jihwang Tang* (Lee Je-ma's
    Schizonepeta, Ledebouriella,
    and Rhemannia Decoction)
    214, 229–30, 246, 263–4
*Hyungbang Peidok San* (Lee Je-ma's
    Schizonepeta and Ledebouriella
    Powder to Overcome Pathogenic
    Influences) 204, 205, 207,
    215, 236, 248, 260–1

*Hyungbang Sabaek San* (Lee Je-ma's
    Schizonepeta and Ledebouriella
    Clear the White Powder)
    208, 214, 215, 232, 261

*I Ching* 10, 11, 27, 32*n*3, 44*n*67,
    57*n*19, 129–30, 242
illness
    categories of 12
    and the *Che/Yong* relationship 18
    four constitutional
        temperaments and 19–20
    location of 97–8
    *see also* Exterior disorders;
        Interior disorders
*In Ryun* (social skills and talents) 33,
    34, 38, 49–50, 68, 69, 71, 88
*In Sa see* Human Affairs, Four
*In Sam Gyeji Buja Tang* (Lee
    Je-ma's Ginseng, Cinnamon
    Twig, and Aconite Decoction)
    105, 122, 191, 192
*In Sam Jinpi Tang* (Lee Je-ma's Ginseng
    and Tangerine Peel Decoction) 199
*In Sam Ohsuyu Tang see Sam Yu Tang*
India 10
*Indongdeng Jigolpi Tang* Lee Je-ma's
    Honeysuckle and Lycium
    Decoction) 239, 249, 265–6
infants, dosage for 22
influenza 9
Interior disorders
    definition 29
    etiology of 12
    *Jung* and 55*n*14
Internal Heat syndrome 212, 235
Internal Heat Yang Ming syndrome *283*
internal illness 98*n*24
Internal liver Heat syndrome 278
Internal Wind 214, 224, 227, 227–8
intestines
    in Chinese medicine 13
    large intestine
        and bone formation *16*
        Cold and 108–9
        Cold nature of 84
        connections 84
        *Ek* in 86, 89
        Yang Ming and 97*n*22
    location 83
    small intestine
        Cool nature of 84
        structure 84
        Tae Yang Individual and 97*n*22
        and tendon formation *16*
        *Yu* in 86, 89
Iron Water Acupuncture technique 172

*Jae Gan* (manners and skills) 37,
    38*n*42, 39, 75*n*55, 82
*Janggan Buyng* 274
Japan, use of local herbs in 10
Japanese Honeysuckle (*Lonicera
    Japonica*) 240
jaundice *144*, 156–7, 161,
    162–3, 166, 185–6, 188
*Ji see* willpower
*Ji Bang* (existence) 32–3, 34, 36*n*25,
    39, 49–50, 69, 70, 71, 88

*Ji Re* syndrome 255
*Jiang Fu Tang* (Ginger Aconite
    Decoction) 149, 175
*Jiang Zhong* syndrome 255
*Jiao*
    correlations 72
    counterparts *58*
    divisions 13
    and locations of *Zhang Fu* organs 83
    Lower 57, 81*n*95, 88, 237,
        242, 266, 320, 345
    Mid-Lower 81*n*92, 88, 345
    Mid-Upper 80*n*89, 87, 152*n*28, 345
    Middle 208, 237, 320
    Upper 57, 80*n*86, 80*n*87, 81*n*98,
        85*n*5, 87, 237, 265, 320, 345
    *see also Cho*
Jie, Emperor 43
Jie Geng (*Radix Platycodi*) 174
*Jie Ke* 278
*Jie Xiong* syndrome 157–9, 205–6,
    207, 208, 209–10, 248, 268
*Jihwang Baekho Tang* (Lee Je-ma's White
    Tiger Decoction with Rhemannia)
    210, 215, 227, 232, 233, 264
*Jin* (clear fluids) *16*, 85, 88, 89, 90
Jin Dynasty 115, 124, 153*n*30
*Jin Gui Shen Qi Wan* (Kidney Qi Pill
    from the Golden Cabinet) 254, 290
*Jin Gui Yao Lue* 94*n*5
*Jin Hei* 85, 87, 88, 91
*Jin Ye* (bodily fluids 107*n*7,
    114, 117*n*28
*Jing Fang Bai Du San* (Schizonepeta
    and Saposhnikoviae Powder
    to Overcome Pathogenic
    Influences) 206–7, 257, 274
Jing Jie (*Herba Schizonepetae*) 163, 247
*Jo* (conduct) 91
*Jogak Daehwang Tang* (Lee Je-ma's
    Honeylocust and Rhubarb
    Decoction) 286, 312
joint adjustment 94*n*10
*Jok Hasuoh Gwanjung Tang* (Lee
    Je-ma's Fleeceflower Smooth the
    Middle Decoction) 158, 197–8
*Jori Peiwon Tang* (Lee Je-ma's
    Regulate the Interior and
    Replenish the lung Source
    Decoction) 279, 280, 310–11
*Joryong Chajonja Tang* (Lee Je-ma's
    Polyporus and Plantago Seed
    Decoction) 214, 232, 262
Joseon Dynasty 338*n*7
*Jowi Sueungchong Tang* (Lee Je-ma's
    Regulate the stomach Support
    and Clear Decoction) 295, 308
joy
    *Dang Yo* and 88
    effects of 60, 61
    flow of 57, 58, 59
    and the Jung emotion of the So Eum
        Individual 56, 61, 63, 65, 69, 72–
        3, 74, 76, 79, 134*n*1, 152, 325
    as one of the four constitutional
        temperaments 12, 13, 17, 28
    as one of the Seven Emotional
        Disorders 12

and the Song nature of the Tae
    Eum Individual 56, 61, 63–4,
    68, 75*n*53, 78*n*72, 325–6
and the Tae Yang Individual 72
*Ju Chek* (profit from loss) 36,
    37*n*31, 38*n*41, 39, 80
*Ju Fang* 183, 185, 187, 255
Ju Hua (*Flos Chrysanthemi Morifolii*) 9
*Jue* 129
*Jue Ni* syndrome 183, 271
*Jue* syndrome *see Han Jue* syndrome
Jue Yin syndrome 97, 98, 100,
    101, 128, 130–2, 152, 153,
    *155*, 165–6, 166, 168, 186
*Jul Shim* (selfishness) 46, 82
*Jung* emotion 88, 90
    anger and 63
    complacency and 63
    definition 12
    effect of imbalanced *61*
    emotional balance and virtue *74*
    imbalance of 98*n*24
    joy and 63
    and the So Eum Individual 56, 76
    and the So Yang Individual 56, 76
    sorrow and 63
    and the Tae Eum Individual
        56, 76, 76–7
    and the Tae Yang Individual 55, 76
*Jung Hei* 86, 88, 88–9, 89, 90, 91
*Jusa Ikwon San* (Lee Je-ma's Cinnabar
    Support the Source Powder) 267
justice 27

kaffa 16
Kaifeng (Da Liang) 285
*Kalgen Bupyong Tang* (Lee Je-ma's Kudzu
    and Spirodela Decoction) 312
*Kalgen Heigi Tang* (Lee Je-ma's
    Kudzu Clear the Flesh
    Decoction) 286, 307
*Kalgen Nabokja Tang* (Lee Je-
    ma's Kudzu Root and Radish
    Seed Decoction) 295
*Kalgen Seunggi Tang* (Lee Je-ma's
    Kudzu Support the Qi Decoction)
    277, 283, 286, 287, 310
*Kamsu Chonil Wan* (Lee Je-ma's Divine
    Gan Sui Pill) 212, 250, 267–8
kidney Heat causing Exterior Heat
    syndrome *see under* So Eum
    (Lesser Yin) Individual
kidneys
    aversion to unpleasant tastes 40
    calmness and 13
    circulation of essence around 71
    distinction and 90
    energy flow to spleen 14
    energy flow towards earth 35
    and the Four Symbols 11
    function 321–2
    herbs for 15, *15*, *16*
    and Human Affairs 38
    *Jung Hei* and 86, 88–9, 91
    kidney group 86
    and Ko Cho 34, 68, 70–1, 79
    location 83
    and the lower abdomen 81*nn*95–6
    and *Minister Fire* 94*n*9

*Pre-Heaven* energy and 13
relationship with the buttocks 75*n*56
So Eum Individual and 97*n*22
stature of 44–7
*see also under* So Eum
kites 50
kiwifruit 320, 344
*Ko Cho* (proper place to reside)
    33, 34–5, 37*n*34, 39, 68,
    70–1, 73, 74, 75*n*52, 75*n*56,
    75*n*58, 79–80, 88, 341
*Konyul Jaejo Tang* (Lee Je-ma's Chestnut
    and Grub Decoction) 296, 313
*Konyul Jogenpi Tang* (Lee Je-ma's
    Chestnut and Ailanthus
    Decoction) 313
Korea
    attitude towards Lee Je-ma 28
    Chinese influence on 9
    hair brushing in 251
    inheritance customs 338*n*7
    in Lee Je-ma's time 26
    lifespan 291*n*15
    use of local herbs in 10
    Western medicine in 20
Ku Shen (*Radix Sophorae*) 215
*Kuan Zhong Tang* (Smooth the
    Middle Decoction) 136, 198
*Kyo Shim* (haughtiness) 40–1, 46, 80
*Kyo Uh* (one on one association)
    33, 34–5, 37*n*32, 38, 67,
    72–3, 74, 78–9, 88, 341
*Kyung Ryun* (government and
    administration of affairs)
    36, 38*n*41, 39, 80
*Kyungbun Kamsu Yongho Dan* (Lee
    Je-ma's Calomel and Kan Sui Root
    Dragon Tiger Pill) 250, 251

*Lao Juan* 181
*Lao Nue* 248
*Lao Tsu* 54
large intestine *see under* intestines
laziness 27, 56, 61, 64, 68, 76*n*62
Lee Je-ma
    approach 10, 11
    *The Attainment of Wisdom through
        Examining the True Nature of All
        Phenomena (Gyeukchigo)* 27
    biography 26–7
    and Chinese medicine 12
    and Confucianism 95*n*11
    *Dongmu Yugo* 14
    formulae 191–202, 260–8,
        328–9, 344
    image *26*
    and temperament imbalance 12
    *see also Dongeui Susei Bowon*;
        The Elder at Mt. Panlong
Lee Shijian 221
leeches 107, 112, 179
Lesser Yang *see* So Yang
Lesser Yin *see* So Eum
Li Chan 95, 120, 154, 157, 162, 185,
    186, 189–90, 256, 303–4, 328
Li Gao (Li Dongyuan) 94, 130,
    149, 181, 188, 240

Li Ting 138, 149, 152, 282
*Li Zhong Tang* (Regulate the Middle
  Decoction) 132, 134, 136, 138
*Li Zhong Wan* (Regulate the
  Middle Pill) 134, 175
Li Zijian 213
*Liang Ge San* (Cool the Diaphragm
  Powder) 241, 254–5
Liang Jiang (*Rhizoma Alpiniae
  Officinarum*) 163
licorice 135, 142, 147, 177, 178
*Ling Shu* 101–2, 284, 290, 317, 347
*Liu Wei Di Huang Tang* (Six Ingredient
  Decoction with Rhemannia) 216
*Liu Wei Di Huang Tang* (Six
  Intgredient Decoction with
  Rehmannia) 224–5, 238, 256
liver
  aversion to unpleasant odors 40
  in Chinese medicine 13
  circulation of blood around 71
  and *Dang Yo* 34, 69, 70,
    74, 78*n*78, 88
  deep thought and 90
  energy flow towards earth 35
  and the Four Symbols 11
  function 323
  herbs for *15*
  and Human Affairs 38
  *Hyul Hei* and 86, 91
  joy and 13
  Jue Yin and 97*n*22
  liver group 86
  and the lower back 75*n*55
  stature of 44–7
  umbilical area and 81*nn*92–3
  *see also under* Tae Eum
liver Heat causing Yang Ming
  syndrome *284*
lockjaw 224, 227
Long Gu (*Os Draconis*) 298
longevity 346
Lou Ying 118
lovage 105, 108, 170, 173, 194
love 27, 33*n*4, 33*n*9, 36*n*25, 37*n*38,
  52, 73*n*47, 78*nn*74–5
Lu Gen (*Rhizoma Phragmitisis*) 327
*Lu Hui Fei Er Wan* (Fat Baby
  Pill) 249, 257–8
lumbar area 60, 71, 83
lung system 270*n*1
lungs
  aversion to unpleasant sounds 40
  in Chinese medicine 13
  and *Chon Shi* 71
  and the Four Symbols 11
  function 323
  herbs for *15*
  and Human Affairs 38
  location 83
  lung energy 13, 14, 35
  lung group 85
  lung tumors 9
  *Ni Hei* and 85, 88, 91
  and *Sa Mu* 34, 70
  sorrow and 13, 19–20
  sorrow and development of 13
  stature of 44–7
  studying and 90
  of the Tae Eum Individual 80*n*86
  Tae Eum Individual and 97*n*22

*Ma Fe San* (Cannabis Boiling
  Powder) 346*n*5
*Ma Huang Ding Chuan Tang* (Ephedra
  Arrest Wheezing Decoction) 306–7
Ma Huang (*Ephedra Sinica*) 136, 147
*Ma Huang Fu Zi Gan Cao Tang*
  (Ephedra, Prepared Aconite, and
  Licorice Decoction) 142, 147, 177
*Ma Huang Fu Zi Xi Xin Tang*
  (Ephedra, Asarum, and Prepared
  Aconite Decoction) 142, 177
Ma Huang (*Herba Ephedrae*) 96*n*17
*Ma Huang Tang* (Ephedra Decoction)
  124, 269, 270, 301
*Ma Ren Tang* (Persica Formula) 179
*Ma Ren Wan* (Hemp Seed Formula) 120
madness 118, 119
*Maekmundong Wonji San* (Lee
  Je-ma's Ophiopogon and
  Senega Powder) 314
*Mahwang Balpyo Tang* (Ma
  Huang Release the Exterior
  Decoction) 270, 311
*Mahwang Jongchun Tang* (Lee Je-ma's
  Ma Huang Ephedra Arrest
  Wheezing Decoction) 295, 308–9
*Mahwang Jongtong Tang* (Lee
  Je-ma's Ephedra Decoction
  for Pain) 296, 309
*Mai Jing* (*The Pulse Classic*) 163, 284–5
Mai Men Dong (*Tuber
  Ophiopogonsis*) 174
*Mak* 87
*Mak Hei* (place where *Gi* resides)
  85, 87, 88, 89, 90, 91
malaria 173, 174, 198, 202,
  231, 241, 248
malevolence 36*n*27, 41*n*60,
  42–3, 45–6, 53, 63
*Man Jing Feng* syndrome 296
*Manbing Huichun* (*Ten Thousand
  Illnesses Return to Spring*)
  95*n*12, 304, 307
Mang Xiao (*Natrii Sulfas*) 117
*Mang Xue* (Blood Collapse) 317
*Mang Yang* syndrome 104*n*1,
  105, 120–3, 125–6, *127*,
  151, 214*n*23, 217–21
*Mang Yin* syndrome 207*n*6, 214,
  217–21, *223*, 231, 234
manliness 76
martial arts 346*n*5
materialistic monism 19
medicine, basic principles 93–102
melancholic temperament 15
Mencius 55
*Mencius* 10, 53*n*7
Meng Shen 96
Mengzi 53*n*7
mercury 190*n*83, 247, 249, 259
meridians 100
metabolic process and organ
  function *323*
metaphysics 15, 18–19,
  29, *41*, *42*, 51*n*1
  *see also* Che
*Mi Dao Fa* (Honey-based
  Purgative Method) 179–80
Mi Hou Tao (*Fructus Actinidiae
  Sinensis*) 327

Mi Hou Teng (*Rhizoma
  Actinidiae Sinensis*) 327
*Mihudeng Ohgapi Tang* (Lee-Je-ma's
  Kiwifruit and Acanthopanax
  Decoction) 344
*Mihudeng Shikhjang Tang* (Lee Je-
  ma's Kiwifruit Vine Support the
  Intestines Decoction) 320, 329
mind/body relationship *see* metaphysics
mind, the, eight components of *91*
Ming Dynasty 95, 180, 254, 302
*Mingli Lun* (*Expounding on
  the Treatise*) 118
Minister Fire 94*n*9
*Mirror of Eastern Medicine
  see Dongeui Bogam*
mission, fulfilling one's *see Sa Mu*
Mo Yao (*Myrrhae*) 249
*Moktong Daean Tang* (Lee Je-
  ma's Akebia Great Relief
  Decoction) 246, 266–7
monism 19
moral behavior 77, 81*n*93, 321, 332–9
mouth
  connection with the esophagus 84
  *Ek Hei* and 91
  *Ek* in 86
  and Heavenly Affairs 38
  and *Ji Bang* 34, 49–50, 70, 88
  as a sensory organ 39–40, 90
  stature of 44
Mu Gua (*Fructus Chaenomelis
  Lagenariae*) 9, 327
Mu Tong (*Caulis Akebiae*) 246
*Mu Xiang Shun Qi San* (Smooth the Qi
  Decoction with Aucklandia) 182
*Muhangon Byung* 274
muscles
  formation 16
  *Hyul Hei* in 86, 89
  twitching 118, 120
*Myung* (conduct) 18, 32–50, 36*n*26,
  37*n*31, 39, 45*n*74, 48, 49, 64
  expanding and fulfilling 67–82

*Na Shim* (laziness) 41–2, 46, 82
nature, ebb and flow of *see Chon Shi*
Negative Tendencies, Four 27
*Nei Jing* 288, 316, 324
neutral temperature 14
*Ni* 87
*Ni Hei* (place were *Shin* resides)
  85, 87, 88, 89, 90, 91
Nirvana 54
*Niu Huang Qing Xin Wan* (cattle
  Gall Stone Pill to Clear
  the Heart) 299, 305–6
*No see* anger
*Nogyung Daebo Tang* (Lee Je-ma's
  Deer Antler Great Tonification
  Decoction) 293, 295, 298, 311
nose
  connection with the esophagus 84
  and Heavenly Affairs 38
  and *In Ryun* 34, 49–50, 69, 88
  as a sensory organ 39–40, 90
  stature of 44
  sweating under 121, 139
  *Yu Hei* and 91
  *Yu* in 86
nosebleeds 112

*Nu Lao* syndrome 161, 163
Nu Rung Ji (glutinous rice) 140

*Ohgapi Jangchok Tang* (Lee Je-ma's
Acanthopanax Strengthern the
Spine Decoction) 317, 328
*Ohsuyu Buja Yijung Tang* (Lee
Je-ma's Evodia Fruit and
Aconite Regulate the Middle
Decoction) 153, 154–5, 200–1
oil, pitta and 16
one on one association *see Kyo Uh*
organs
Chinese medical organ system *13*
Five Yin and Six Fu 13
imbalance of 12
influence on bodily fluids *90*
metabolic process and
organ function *323*
metaphysics and 19
organ energy 16
organ groups and associations *87*
Sasand medicine organ system *14*
sizes *51*, 53, 55–6, 64
stronger and weaker organs 14
Organs, Four Major *Fu 52n4, 58*,
83–92, *84*, 97*n22*, 269*n50*
*see also* esophagus;
intestines; stomach
Organs, Four Major *Zhang* 13, 17, 19,
35, 52*n4*, 54, 55–7, *58*, 59, 60,
64, 83–92, 97*n22*, 166, 269*n50*
*see also* kidneys; liver; lungs; spleen
overreaction, prevention of 36

*Padu Dan* (Lee Je-ma's Croton Seed
Pill) 109, 117, 131, 158, 160, 199
*Padu Yeowi Dan* (Lee Je-ma's
Croton Seed Invigorate the
Willpower Pill) 139, 159
*Paduk* strategy 347
*Palmul Gunja Tang* (Lee Je-ma's Eight
Ingredient Gentlemen Decoction)
108–9, 113, 117, 119, 131, 195
pancreas 19
Pang An Jiao 96
pheasant 226
philosophy 10, 15, 17, 18, 20, 27, 29
phlegmatic temperament 15
physiology 15, 20, 27
*Pi Li San* (Thunderbolt
Powder) 154, 186
*Pi Wei Lun* 94*n7*
pitta 16
Plato 18
pneumonia 21
posterior body *42*
*Pre-Heaven* energy 13
pride, prevention of 36
psychology 15, 20
psychosis 107–8, 110, 224, 227, 229
Psychosis and Delirium syndrome 228
pubic hair 86
*Puji Ben Shi Fang* (*Practical Formulae
for Universal Benefit*) 117
pulse diagnosis 97

*Qi*, remedies for supporting 310
Qi Bo 93*n3*, 99, 101*n32*, 102
Qi Cao (*Holotrichia*) 275

*Qi* (energy, life force) 19, 85, 90
Agastache Powder to Rectify
105, 109, 113, 136, 164
distribution of 323–4
and the kidneys 81*n95*
and the liver 57, 81*n92*
and the lungs 57, 80*n86*, 323
remedies 96*n17*, 112, 115–16,
117–18, 119, 120, 124, 128,
129, 130, 134, 148, 180,
182, 184, 195, 274, 301
and the sensory organs 40
and the spleen 80*n89*
and *Ye Ge Fan Wei* syndrome 320
*Qi Yu* syndrome 183
*Qian Jin Fang* (*Thousand Golden
Essential Prescriptions*) 302
Qin Dynasty 10, 48, 94, 95
Qin, Emperor 48
Qing Fen (*Calomelas*) 249, 250
Qing Pi (*Pericarpium Citri
Ret. Viridae*) 163
Quiang Huo (*Rhizoma et Radix
Notoperygii*) 163, 227
*Quianjin Fang* (*One Thousand
Golden Formulae*) 242

*Rak see* calmness
rashness 27
Ren Dong Teng (*Caulis Lonicerae*) 240
*Ren Shen Gui Zhi Tang* (Cinnamon
Twig Decoction with Ginseng)
108, 112, 116, 138
Ren Shen (*Radix Ginseng*) 96*n17*,
118, 119, 122, 138, 141, 174
residence, proper place to
reside *see Ko Cho*
respect 27
*Revised Collection of Baekje Formulas* 9
rhubarb 107, 112, 179, 286, 312
*Ri Hua Zi Ben Cao* 96
righteousness 17, 33*n5*, 33*n10*,
37*n37*, 52, 78*nn72–3*
*Rong* (pure energy of blood) 269
*Rong Xue* (nutrition) 269*n51*
Rou Gui (*Cortex Cinnamomi*)
118, 132, 141, 148
Ru Xiang (*Resina Olibani*) 249
*Ru Yi Dan* (Invigorate the
Willpower Pill) 190
rudeness 47
*Ryuh* (consideration) 91

*Sa Dan* (Four Basic
Characteristics) 51–66
*Sa Mu* (fulfilling one's mission and
work) 33, 34–5, 37*n31*, 38, 68, 70–
1, 73, 74, 75*n53*, 79–80, 88, 341
sadness *see* sorrow
Saejeong, King 10
Sage, the 52–5
*Sahyang San* (Moschus Powder) 314
salt 260
salt water 171
salty flavor 14
*Sam Yu Tang* (Lee Je-ma's
Ginseng and Evodia Fruit
Decoction) 131, 153, 200
*Samgye Palmul Tang* (Lee Je-ma's
Ginsend and Cinnamon Twig
Eight Ingredient Decoction) 344

*San Leng Xiao Ji Wan* (*Scirpus Eliminate
the Accumulation Decoction*) 188
San Miao (You Miao) 62
*San Wei Shen Yu Tang* (Three Flavors
Ginseng and Evodia Fruit
Decoction) 130, 131, 152, 186
*San Wu Bai San* (Three Ingredients
White Powder) 157, 158, 189
sanguine temperament 15
Sasang medicine
birth of 11, 12
compared with Chinese medicine
11–14, *13*, *14*, *15*
description of 10
herb affiliation *15*
organ system *14*
*Sashipil Byung* 274
scents, pleasant and unpleasant 40
scrofula 250
*Sei Wei* (society) 33, 34–5, 36*n23*, 38,
49–50, 68, 70, 71, 72, 77*n70*, 87
self-conceit, prevention of 36
self-praise, prevention of 36
self-reflection 17, *38*, 40*n49*, 50
selfishness 36*n27*, 37*nn35–38*, 46, 48,
52, 53, 54, 55, 63, 75, *77*, 153, 292
senses 49–50
sensory organs 39–40
*Seungyang Ikgi Buja Tang* (Lee Je-ma's
Raise the Yang and Benefit the Qi
Decoction with Aconite) 105, 192
*Seungyang Ikgi Tang* (Lee Ja-ma's
Raise the Yang and Benefit the
Qi Decoction) 105, 117, 193
sexual attraction 334
sexual intercourse 94*n9*, 238,
242, 292, 296, 335, 338
Sha Ren (*Fructus Amomi*) 141
shamans 101–2
Shan Zhu Yu (*Fructus Corni
Officinalis*) 293
Shang Dynasty 43, 44*n67*, 93, 96
Shang Han
*Bi* syndrome and 135, 158
Cold and 134
Exterior Cold syndrome 207
and females 112
Greater Cold and Lesser Heat
syndrome 224, 226–7
Heat and 113
illness associations 98, 107,
138–9, 162, 172, 269
*Jue* syndrome 270–1
and Jue Yin 128–9, 131
outcomes 115
remedies 257
stages of influence 99–101
treatments 105, 117–18, 119, 269
Yang Pattern Shang Han
syndrome 213, 222
*Shang Han Lun* 10, 12, 94*nn5–6*,
97*n22*, 98, 99, 104*n1*,
106*n4*, 108*n9*, 114, 175–80,
252–4, 290, 317*n3*
*Shang Han Shi Quan* (*The Ten Teachings
of the Shang Han Lun*) 213
*Shang Xiao* syndrome 237–9,
*239*, 241, 242
Shao Dynasty 335
Shao Yang 97, 98, 100, 101,
123–5, *211*, 223, 232, 302
*see also* So Yang

Shao Yang *Shang Feng* syndrome
204, 206, *206*
Shao Yin syndrome 97, 98, 100, 101,
125, 126, 136, 141–2, *150*, 155–6,
156, 164, 165, 166, 167–8, 186
illness associations 146–9, *147*
*see also* So Eum
She Xiang (*Moschus*) 301
Shen Nong 93, 95
Sheng Di Huang (*Radix
Rehmanniae*) 229
*Sheng Jian* (*Rhizoma Zingiberis
Recens*) 137n7
Sheng Jiang (*Rhizoma
Zingiberis*) 141, 182
*Sheng Jiang Xie Xin Tang* (Ginger
Decoction to Drain the
Epigastrium) 135, 178
Sheng Ma (*Rhizoma
Cimicifugae*) 277, 286
*Sheng Mai San* (Generate the
Pulse Powder) 303–4
*Sheng Shu Di Huang Wan*
(Combined Raw and Prepared
Rehmannia Decoction) 256
*Shennong Bencaojing* (*The Classic
of Herbal Medicine*) 93, 95
Shi Chang Pu (*Rhizoma Acori
Graminei*) 300
*Shi Chang Pu Yuan Zhi San* (Sweetflag
and Senega Powder) 302
Shi Gao (*Gypsum Fibrosum*) 212,
215, 225, 226, 227, 229, 230
*Shi Quan Da Bu Tang* (All-inclusive
Great Tonifying Decoction) 180–1
*Shi Yi De Xiao Fang* (*De Xiao Fang*) 105
*Shi Zao Tang* (Ten Jujube
Decoction) 208, 212, 254
Shie gao (*Gypsum Fibrosum*) 10
*Shijing* (*Classic of Poetry*) 49
*Shik Kyun* (right time to take
action) 37, 38n42, 39, 81
*Shin Ji Dang* (kidney group) 110n14
*Shin* (spirit) 85, 87, 90
*Shipimi Jihwang Tang* (Lee Je-ma's
Twelve Ingredient Rehmannia
Decoction) 242, 245, 264
*Shiyi Dexiaofang* 94n10
shock 12
shoulders, stature of 44–7
*Shui Jie Xiong* syndrome 157, 158, 196
*Shuiyin Xunbi Fang* (Inhaled Mercury
Formula) 249, 259–60
Shun, Emperor 43, 44–5,
55, 62, 335, 347
*Si Ni San* (Frigid Extremities
Powder) 176
*Si Ni Tang* (Frigid Extremities
Decoction) 134, 138,
142, 152, 153
*Si Shun Li Zhong Tang* (Four Ingredients
Decoction to Smooth and
Regulate the Middle) 134, 175
*Si Shun Tang* (Four Ingredients
Decoction to Smooth the Qi) 130
Silla Dynasty 10
Six Channel theory 98
Six Stages of Illness 97n22
skin
formation of *16*
in the lung group 85

small intestine *see under* intestines
"smelling" 34, 39, 49–50, 68, 71
snakes 171
So Eum (Lesser Yin) Individual
13 formulae presented by doctors
of the Song, Yuan, and
Ming Dynasties—with six
containing Ba Dou 180–90
23 formulae from Zhang Zhongjing's
*Shang Han Lun* 175–80
24 newly discovered
formulae 191–202
anger and 72–3
bladder of 110
calmness and 56, 61, *63*,
69, 75n54, 78
complacency and 325
*Dang Yo* and 79
desire to dwell in a
familiar setting 75
eyes of 70, 71–2
*Gung Shim* and 80
headaches 217
herbs for 14, 15, 16
illness 104–202
joy and 56, 61, 63, 65, 69,
72–3, 74, 76, 79, 325
*Jung* emotion 76
kidney Heat causing Exterior
Heat syndrome 104–33, *106*
comparison between False Heat
and False Cold-related
symptoms of the So Eum
and So Yang Individual *127*
comparison between the three
kidney Heat-induced
Exterior syndromes *133*
*Daejang Pahan* and *Ulchuk
Panggwang* syndromes
*109, 110, 111*
Mang Yang syndrome *127*
Tai Yang/Yang Ming
syndrome *113*
Wei Jia Shi syndrome *114*
*Ko Cho* and 75n58
*Kyung Ryun* and 80
liver of 70, 74
love and 78nn74–5
lungs of 81n99
moral behavior 78
mouth of 70, 71
need for vigilance 66
as one of the four constitutions 11
selfish tendencies 76, *77*
selfishness and 52
*Shik Kyun* and 81
smaller and larger organs *51*
*Song* nature of 75
spleen of 70, 79, 80nn89–90,
99, 110, 136
stomach Cold causing Interior
Cold syndrome 134–63
combined three stage
syndromes *160*
general treatment strategy for
bluish-green diarrhea *149*
Jue Yin syndrome *155*
Shao Yin syndrome *147, 150*
Tai Yin syndrome *137, 143–5*
stomach of 99
synopsis of illness 164–202

Tai Yang sickness and 99
*Tal Shim* in 81
*Wei Jia Shi* syndrome 220
Yang Ming sickness and 99
Yin illness and 99
Zhang Zhongjing and 96
*So In* (uncultivated) 52n2
So Yang (Lesser Yang) Individual
anger and 56, 61, 63, 68,
75n52, 75n56, 77n70
*Bi Ying* syndrome 108n10
calmness and 73
desire to grasp 75
*Do Ryang* and 81
eyes of 70, 71
*Gwa Shim* in 81
headaches 235
herbs for 15, 15, 16
humility and 77n70, 78n71
illness 203–68
Internal Heat 126
*Jie Xiong* syndrome 158
*Jung* emotion 76
kidneys of 70, 74, 81nn95–6
*Ko Cho* and 75n52, 79
liver of 82n106
lungs of 70
moral behavior 77–8
mouth of 70, 71
*Na Shim* and 82
need for vigilance 65, 66
as one of the four constitutions 11
*Sa Mu* and 79
selfish tendencies 76, 77
selfishness and 52
Shao Yang illness and 99
smaller and larger organs 51
*Song* nature of 75
sorrow and 56, 61, 63, 65,
68, 73, 74, 76, 325
spleen Cold causing Exterior
Cold syndrome 203–30
*Mang Yin* syndrome *223*
Shao Yang Shang Feng
syndrome *206*
Shao Yang stage external
syndrome *211*
Tai Yang stage syndrome *204*
Yang Pattern Shang Han
syndrome *222*
stomach Heat causing Interior
Heat syndrome 231–43
Shang Xiao, Zhong Xiao, and
Xia Xiao syndromes *239*
thirsting disorder syndromes *243*
Yang Ming and three Yang
stage syndromes *236*
stomach of 99
synopsis of illness 244–68
17 newly discovered
formulae formulated
by Lee Je-ma 260–8
nine formulae presented by
doctors of the Yuan and
Ming Dynasties 254–60
ten formulae from Zhang
Zhongjing's *Shang
Han Lun* 252–4
Tai Yang sickness and 99
Yang Ming sickness and 99
Zhang Zhongjing and 96
social skills *see In Ryun*

society *see Sei Wei*
*Sokchangpo Wonji San* (Lee Je-ma's Sweetflag and Senega Powder) 313, 314
solid organs *see* Organs, Four Major, *Zhang*
Song Dynasty 94, 95, 96, 180, 208n10, 213n18, 302
*Song* (human nature) 32–50, 39, 45n74, 47
    anger and 63
    calmness and 63
    as *Che* 18
    definition 12
    imbalance of 98n24
    joy and 63
    and the So Eum Individual 56
    and the So Yang Individual 56
    sorrow and 63
    and the Tae Eum Individual 56
    and the Tae Yang Individual 55
    wisdom and 49
sorrow 63, 64, 67
    and the *Che/Yong* relationship 18
    effects of 60, *61*
    flow of 57, *58*, 59
    and the *Jung* emotion of the So Yang Individual 56, 63, 65, 68, 73, 74, 76, 325
    and the *Jung* emotion of the Tae Yang Individual 76
    as one of the four constitutional temperaments 12, 13, 17, 19–20, 28
    as one of the Seven Emotional Disorders 12
    and *Sa Mu* 88
    as the *Song* nature of the Tae Yang Individual 55, 63, 67, 75
    and the Song nature of the Tae Yang Individual 77n67, 325
    and the Tae Eum Individual 73
sounds, pleasant and unpleasant 40
Southern and Northern Dynasties 94
Southern Zhou Dynasty 335
soy sauce 260
spine 83
    lower 86, 88
    upper 85, 87, 91
spleen
    anger and 13, 20, 67
    aversion to unpleasant colors 40
    in Chinese medicine 13
    energy flow from kidneys to 14
    energy flow towards heaven 35
    and the Four Symbols 11
    function 321–2
    herbs for 14, 15, *15*, *16*
    and Human Affairs 38
    inquiry and 90
    and *Kyo Uh* 34, 70, 74, 79
    location 83
    *Mak Hei* and 91
    *Mak Hei* in 85, 88
    and *Sei Wei* 71–2
    of the So Eum Individual 80nn89–90, 136
    spleen group 85

stature of 44–7
Tae Eum Individual and 97n22
    and Yin Fire 94n7
    *see also under* So Yang
stomach
    in Chinese medicine 13
    Go in 85, 89
    location 83
    and muscle formation 16
    structure 84
    Yang Ming and 97n22
    *see also under* So Eum;
        *under* So Yang
strokes 244, 245, 250, 300–1, *300*, 313
stupidity 47
*Su Gok* (ingested food and drink) 84–6, *84*, *87*
*Su He Xiang Wan* (Liquid Styrax Pill) 136, 183–4, 228
*Su Wen see Huang Di Neijing* 93
Sui Dynasty 94, 95
*Sui Ni* 208
*Sukjihwang Gosam Tang* (Lee Je-ma's Processed Rhemannia and Sophora Decoction) 216, 239, 266
Summer Heat 12
*Sun* (downward flow of energy) 40n49
Sun Si Miao 242, 302
*Supplementation to the Ben Cao Shi Yi* 96
sweet flavor 14
Symbols, Four 11, 32n3

Tae Eum (Greater Yin) Individual 136, 282n18
    calmness and 73, 76
    *Chi Shim* and 82
    complacency and 65, 68, 74
    desire for peace and quiet 75
    ears of 69, 71
    esophagal Cold causing Exterior Cold Syndrome 269–81
        *Han Jue* syndrome *276*
        Tai Yang syndrome *270*
        Warm Febrile syndrome *280*
    hair brushing 251
    herbs for 14, *15*
    illness 269–315
    joy and 56, 61, 63–4, 68, 75n53, 325–6
    *Ju Chek* and 80
    *Jung* emotion 76–7, 77n66
    kidneys of 71
    *Ko Cho* and 80
    *Kyo Shim* and 80
    laziness and 61, 64
    liver Heat causing Interior Heat syndrome 282–94
        Internal Heat Warm Febrile disease syndrome *288*
        Internal Heat *Yang Ming* syndrome *283*
        Internal Heat *Zao Re* syndrome *294*
        liver Heat causing *Fei Zao* syndrome *292*
        liver Heat causing *Yang Ming* syndrome *284*
    lungs of 71, 74, 80n86
    moral behavior 78
    need for vigilance 66

nose of 69, 71
    as one of the four constitutions 11
    righteousness and 78nn72–3
    *Sa Mu* and 75n53, 80
    selfish tendencies 76–7, 77
    selfishness and 52
    shoulders of 82
    smaller and larger organs 51
    *Song* nature of 75, 78n72
    sorrow and 73
    *Su He Xiang Wan* 184
    synopsis of Tae Eum illness 295–315
        24 newly discovered formulae (formulated by Lee Je-ma) 307–15
        esophageal Cold syndrome *297–8*
        four formulae from Zhang Zhongjing's *Shang Han Lun* 301–2
        Internal Heat *Zhong Feng* (stroke) syndrome *300*
        nine formulae presented by doctors of the Tang, Song, and Ming Dynasties 302–7
        treatment according to everyday complexion before the onset of *Zhong Feng* (stroke) syndrome *300*
    Tai Yang sickness and 99
    wisdom and 75
    Yang Ming sickness and 99
    Zhang Zhongjing and 96
*Tae Eum Jowi Tang* (Lee Je-ma's Regulate the stomach Decoction for the Tae Eum Individual) 277, 286, 295, 307
Tae Yang (Greater Yang) Individual
    anger and 55, 61, 63, 65, 67, 72, 74, 76, 319n1, 324–5
    *Bol Shim* and 81
    *Dang Yo* and 75n51, 78
    desire to advance 75
    ears of 69, 71
    Externally contracted illness affecting the lumbar spine 316–18, 318
        *Xie Yi* syndrome *318*
    *Heng Gom* and 81
    herbs for *15*
    illness 316–29
    Internally contracted illness affecting the small intestine 319–26, 326
        metabolic process and organ function *323*
        *Ye Ge Fan Wei* syndrome *326*
    joy and 72
    *Jul Shim* and 82
    *Jung* emotion 76
    kidneys of 82n109
    Kyo Uh and 78
    liver of 70, 74, 75n55, 78n78, 81nn92–3
    moral behavior 77
    need for vigilance 65, 66
    nose of 69
    as one of the four constitutions 11
    selfish tendencies 76, *77*
    selfishness and 52
    smaller and larger organs *51*
    *Song* nature of 75

sorrow and 19–20, 55, 61, 63, 67, 75, 76, 325
spleen of 70
ten herbs from the Ben Cao Lun, and two introduced by Li Chan and Gong Xin 327–8
two newly discovered formulae (formulated by Lee Je-ma) 328–9
wisdom and 77*nn*67–8
Zhu Zhenheng and 97
*Tai Chi* 11, 32*n*3, 52
*Tai Qi* 11
Tai Yang *Shang Feng* syndrome *see* So Eum (Lesser Yin) Individual: kidney Heat causing Exterior Heat syndrome 131
Tai Yang syndrome 97, 98, 99, 101, 104, 125, 164, 165–6, 167–8, 203, *204*, 231, 232
of the Tae Eum Individual 270
*see also* Tae Yang
Tai Yang/Yang Ming syndrome *113*
Tai Yin syndrome 97, 98, 100, 101, 125, 126, 134, 135, *137*, *143*–5, 146, 158, 164, 165–6, 166, 167–8
*see also* Tae Eum
*Tal Shim* (desire to take from others) 81
Tang Dynasty 94, 95, 96, 302
tangerine 140, 157, 162, 163, 168, 186, 199
*Tangye Bencao* 95–6
*Tao Ren Cheng Qi Tang* (Guide the Qi Formula with Persica) 179
*Tao ren Cheng Qi Tang* (Peach Pit Decoction to Order the Qi) 108
taste
lack of 71
sense of 69
tastes, pleasant and unpleasant 40
tea
green 256
herbal 21, 22, 132, 228, 313, 327
temperament imbalance 12
temperaments, four constitutional 12, 13, 19–20, 28, 98*n*23
temperature-related effects of the spleen and kidneys *16*
Temperatures, Five 14
*see also under* So Eum; *under* So Yang; *under* Tae Eum
*Ten Wings* 32*n*3
tendon formation *16*
tendons, *Mak Hei* in 85, 89
thirsting disorder syndromes 236–43, *236*, *243*
*see also Xiao Ge*; *Xiao Shen*; *Xiao Zhong*
thoracic area 60, 71
location 83
thoracic-spine, location 83
Three Kingdoms Period 48
Three Poles Theory (San Ji Zhi Dao) 35, 40*n*49
Three Yin and Three Yang method 97
throat disorders 235, 248–9, 250, 302
*Tiao Wei Cheng Qi Tang* (Regulate the stomach Order the Qi Decoction) 282, 301
*Tiao Zhong Tang* (Regulate the Middle Decoction) 302–3

tidal fever 115, 116, 117, 118–19, 125, 128
tigers 9
tinnitus 100
Tong Cao (*Medulla Tetrapanacis*) 96*n*17
tongue 50*n*88, 85, 91
Tridosha Theory 16
Triple Burner, So Yang Individual and 97*n*22
tumors 9, 96*n*18, 235, 240–1, 249
Two Yang Energies 290

*Uhwang Chongshim Wan* (Lee Je-ma's Cattle Gall Stone Pill to Clear the Heart) 299, 300, 314–15
*Ul Kwang* syndrome 107, 125–6
ulcers 289
*Ulchuk Panggwang* syndrome *109*, 110*n*14, *111*
umbilical area/umbilicus
*Bol Shim* in 40, 81
*Heng Gom* in 36, 81*n*93
location 83
stature of 44–7
wisdom and 38
*Yu Hei* and 91
*Yu* in 86
*Ungdam San* (Bear Gallbladder Powder) 313
Uterine Heat 112

vata 16
virtue 48, 49, 55*n*14
Virtues, Four 17, 27, 32*n*1
*see also* humility; love; righteousness; wisdom
The Virtuous Path—Advice for Everyday Life 332–9

*Wan Bing Hui Chun* (Restoring Health from Tens of Thousands of Diseases) 182, 257, 285*n*7
Wang Hao Gu (Hai Zang) 94, 96, 118*n*29, 162, 236–7, 241
*Wang Hao Gu Tangye Bencao* 96
Wang Shu He 94*n*5, 163, 284
Warm
nature of esophagus 84
as one of the five temperatures 14
Tae Yang Individual and 323
Warm Febrile disease 96*n*18, 275, 277–80, *280*, *281*, 286–8, *288*, 302, 304
Warm Yang *Qi* 247
Warm Yin *Qi* 247
Warring States period 124
water, in Chinese philosophy 34*n*14
Wei Dynasty 95
*Wei Han* 129
*Wei Jia Shi* syndrome 113, *113*, 114, *114*, 118–19, 123–5, 125, 128, 166, 167, 220
Wei Yilin 94, 105, 183, 185, 188, 238, 240, 255, 293
*Wen Bai Yuan* (Warm the White Pill) 187
Wen (founder of Zhou Dynasty) 44, 57*n*19
*Wen Huang see* jaundice
Western medicine 15, 20
Western patients 21
wheat flour, avoiding 242

wheezing 295, 299, 306–7, 309, 313
*Wi Eui* (respect) 37, 38*n*42, 39, 82
Wild Ginseng (*Radix Ginseng*) 171
willpower 41, 91, 139, 159, 190, 321, 322
Wind
as a cause of illness 99
as one of the Six Climatic Factors 12
wisdom
blocking and attaining 46–8
and humility 78*n*71
inner 38
as one of the four virtues 17, 27, 33*n*7, 33*n*12, 36*n*22, 37*n*35, 52, 73*n*44
and Song 49
and the Tae Eum Individual 75
and the Tae Yang Individual 75*n*51, 77*nn*67–8
and virtuous action 38*n*43
*see also* Sage, the
womanliness 76
worry 12
Wu, Emperor 48*n*84
Wu Jia Pi (*Cortex Acanthopanacis*) 327
Wu, King 44
*Wu Ling San* (Five Ingredients Powder with Poria) 252
*Wu Wei* 10
Wu Wei Zi (*Fructus Shizandrae*) 174
*Wuhwang Chongshim Tang* (Lee Je-ma's Cattle Gall Stone Ill to Clear the Heart) 313

*Xia Jiao* 242
*Xia Xiao* syndrome 239, *239*, 241
*Xian Xiong Tang* (Sinking into the Chest Decoction) 212
Xiang Fu (*Rhizoma Cyperi*) 137*n*7
Xiang Fu Zi (*Rhizoma Cyperi*) 163
*Xiang Sha Liu Jun Zi Tang* (Six Gentlement Decoction with Aucklandia and Amomum) 136, 181–2
*Xiang Su San* (Cyperus and Perilla Leaf Powder) 105, 184–5
*Xiao Ban Xia Tang* (Minor Pinellia Decoction) 157
*Xiao Chai Hu Tang* (Minor Bupleurum Decoction) 204, 205, 206, 223, 252
*Xiao Cheng Qi Tang* (Minor Order the Qi Decoction) 117–18, 149, 180
*Xiao Du Yin* (Decoction to Eliminate Toxins) 258
*Xiao Ge* syndrome 236–7, 265, 290
*Xiao Jie Xiong* syndrome 212
*Xiao Ke* 132
*Xiao Shen* 236–7
*Xiao Xian Xiong Tang* (Minor Sining into the Chest Decoction) 209, 253
*Xiao Zhong see Zhong Xiao*
*Xie Xin Tang* (Drain the Epigastrium Decoction) 135, 136
*Xie Yi* syndrome 316–18, *318*, 321, 324–5, 341
Xiong Dan Powder (*Vesica Fellea Ursi*) 171–2, 274, 275, 279
*Xiong Ge Re* syndrome 235
Xu Shu-wei 117–18, 183

*Xue* (blood) 269
Xue Ji 130*n*48

Yang
    Clear Yang 234 238–40, 241, 247
    floating 104
    Two Yang Energies 290
    *see also Mang Yang* syndrome
*Yang Dok Baek Ho Tang* (Lee Je-ma's
    White Tiger Decoction to
    Eliminate Yang Toxin) 265
*Yang Jue* syndrome 233
Yang Ming syndrome 97, *113*
    formulae for 186
    illness associations 98, 99–100,
        101, 112–17, 118–20, 164,
        165, 166, 167–8, 232
    laxatives 149
    treatments 283, 302, 304–5
    *see also Bi Yao* syndrome; *Shao*
        *Yang*; *Wei Jia Shi* syndrome
Yang Pattern Shang Han
    syndrome 213, *222*
Yang toxin 282, 303
Yang Tse River 62*n*44
*Yangdok Baekho Tang* (Lee Je-ma's
    White Tiger Decoction to
    Eliminate Yang Toxin) 249
*Yanggyuk Sanhwa Tang* (Lee Ja-ma's
    Cool the Diaphragm and Disperse
    Heat Decoction) 239, 249, 265
Yao, Emperor 43, 44–5, 55, 62, 335
*Ye Ge Fan Wei* syndrome 319–22,
    324–5, *326*, 341, 345
*Ye* syndrome *see Ye Ge Fan*
    *Wei* syndrome
yellow bile 15
*The Yellow Emperor's Classic* 10, 12
*Yellow Emperor's Inner Canon*
    *see Huang Di Neijing*
*Yellow Songs* (*Huang Ge*) 307
*Yi Ching see I Ching*
*Yi* (justification) 91
*Yi Xue Zheng Zhuan* (*True*
    *Lineage of Medicine*) 256
*Yi Yao Fa Fang* 99
Yi Yi Ren (*Semen Coicis*) 275
Yi Zhi Ren (*Fructus Alpiniae*
    *Oxyphyllae*) 163
*Yijianshu* (*Mirror of Eastern Medicine*)
    182, 184, 187, 257–8, 304–6

Yin
    *Clear Yin* 234
    deficient 104
    exhaustion of 293
    *see also Mang Yin* syndrome
Yin and Yang theory 10, 11, *13*, 14,
    *14*, 52*n*4, 74*n*50, 82*n*102, 82*n*105,
    82*n*108, 94*n*8, 98, 213, 242
    *see also Che; Yong*
*Yin Chen Fu Zi Tang* (Artemisia
    Yinchenhao and Poria
    Decoction) 157, 162, 185
*Yin Chen Hao Tang* (Artemisia
    Yinchenchao Decoction)
    156, 158, 162, 178–9
*Yin Chen Ju Pi Tang* (Artemisia
    Yinchenhao and Tangerine Peel
    Decoction) 157, 163, 186
*Yin Chen Si Ni Tang* (Artemisia
    Yinchenhao Decoction for Frigid
    Extremities) 157, 162, 163, 185
*Yin Chen Wan* (Artemisia Pill) 188
*Yin Duo 137*, 138, 165, 166, 168
*Yin Duo Man Feng* syndrome 199
Yin Dynasty *see* Shang Dynasty 96
Yin Excess Overwhelming
    Yang syndrome 153–5
*Yin Fire* concept 94*n*7
*Yin Huang* 162
*Yixue Gangmu* (*Compendium*
    *of Medicine*) 118, 157,
    158, 162, 238, 256
*Yixue Rumen* (*Introduction to*
    *Medicine*) 95*n*11, 120
*Yixuefang* (*Introduction to Medicine*) 185
*Yok Shim* (selfishness) 41–2
*Yok* (upward flow of energy) 40*n*49
*Yong see Che/Yong* relationship
You Miao (San Miao) 62
Yu, Emperor 62
*Yu Hei* 86, 88, 91
*Yu* (oily fluids) 16, *16*, 86, 88, 89, 90
Yu Tuan 256
Yuan Dynasty 10, 94, 95, 96, 180, 254
*Yuan Qi* 293
Yuan Zhi (*Radix Polygoni*) 300
*Yulda Hanso Tang* (Lee Je-ma's Greater
    Heat and Lesser Cold Decoction)
    287, 289, 290, 291, 298, 309–10
*Yuxuerumen* (*Introduction to*
    *Medicine*) 186, 189–90, 303–4

Zao Jiao (*Gleditsia Sinensis*) 285, 300
*Zao Re* syndrome 290–2, *294*
*Zao* syndrome 288–9
*Zao Yi* syndrome 302
Ze Xie (*Rhizoma Alismatis*) 163, 210
*Zhang Dan Wan* (Epidemic
    Jaundice Pill) 157, 188
*Zhang Gan Bing* 270–3, 275
Zhang Ji Feng 320
*Zhang Jie* syndrome 158–60, 247
*Zhang Jue* syndrome 151–2, 154–5
*Zhang* organs 52
    *see also* kidneys; liver; lungs; spleen
Zhang Zhongjing 12, 94, 95, 96,
    98, 105, 107–10, 112–16, 117,
    119–20, 123–5, 128, 131,
    134–7, 138, 141–2, 152, 156,
    158–9, 161, 175–80, 203, 204,
    206, 208, 212, 223, 231–2,
    252–4, 269–71, 274, 275, 290
*Zhen Qi* 237, 293
*Zhen Yin* 264*n*47
*Zhen Zhang Qi see Zhang Jue* syndrome
*Zheng Qi* 131, 166, 167, 170, 213,
    220, 238, 259, 272, 273
*Zhi Mu Bai Hu Tang* (White
    Tiger Decoction with Added
    Anemarrhena) 229
Zhi Mu (*Rhizoma Anemarrhenae*) 229
Zhi Shi (*Fructus Aurantii*
    *Immaturus*) 117
Zhi Zi (*Fructus Gardeniae*
    *Jasminoidis*) 156
*Zhong Feng* (stroke) syndrome
    183, 299, 300–1, *300*
*Zhong Qi* syndrome 174, 182, 183
*Zhong Xiao* syndrome 170*n*66,
    236–9, *239*, 241, 242, 247
Zhou Dynasty 44, 94
Zhou, Emperor 43, 44*n*67
Zhu Danxi, Master (Zhu Zhenheng)
    *see* Zhu Zhenheng
Zhu Gong 44, 94, 95, 129–30,
    132, 148, 151, 153, 159, 162,
    185–6, 207, 233, 282, 302–3
*Zhu Ling Tang* (Polyporus
    Decoction) 124, 232, 252
Zhu Zhenheng (Master Zhu Danxi)
    94, 119, 162, 163, 189, 213, 221,
    237–8, 259, 319–20, 321–2, 324